D1560721

THE ENCYCLOPAEDIA
OF
MEDICAL IGNORANCE

Also edited by Duncan and Weston-Smith

THE ENCYCLOPAEDIA OF IGNORANCE
Everything you ever wanted to know about the unknown

LYING TRUTHS

THE ENCYCLOPAEDIA
OF
MEDICAL IGNORANCE

Exploring the frontiers of medical knowledge

Edited by

RONALD DUNCAN

and

MIRANDA WESTON-SMITH

PERGAMON PRESS

OXFORD · NEW YORK · TORONTO · SYDNEY · PARIS · FRANKFURT

U.K.	Pergamon Press Ltd., Headington Hill Hall, Oxford OX3 0BW, England
U.S.A.	Pergamon Press Inc., Maxwell House, Fairview Park, Elmsford, New York 10523, U.S.A.
CANADA	Pergamon Press Canada Ltd., Suite 104, 150 Consumers Road, Willowdale, Ontario M2J 1P9, Canada
AUSTRALIA	Pergamon Press (Aust.) Pty. Ltd., P.O. Box 544, Potts Point, N.S.W. 2011, Australia
FRANCE	Pergamon Press SARL, 24 rue des Ecoles, 75240 Paris, Cedex 05, France
FEDERAL REPUBLIC OF GERMANY	Pergamon Press GmbH, Hammerweg 6, D-6242 Kronberg-Taunus, Federal Republic of Germany

First edition 1984

Library of Congress Cataloging in Publication Data

Main entry under title:
The Encyclopaedia of medical ignorance.
Includes index.
1. Medicine—Philosophy—Addresses, essays, lectures.
I. Duncan, Ronald Frederick Henry, 1914-
II. Weston-Smith, Miranda. [DNLM: 1. Medicine—Trends.
WB 100 P445]
R723.E53   1983   616   83-4785

British Library Cataloguing in Publication Data

The Encyclopaedia of medical ignorance.
1. Medicine
I. Duncan, Ronald   II. Weston-Smith, Miranda
610   R130
ISBN 0-08-024515-3

Printed and bound in Great Britain by
William Clowes Limited, Beccles and London

CONTENTS

INTRODUCTION

Like the previous two volumes in this series this book focuses on ignorance not knowledge. We have asked scientists to state what it is they do not know in their own particular field, and where they would like to see research directed. The articles are concerned with ignorance of how our bodies and minds function in health and disease. They range from papers on transplantation biology to psychotherapy and from multiple sclerosis to depression.

The reason for inviting contributors to take this approach to their subject was the belief that examining a topic from a new perspective might provide new insight on old problems. We think that the articulation of a problem is a major step towards its solution. Here medical scientists are outlining important questions in a new way.

We hope that this book will enjoy a wide readership and we have attempted to ensure that the essays are intelligible to the scientifically literate layman. Human medicine is everyone's concern and yet there is more ignorance in this field than in many others. Indeed the ignorance is so great that in compiling this book we have not sought to include entries on every subject, but have rather chosen to pick out those areas which highlight current problems. We hope that future volumes in this series will cover other aspects of this subject.

It has been an exciting pleasure compiling this book, greatly saddened by the death in June 1982 of the poet and playwright Ronald Duncan, my co-editor and originator of these volumes.

Miranda Weston-Smith

PSYCHOTHERAPY

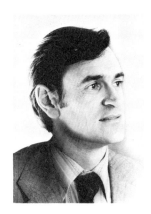

Anthony W. Clare

Senior Lecturer, Institute of Psychiatry, London.

Honorary Consultant Psychiatrist, Bethlem Royal and Maudsley Hospitals, London and he is also an adviser to the World Health Organization. He is the author of *Psychiatry in Dissent*.

In the forty years and more since Freud's death, psychoanalysis has flourished both as a theory of psychological development and as a treatment for the mentally ill. In the United States, psychotherapies derived from Freudian theories have become a major lucrative industry catering to the needs of millions of consumers (Clare and Thompson, 1981). Not surprisingly, many people inside and outside psychiatry assume that a training in psychoanalysis is a *sine qua non* for any budding recruit and the idea has grown up over the years that psychoanalytic treatment is the treatment which every mentally ill patient would have in an ideal world but, sadly, many have to make do with inferior treatments such as drugs and behavioural approaches.

In fact, however, solidly based and objective information as to the nature and efficacy of psychoanalysis and the psychotherapies derived from it is notable for its absence. Nearly a century after Freud's initial speculations concerning the nature and treatment of mental disorder, we still do not know whether talking actually does cure. This is not to suggest that there have not been attempts to establish the efficacy of such treatments. On the contrary, there have been many such studies published in the professional literature, but the majority of them are seriously flawed and repetition here would serve little purpose. There has also been a handful of attempts in recent years which has served to cast some light on a number of interesting features of this area, which otherwise tends to be neglected.

One of the earliest intensive studies was undertaken at the famous Menninger Clinic in Topeka, Kansas. The purpose of this study was to explore changes in patients brought about by 'psychoanalytically-oriented psychotherapies and psychoanalysis'. Psychoanalysis was defined in this study as 'a technique employed by a neutral analyst resulting in the development of a regressive transference neurosis. The ultimate resolution of this neurosis is achieved by techniques of interpretation alone' (Bulletin of the Menninger Clinic, 1972).

In contrast, psychotherapy includes approaches derived from the theory of psychoanalysis, but which do not aim to induce a full transference neurosis. ('Transference neurosis' refers to the process which is said to occur during analysis by which the patient displaces on to his analyst the feelings, ideas and beliefs which derive from previous figures and experiences in his life.) In psychoanalysis, interpretation, confrontation and clarification are used as the main therapeutic interventions, whereas in other forms of psychotherapy other interventions are used, such as suggestion, advice, reassurance, prohibitions and persuasion based on rational factors.

On the basis of the Menninger study, the authors of the report concluded that for patients with what they termed 'high Ego strength, high Motivation, high Anxiety Tolerance and high Quality of Interpersonal Relationships' psychoanalysis is the treatment of choice. 'Ego strength' was defined in this study as a combination of the degree of integration, stability and flexibility of the personality, the degree to which relationships with others are 'adaptive, deep and gratifying of normal instinctual needs' and the degree to which the individual's disturbance is manifested by symptoms. Stripped of the technical

jargon, what the study revealed was that psychoanalysis is indeed useful, but for patients who are already reasonably healthy, well-motivated, socially functioning and generally personable! More recent studies, conducted in the main by researchers favourably disposed towards analysis, have demonstrated similar findings.

Even more intriguing were the results of a study conducted by a group of researchers at Temple University in Philadelphia. In this study ninety-four patients presenting at a psychiatric outpatients department and diagnosed as suffering from moderately severe neurotic disturbances or personality disorders were randomly assigned to one of three groups. One group was treated by psychoanalytically trained psychotherapists. Another group was treated by experienced behaviour therapists, while the third group had no formal treatment at all other than the initial 'indepth' assessment interview common to all three groups and a monthly telephone call assuring them that they had not been forgotten and would be assigned to active treatment as soon as possible. The three groups of patients were assessed at four months, twelve months and two years. At four months, all three groups had improved significantly in so-called 'target symptoms', that is to say those particular symptoms which the patient himself spontaneously identified as being a specific problem at the outset of the study. Both the treatment groups improved significantly more than those on the waiting list, but there was no significant difference in the amount of symptomatic improvement, social adjustment and work ability between the psychotherapy and the behaviour therapy groups.

The results of this study, as the analyst Judd Marmor pointed out in a foreword (Sloane et al., 1975), 'offer little comfort to those adherents of either group (psychoanalytically derived psychotherapy and behaviour therapy) who are involved in passionately proclaiming the inherent superiority of this particular brand of therapy over all others'. Indeed, this study suggested that despite their mutual antagonism, there was a remarkable overlap in the approaches of the psychotherapists and behaviour therapists, suggesting that any differences may be more matters of degree than substance. Behaviour therapists tended to be more directive, more concerned with symptoms, less concerned with childhood memories and, despite their reputation for coldness and lack of clinical involvement, warmer and more active therapists. Tape-recorded interview analysis showed that they made as many interpretative statements as did the psychoanalysts. Given the similarities between the two approaches in practice, it is not clear from the study whether the behaviourists and the psychoanalysts did actually use fundamentally different approaches to reach the same therapeutic end or whether the effectiveness of their treatments was due to factors common to two very different schools of thought. The patients themselves, however, were in less doubt. Those who improved attributed their response less to the theoretical framework within which they had been treated and more to the personality, enthusiasm and involvement of the therapists.

A similar picture emerged from an extensive study undertaken by a group of American researchers and entitled provocatively 'Comparative Studies of Psychotherapies: is it True that "Everyone has Won and All Must have Prizes"?' These authors compared various psychotherapeutic approaches: individual psychotherapy versus group psychotherapy, time limited versus time-unlimited, simple here-and-now based treatments versus treatments which emphasized unearthing and working through material from childhood and so on. The major conclusion of this review was that the different forms of psychotherapy do not make significant differences in the proportion of patients improving by the end of therapy. The other conclusion of note was that most patients who go through any form of psychotherapy gain from it (Luborsky, Singer and Luborsky, 1975).

What has emerged in recent years is that talking about problems appears to help, but that there is no difference between the kind of talking that is employed. Relatively simple approaches, such as those pioneered by psychologist Carl Rogers and which lay considerable emphasis on personal characteristics of the therapist, including his ability to care, his empathic skills and his 'genuineness', appear to be every bit as effective as much more complicated, time-consuming and expensive approaches such as psychoanalysis.

Perhaps psychoanalysts treat more difficult and disordered individuals than less trained and less skilled therapists and hence their results are no better? There is little evidence that this is so. Indeed, despite the fact that Freud and his followers appeared to regard psychoanalysis as a suitable treatment for the majority of mental disorders, it is in fact reserved for those who, like the patients in the Menninger Study referred to earlier, are only minimally impaired. A celebrated study in Britain, which collapsed in mid-stream, casts interesting light on this selectivity in action. A carefully designed trial of psychotherapy involving therapists from the Tavistock Clinic and the Maudsley Hospital in London was set up in the early 1970s (Candy *et al.*, 1972). It was agreed from the outset that the aim should be to include only those patients who appeared to be highly suitable for the particular form of psychotherapy to be used. Selection of possible participants took place in three stages. First, psychiatrists working within a reasonable distance of the two centres referred patients who appeared to them to fulfil particular criteria for psychotherapy. These criteria included:

1. No evidence of serious physical or psychotic illness.
2. No serious drug addiction, sexual deviation or sociopathic disorder.
3. Discernible and lasting problems in interpersonal relationships.

4. No evidence suggesting the need for hospital admission.
5. Average intelligence at least.
6. No previous formal psychotherapy.
7. Active motivation for treatment.
8. Willingness to participate in a research programme.
9. Age between 18 and 45.
10. Willing for a relative to be seen.

One hundred and thirteen patients were referred. Of these, twenty-three failed to return the screening questionnaires (which asked for details of the individual's difficulties, family circumstances and history, sexual experience and occupation). Ninety patients were left. However, on the basis of the Tavistock psychotherapists' assessments of the question-naire responses, only twenty-seven of the ninety were accepted to pass on to the third stage of selection. Each of the twenty-seven was given an interview with one of the four Tavistock participants, an interview which lasted at least one-and-a-half hours and which was tape-recorded. The Tavistock participants then met and discussed each case and agreed to accept eight into the study. These eight represent approximately nine per cent of those who had completed screening question-naires and seven per cent of the patients identified as candidates for psychotherapy by sympathetic psychiatrists. A more dramatic example of the selectivity of contemporary psychotherapists would be hard to come by.

However, if psychoanalysis applied to minimally ill patients is no better than less complicated approaches, what is the price of the intricate techniques of interpretation, analysis and resolution? If simpler approaches are indeed effective, how do they bring about their effects? Here is where we remain woefully ignorant. The talking therapies may indeed be effective, but why and in what way seems unclear. What does not seem important is the expertise of the therapist. (Expertise of a therapist may well be important when it comes to the diagnosis and treatment of the more seriously mentally ill, but in this group psychotherapy is less and less considered a major therapeutic intervention of worth and, when it is used, it is almost always as an adjunct to other treatment such as drugs and social manipulations.) In 1979 a study was published claiming to clarify the extent to which such therapeutic effects as do occur are due to specific techniques as opposed to so-called non-specific factors in any benign human relationship. 'Highly experienced' psychotherapists treated fifteen male college students because of their high scores on a personality inventory designed to identify disturbed individuals. A comparable sample was treated by a group comprising 'professors of English, history, mathematics and philo-sophy', while another comparable group underwent no therapy but was merely tested at intervals for comparison with those in treatment. On average, the young men treated by the professors showed as much improve-ment as those treated by the professional therapists, despite the fact that the five professional therapists had on average twenty-five years of experience and had been selected on the basis of their reputation in the pro-fessional and academic community for their clinical expertise. More sobering still is the fact that the group of young men who receiv-ed no treatment at all did almost as well.

As one might expect, the analytically-trained psychotherapists and the college professors behaved differently with their respective patients. The analytically-oriented therapists fostered a 'professional' relation-ship characterized by respectful listening, questioning, making psychoanalytic interpre-tations (on the basis of such notions as trans-ference, oedipal conflicts etc.) and maintain-ing a notable interpersonal distance. The college professors, whose behaviour resembled so-called 'experiential' psychotherapists, tend-ed to be more relaxed, more willing to engage in free-and-easy exchange with their patients, more ready to provide direct advice and guid-ance and more likely to discuss issues other than feelings, conflicts and difficulties. In the words of the authors of this study,

> 'the professional therapist's unique contribution to treatment outcomes . . . . did not appear to be linked with specific skills in dealing with resistances or in interpreting neurotic patterns but rather with his ability to potentiate therapeutic gains in individuals who appeared to be highly motivated for therapy and whose resistance to change is low' (Strupp and Hadley, 1979).

In the light of this and other evidence which suggests that psychoanalysis has little to offer over and above less complicated and demanding treatments, the growth of much simpler forms of talking treatment is more readily understandable. The rise of these psychotherapies has served to sharpen the debate over the efficacy of psychoanalysis, a debate given an extra twist by growing concern regarding the financial cost of analytic treatment and training. A recent review of the length of the average training analysis of all the applicants to the American Psycho-analytical Association indicated that only three of the 191 applicants over a four-year period underwent a training analysis lasting less than four hundred hours. Eighty-seven had analyses lasting more than a thousand hours, thirty-three of more than fifteen hundred hours and six of more than two thousand hours. The overall average for the sample was just over one thousand hours. It is therefore hardly surprising that another study of some 850 analytic candidates and their spouses reported that the psychoanalytic training was creating a strain on their relationship with their children and spouses, leaving out the impact of the financial burden of paying the training fees, a burden that eighty per cent of the respondents found either 'substantial' or 'horrendous'. Perhaps we whould not be surprised that professionals, having negotiated a training experience surpassed in length and intensity only by the Jesuit novitiate, should prove somewhat

reluctant to embark on research exercises aimed at discovering whether the whole business amounts to anything truly significant.

Thus we find ourselves confronted by a number of nagging questions to which answers remain elusive. There is no general agreement as yet on what constitutes a valid psychotherapeutic training. There is no good evidence that patients benefit from treatment by most qualified psychotherapists. There is no evidence, either, that the proliferation of ersatz and superficial psychotherapies such as primal therapy, rolfing, est, marathon nude groups and the rest of what one critic has referred to as the 'transatlantic psychotherapy zoo' represents a threat or a boon to the mental health of potential consumers. As Sir John Foster pointed out in his report on Scientology, the worry is that the individuals who flock to psychotherapy, orthodox and unorthodox, tend to be the very people 'who are most easily exploited' and include the weak, the insecure, the nervous, the lonely, the inadequate and the depressed 'whose desperation is often such that they are willing to do and pay anything for some improvement of their condition' (Foster, 1971).

'A great many of us', declared Bishop Latimer in 1553, 'when we be in trouble, or sickness, or lose anything, we run hither and thither to witches, or sorcerers, who we call wise men . . . seeking aid and comfort at their hands.' In four hundred years, little has changed. The mentally distressed, like the poor, are always with us and the wizards, the witches, the sorcerers, wise men and sages are with us too, purveying the same potent or impotent brew of medicine, magic and myth. Attempts to distinguish the potent from the impotent and the charlatan from the genuine continue, but these are dogged by many problems, not least being the fact that in psychotherapy, more than in any other form of treatment, the charismatic personality of the therapist may be one of the most important elements in the overall efficacy. In this respect, it is worth noting that in a study of encounter groups undertaken by researchers at Stanford University it was found that those therapists who seemed to possess particularly powerful, even invasive personalities, appeared to wield the most therapeutic influence — in both beneficial and harmful directions.

It is, of course, fashionable to attribute the growth of psychoanalysis and psychotherapy to affluence, easy living and boredom. A more relevant factor may be the extent to which psychotherapy flourishes in societies in which traditional personal, family, social and communal supports have been eroded. It is interesting to note in this regard that Foster's scientology report distinguished between psychotherapy practised for fee or reward and 'the kind of psychotherapy we all practise on each other in our personal relationships' and that provided by many organizations involved in 'counselling'. The first and third are needed when the second is less available. Burgeoning self-help movements reflect a growing dissatisfaction with the tendency to assume that all manner of problems of life and living require appropriate experts, be they trained, partly trained or untrained, to provide solutions. The characteristics of self-help groups include the mutual help and support members provide, the notion that it may be the helper who benefits most from the therapeutic exchange, the valuable notion of normality which such groups foster, the promotion of greater factual understanding, the action-orientated philosophy (the notion that members learn by doing and are changed by doing, rather than by developing intrapsychic understanding) and the collective will-power and belief which enables each person to look to others in the group for validation of his feelings and attitudes. The self-help movement, in short, may represent a significant alternative response to what hitherto has been an assumption at the heart of the psychotherapies, both old and new, that life's problems require a system, a technique, a body of skill, be it Freudian, Rogerian, trans-actional, primal or psychodrama theory.

In the face of these developments, the protagonists of psychotherapy have not stayed still. Confronted by evidence which suggests that their effectiveness is not much better than relatively untrained practitioners using personal characteristics of charisma, empathy and concern, some have responded by suggesting that psychotherapy, particularly psychoanalysis, is not concerned with symptomatic behaviour or cure or even change so much as with meaning. It is true that many of the people who flock to treatment are better categorized as unhappy, bewildered and demoralized than as ill and that the questions they ask are often ultimate questions concerning existence, purpose, meaning, happiness, pain, evil and death. Psychotherapists are increasingly willing to provide answers — which may not be surprising given that Freud, asked to define the new worker he had created, answered 'secular pastoral counsellor'.

Should psychotherapy frankly acknowledge its secular religious role and turn away from any pretence of being scientific, the question of efficacy, about which we are still so ignorant, may well become largely redundant. One does not ask whether prayer or religious faith 'works' in the sense that we ask whether penicillin or an antidepressant or aversion therapy works. There is, of course, an element of faith involved in every medical treatment. However, when that element becomes the only element then the 'treatment' concerned moves from the realm of science to the realm of faith. It could be argued that our remarkable ignorance concerning the actual effectiveness of psychoanalysis and psychotherapy persisting well into the last decades of this century owes something to the fact that such activities belong more properly to religion than medicine. If that is the case, it would seem unwise to expect a speedy resolution.

References

BULLETIN of the Menninger Clinic (1972) *Psychotherapy and Psychoanalysis.* Final Report of the Menninger Foundation' Psychotherapy Research Project. Vol. 36 ,Nos 1—2.

CANDY, J., BALBOUR, F.H.G., CAWLEY, R.H., HILDEBRAND, H.P., MALAN, D.H., MARKS, I.M. and WILSON, J. (1972) A feasibility study for a controlled trial of formal psychotherapy. *Psychological Medicine,* 2, 345—362.

CLARE, A.W. and THOMPSON, S. (1981) *Let's Talk About Me: A Critical Examination of the New Psycho-therapies.* BBC, London.

FOSTER, J.G. (1971) *Enquiry into the Practice and Effects of Scientology.* HMSO, London.

LUBORSKY, L., SINGER, B. and LUBORSKY, L. (1975) Comparative studies of psychotherapies: is it true that 'everyone has won and all must have prizes'? *Archives of General Psychiatry,* 32, 995—1008.

SLOANE, R.B., STAPLES, F.R., CRISTOL, A.H., YORKSTON, N.J. and WHIPPLE, K. (1975) *Psychotherapy Versus Behaviour Therapy.* Harvard University Press, Boston.

STRUPP, H. and HADLEY, S.W. (1979) Specific versus non-specific factors in psychotherapy. *Archives of General Psychiatry,* 36, 1125—1136.

THE NEGLECT OF ADVANCES IN THE NEUROLOGY OF BEHAVIOR

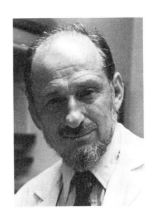

Norman Geschwind

James Jackson Putnam Professor of Neurology, Harvard Medical School, Chief of Neurology, Beth Israel Hospital, Boston*, and Professor of Health Sciences and Technology and Psychology, Massachusetts Institute of Technology, USA.

Formerly Professor of Neurology at the Boston University School of Medicine. His major interests have been in the relationships of brain to behaviour. He has written on the organization and pathological disruptions of the language systems in the brain, on callosal syndromes and the effects of disconnections of various brain regions from each other on the anatomical asymmetries of the human and other animals, and on the history of ideas in the study of brain and behaviour.

The state of ignorance can have many causes. The most challenging to the scientist is the actual lack of data. In many cases, however, some individuals may be unaware of the existence of important findings either as a result of lack of exposure, failure to understand, or failure of memory. In other instances ignorance may be widespread even among those who are informed, intelligent, and retentive simply because the existing knowledge is unavailable, either through lack of publication, publication in a foreign language (especially one that is little known), or because of publication in journals or books that are, for other than linguistic reasons, either unobtainable or rarely consulted. Ignorance which results from these causes is well recognized and the scientific world has devised many effective corrective stratagems: expansion of research, improved education, free exchange of reprints, abstracting and translating services, and the creation of review journals. There are, however, other causes of ignorance of existing knowledge which are much more difficult to

* From the Charles A. Dana Laboratories, Beth Israel Hospital, Boston and the Boston University Aphasia Research Center. Some of the work was supported by grants from The Essel Foundation, The Orton Fund, The National Institutes of Health (NINCDS 14018, NINCDS 06209) and the National Science Foundation (NSF BNS–77–05674).

9

correct and therefore more pernicious. There may be neglect of correct existing facts or theories, either through deliberate suppression or through widespread acceptance of incorrect data or erroneous criticisms. Furthermore, although the actual lack of data in an important area should be a powerful stimulus to scientific curiosity, there are cases in which research is not carried out either because of the erroneous belief that there are no suitable investigative methods or because well established scientists and administrators are unwilling to allocate resources to innovative areas because of prejudice, timidity, or simple desire to support their own fields at the expense of newer less influential ones. Finally, ignorance may result from the deliberate publication of false data, or the prevention of publication by rivals, or the willful withholding of information that might enable others to move ahead.

There is a powerful implicit belief that science advances inexorably. Inherent in this view is the idea that errors in data or theory cannot persist for any length of time, and that potentially fruitful areas of investigation will inevitably be pursued actively. There is a widely held supposition that one's scientific peers are honest, well informed, not swayed by prejudices, and open to imaginative ventures into the unknown. The most common assumption among scientists is that ignorance is almost always the result of an actual lack of knowledge about a given field and that in a minority of instances it is due to inadvertent failure to be aware of obscure publications, such as Mendel's original work on heredity. This utopian faith in scientific advance persists despite many occurrences which demonstrate that although science has replaced religion in the minds of many educated people, the unquestioned belief in the virtues of scientists may be as misinformed as the older faith that the clergy were always the true repository of spiritual values.

We need only to recall the many instances of deliberate falsification of data. There is a vehement reaction against what are construed to be anti- or pseudo-scientific activities such as the creationist movement or the writings of Velikovsky, yet instances of scientific fakery are typically regarded as random aberrations which lead to unfavorable publicity. This is comparable with the reluctance of many scientists to discuss the wasteful use of research funds for fear that the public might be prepared to withdraw its support. Yet examples of scientific chicanery have been so common that one can hardly neglect them, especially when many have occurred in what were considered to be the most advanced scientific communities in the world. Thus, in England we find the Piltdown Man, and the deliberate distortion of data by Cyril Burt who was the leading psychometrician of his day. In the most widely read weekly scientific journals, *Nature* and *Science*, we find repeated descriptions of plagiarized or invented data. Thus within the last several years researchers at the medical schools of Harvard, Yale, Cornell, and Boston University have been dismissed as the result of invented or plagiarized data (Broad, 1981; Gillie, 1979).

Furthermore, it has become increasingly clear that scientists, even when honest, may engage in destructive competition and backbiting, often at the expense of vulnerable and junior people. The revelations of the discovery of the double helix were regarded as unfortunate reflections on scientific behavior by some, but were justified by a very large number of scientists on the basis of a morality that some regard as reflecting the most seedy aspects of the business world, i.e. success is its own justification. There is, furthermore, widespread acceptance in many scientific communities of the custom of chiefs of units placing their names on every paper, even when they have in no way been involved in the research.

It is my purpose here to point out that in the field of the neurology of behaviour, major advances were neglected, not for a few years, but for nearly half a century because of a series of factors which had nothing to do with the quality of the investigations, the distinction of the researchers, or the journals in which the data were published. As I will try to show, the neglect of these important data resulted from influences which were essentially non-scientific. I will furthermore argue that just as in our naivete we have been prepared to accept gross scholarly deceit, failure to take account of these non-scientific influences will leave us open in the future to making similar errors repetitively.

In order to make this account more vivid let me begin by telling you about a particular patient. A 57 year old woman exhibited some rather remarkable behaviour with her left hand, which she claimed was beyond her control. It would come up to her neck and apparently tried to strangle her so that she had to pull it away with the right hand, or would rip the sheets off the bed. The right hand showed no such behaviour. She was examined by a young neurologist who found that she was awake and attentive and spoke and understood written and spoken language normally. Her left leg was paralyzed, but the left arm was not. Her right hand carried out all requested movements correctly. On the other hand, when a pen was placed in her left hand she would write illegibly, producing only strokes or rings. She did not carry out on request even simple movements, e.g. raising the hand, with the left arm. She failed with the left hand to imitate movements made by the examiner. When objects were placed in the left hand she often manipulated them incorrectly, although right hand manipulation of objects was faultless. Thus the left hand carried a comb to a position under her nose and brushed her hair with the back of a brush. Yet in the course of a day the left hand might pick up one of the very same objects spontaneously and use it correctly. If, when the patient was blindfolded, the right arm was placed in a particular position, she could not imitate this with her left arm.

After detailed study the examiner con-

cluded that the patient had suffered damage to the corpus callosum in the brain on the basis of a loss of its blood supply as a result of occlusion of the major artery which supplied this structure. He was able to make this diagnosis because he recognized that the patient showed several of the typical features of disconnection of the cerebral hemispheres which had already been established on the basis of earlier studies. This diagnosis made in life was fully confirmed, since the patient subsequently died and the brain was subjected to careful examination. The whole fixed brain was cut in serial sections and the full extent of the damage was mapped. She had, as predicted, suffered from destruction of most of the extent of the corpus callosum.

This case is a dramatic example of the syndrome of disconnection of the corpus callosum. But perhaps the most dramatic aspect of this case report is that it was published in 1908 (Goldstein, 1908) and the final complete report of the pathological findings was published in 1912. Furthermore, the author of this article was not an obscure figure but, in fact, an individual who was later to achieve a major international reputation: Kurt Goldstein, who came to the United States as a refugee in the 1930s and who was to become one of the leading figures in American psychology. His publications were read by thousands of American students and many of his pupils and associates became important leaders of American psychology.

Furthermore, Goldstein's conclusions about this patient were based on his knowledge of the very first description of the syndrome of the anterior four-fifths of the corpus callosum by Hugo Karl Liepmann (1900) whose diagnosis had also been subsequently fully confirmed anatomically. There had also been earlier descriptions of cases in which the posterior fifth of the corpus callosum, rather than the anterior four-fifths, was damaged, producing a failure to transmit information between the hemispheres. Damage of this type is characteristic of the condition called pure alexia without agraphia, the first description of the brain changes being that of the French neurologist, Jules Dejerine (1892).

The syndromes of hemispheric disconnection resulting from lesions of the corpus callosum were described in many other papers and were well known before World War I. Furthermore, several books on the subject were published by German, French and Italian authors. The English neurologist Kinnier Wilson published an account of these studies in *Brain*, the most distinguished neurological journal of that period, in 1913. The callosal syndromes became a standard part of German neurological teaching, and were, for example, discussed extensively in the monumental multivolume *Handbuch der Neurologie* published in the 1930s.

The remarkable fact is that despite these superb descriptions of the clinical picture of callosal disconnection by master observers, and the confirmation of the location of the damage at post-mortem examination, almost every bit of this fundamental knowledge disappeared from the neurological literature in England, France, and the United States. Even more striking than the neglect of this original knowledge concerning the functions of the corpus callosum and its disorders was the appearance in the literature of incorrect descriptions or bold statements that nothing was known about the callosum and its functions. Walter Dandy, the distinguished neurosurgical pioneer at Johns Hopkins, went so far as to state that, on the basis of his own experience, he could dismiss all the fantastic claims which had been made for the functions of the great cerebral commissure. Warren McCulloch, a distinguished neuroscientist at Yale, Illinois, and MIT, once told me that in that period between the wars there were two views about the corpus callosum which expressed humorously the positive certainty of ignorance. One was that the only function of this structure was to facilitate the propagation of epilepsy between the two cerebral

hemispheres, and the other, even more facetious, was that its only role was to keep the hemispheres from falling apart!

How is one to account for this state of affairs? Obviously, this important work was either totally neglected or misquoted, or, even when read, studied so incompletely that the evidence and the methods of examination were simply not adequately learned. Even the occasional well-documented observation which ran counter to the general views was disregarded. Thus, after Walter Dandy had announced that he found no effects from cutting the posterior end of the corpus callosum, two colleagues in the same institution, John Trescher and Frank Ford (1937) published a paper demonstrating signs of callosal disconnection in one of Dandy's own patients! This publication was also the first demonstration of callosal disconnection in humans as the result of surgery, the earlier cases having been the result of spontaneous disease processes, most often obstructions of a vessel supplying a part of the corpus callosum. When some years later Paolo Maspes, a neurosurgeon at the University of Milan, confirmed the findings of Trescher and Ford in several cases, his work was also disregarded. When Andrew Akelaitis, of the University of Rochester, studied the cases in whom the neurosurgeon Van Wagenen had carried out a section of the corpus callosum for treatment of epilepsy, he also denied finding signs of disconnection. Yet, several of his cases showed the same phenomenon of the uncontrollable left hand that had been described by Goldstein. Since subsequent experience has confirmed that surgery of the callosum in humans, as reported by Gazzaniga and Sperry and others, does indeed produce signs of disconnection, one suspects that the investigators in Rochester had not adequately learned the methods of examination of the earlier clinical masters.

A major factor in the failure to read the older literature at all, or to misread it, was almost certainly the fact that most of the classical papers in this area were by German authors. Before the First World War German neurological literature clearly dominated that of all other nations, and was avidly read and studied. German was the major language of science not only in Germany, Austria, and Switzerland, but also in the major centers of the Austro-Hungarian empire outside of Austria itself, i.e. in the regions which today include most of Eastern Europe and part of Italy. Furthermore, most Dutch and Scandinavian researchers published in German as did those within the Russian empire. The major affiliations of American neurological science at this period were to German investigations and publications. The First World War led not only to the political defeat of Germany and the dissolution of the Austrian empire, but also to a major decline in German prestige and continued hostility toward German science. These anti-German feelings persisted, curious as it may seem today, much longer after the first World War than after the second. Just as the prestige of German science had increased greatly as a result of the victory over the French in the Franco-Prussian War, so the defeat of Germany in World War I led to a corresponding rise in the prestige of the English speaking countries. Articles or books on the higher functions in English or French after 1918 show a remarkable tendency to omit or misquote German references.

Another major factor in this neglect of the early work was the simultaneous growth of dynamic psychiatry and holistic psychologies. Despite Freud's own background in neurology and the constant assertion of his biological interest, references to the brain are almost totally lacking in the literature of psychoanalysis in that period. Neurological aspects of behaviour were almost totally lacking in British academic psychology and the tremendous growth of psychology as a discipline in the United States was accompanied by a strong aversion to the belief that the structure of the brain could help to account for behaviour.

Certain influential individuals had an enormous influence on thinking in this period. Percival Bailey, Warren McCulloch, and Gerhard von Bonin spent many years mapping the connections of the cerebral cortex in non-human primates, but explicitly stated that these connections were known to be without functional significance. As McCulloch later told me they were all so hypnotized by the theoretical arguments of the distinguished American psychologist Karl Lashley who had argued against the importance of the cortical connections in behaviour that they did not realize how bizarre their position was. Even more curious was the influence of Kurt Goldstein, who had himself described so brilliantly one of the early cases of callosal disconnection quoted above. His major influence on American psychology and neurology was as a leading exponent of the view that analyses of behavior in terms of localized brain structures and connections were naive and erroneous. Oddly enough, it was apparently totally unrecognized that there was a major contradiction between these theoretical statements and his own substantive publications (Geschwind, 1964). It cannot be argued that he had abandoned his belief in this earlier work, since the second half of one of his later books (published in 1948) contains detailed discussions of the importance of localized brain lesions and the connections of the cerebral cortex. Indeed, he continued to point with pride in this book to his own early work on the callosal disconnection syndromes. That so major a public figure could have succeeded over so many years in leading the life of an intellectual double agent unbeknownst even to his closest students is astonishing. Even after his death the French journal *Neuropsychologia* carried a series of articles on him, none of which pointed out these glaring contradictions or even acknowledged the existence of a published critique of his curiously paradoxical position.

A similar major influence was the work of the English neurologist Henry Head (1926), which also led neurologists throughout the world to essentially the same positions as those supported by Lashley and Goldstein. The fact that this widely read work was also self-contradictory appears to have attracted no attention at the time of its publication. This effect of Lashley, Goldstein and Head reminds one of the cynical statement that the real greatness of a man is measured by how long he manages to hold up progress.

In addition, the study of the brain as related to behaviour was almost entirely neglected in the period between the wars. Thus, despite the distinguished accomplishments of British neurophysiology in the period between the wars, one looks almost in vain for any work on neural foundations of behaviour in either animals or humans. This strongly suggests that the small number of powerful figures who controlled English research simply regarded this field as without promise.

What is the moral of this story? It would be easy to dismiss it on the grounds that this could not happen today, and that these stories belong with those of the unfortunate influences of Aristotelian science, Ptolemaic astronomy, the phlogiston theory, or bloodletting. Unfortunately, I believe that this is wishful thinking of the kind which has led to the many abuses I mentioned at the beginning of this article. The fact that science is constantly changing leads most scientists to have short memories, and to the too-ready assumption that once a situation like this is corrected, or indeed only partially corrected, science is back on the correct track of honesty and inevitable advance. Yet the history recounted here shows us how readily highly intelligent and powerful people are caught up in scientific fads, in unwitting agreement with false data or theories, and in the suppression of true knowledge for long periods. Many, if not most, of those who are aware of the situation while it is going on are reluctant to speak up because of the unpleasantness of public attack or fears for their academic futures: they often

fail to get their ideas or investigations published. Their work, when published, is often relegated to the category of naivete or ignorance. I have already referred to the failure of Bailey, McCulloch, and Bonin to assess properly the significance of their own work. Another dramatic example was the publication by one neurosurgeon of a case of obvious callosal disconnection which was correctly interpreted. While the paper was in press he added a footnote at the end saying that he realized that his interpretation must of course be wrong!

The account I have given here is only one example of the failure in advances in the neurology of behaviour to be appreciated for long periods. There are other cases, for example, in the history of the study of aphasia, but I will not go on to discuss these since they only serve to illustrate again the points already made. Furthermore, even today there are similar instances which I will not discuss.

In brief, the lessons to be learned are clear. Science is clearly one of the outstanding achievements of humanity, but like any other great accomplishment it suffers the risk of being distorted by the failings of human beings. It should indeed be part of the training of every young scientist to be aware how non-scientific influences can positively block the forward advance of science. Nationalism is one source of error. Strongly held political views, especially those which view science as an expression of politics, are also potent sources of obstruction of the search for the truth. The implication by some writers that science is distorted only by political conservatives is remarkable for the failure to appreciate that almost all political dogmas whether of the left, right, or centre have been instrumental in distorting science. This is particularly true in any field dealing with behaviour since political dogmas of any color usually embody an implicit or explicit theory of behaviour.

Another major source of difficulty is

professional chauvinism, i.e. the strong patriotic attachment to one's own discipline with contempt for work carried out by those in other fields. Excessive control of any scientific endeavour by a small number of powerful individuals is a danger, however distinguished these persons may be. To this sorry list we must add personal failings, such as excessive ambition and envy which may lead to the unfair criticism of known work, the failure to provide support or to permit publication of the work of rivals, and indeed even plagiarism, concealment of one's own work, and deliberate falsification. Finally, we should recall that while modern science advanced only when free investigation was liberated from the shackles of all-embracing philosophies, there is still a powerful tendency, especially in fields related to human behaviour which have such broad implications for politics and morality, for individuals to adopt universal philosophical positions that blind them to the actual data, even when, as is usually the case, these data have no political implications.

References

BROAD, W.J. (1981) Fraud and the structure of science, *Science*, **212**, 137—141.

DEJERINE, J. (1892) Contribution a l'étude anatomo-pathologique et clinique des différentes variétés de cécité verbale, *Bulletin et mémoires de la Société de Biologie*, **4**, 61—90.

GESCHWIND, N. (1964) The paradoxical position of Kurt Goldstein in the history of aphasia, *Cortex*, **1**, 214—224.

GILLIE, O. (1979) Burt's missing ladies, *Science*, **204**, 1035—1039.

GOLDSTEIN, K. (1908) Zur Lehre von der motorischen Apraxie, *Journal für Psychologie und Neurologie*, **11**, 169—187 and 270—283.

HEAD, H. (1926) *Aphasia and Kindred Disorders of Speech*, Cambridge University Press, Cambridge.

LIEPMANN, H. (1900) *Das Krankheitsbild der Apraxie*, S. Karger, Berlin.

TRESCHER, J. and FORD, F. (1937) Colloid cyst of the third ventricle, *Archives of Neurology and Psychiatry*, **37**, 959—973.

SCHIZOPHRENIA – THE PROBLEM OF THE MECHANISM OF THE DISTURBANCE AND ITS CAUSATION

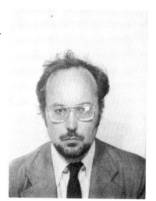

T.J. Crow

Head of the Division of Psychiatry, Clinical Research Centre, Northwick Park Hospital, Middlesex.

He is an honorary consultant psychiatrist to Northwick Park and Shenley Hospitals and was previously senior lecturer in Psychiatry at the University of Manchester and lecturer in Mental Health and Physiology at the University of Aberdeen. His research interests are in the physiology of monoamine neurones, with particular reference to reward mechanisms, neurochemical studies of schizophrenia and Alzheimer's disease, the pharmacology of neuroleptic drugs, and the possible role of viruses in the aetiology of psychiatric illness.

Schizophrenia as a concept is a focus for the controversies of psychiatry. That there are diseases whose only manifestations are mental and that predictions concerning outcome and response to treatment can be based upon an analysis of subjective phenomena, are notions from which some dissent. Whether specific symptoms reliably demarcate the group of illnesses labelled schizophrenias from manic-depressive illness, that other major group of functional psychoses on the one hand, and the organic states on the other, are questions which academic psychiatrists continue to debate. Yet since one per cent of the general population at some point in a lifetime is estimated to be at risk of an illness which will be diagnosed schizophrenic, and a majority of the occupants of long-stay mental hospital beds have this diagnosis, these issues are not esoteric.

The concept originates from Kraepelin's delineation of dementia praecox from manic-depressive psychosis. Kraepelin argued that the earlier descriptive categories of paranoia, hebephrenia and catatonia were related to each other by an overlap in symptoms and some uniformity of outcome; these patients did badly in that symptoms often tended to persist. By contrast in manic-depressive psychosis relapses might occur, but complete recovery (*'restitutio ad integrum'*) was to be expected. Dementia praecox and manic-depressive insanity together, according to Kraepelin, were to be distinguished from the organic psychoses, a point emphasised by E. Bleuler, who enlarged Kraepelin's concept of dementia praecox to include some cases with less obvious symptoms, and relabelled it schizophrenia. According to Bleuler, in schizophrenia true intellectual deterioration does not occur. With some equivocation Kraepelin appears to have agreed that the same was true of dementia praecox. In this way schizophrenia was to be distinguished from the organic psychoses.

Within the group of the functional psychoses the primary criterion by which Kraepelin considered the disease was to be distinguished from manic-depressive insanity was outcome. Yet, although of historical significance, the criterion of outcome is unsatisfactory as a diagnostic rule, not least because the role of diagnosis in predicting outcome is undermined. In practice diagnosis is based upon the phenomena of the presenting illness, and the presence or absence of affective disturbance assumes a crucial role. If there is affective disturbance (i.e. depression or elation) and such other psychotic phenomena (e.g. delusions or hallucinations) as are present can be seen to congruent with and possibly secondary to such affective disturbance the rule is that the diagnosis is manic-depressive illness. If affective disturbance is absent, or the psychotic phenomena cannot be understood in this way, and organic illness can be excluded, the diagnosis is schizophrenia. While there is little doubt that illnesses in which the primary disturbance is affective have as Kraepelin supposed a better outcome than those with symptoms of the dementia praecox type, there is yet considerable overlap both with respect to symptoms and outcome. Thus there is doubt as to whether either outcome or the relationship of the affective to other psychotic symptoms can be used as a criterion for demarcating a group of illnesses which can be exptected to be of uniform pathogenesis. Moreover the significance of the discrepancy between the affective and non-affective symptoms, indeed the nature of the characteristically schizophrenic component, remains to be elucidated.

The Nature of the Symptoms

The schizophrenic symptoms themselves may provide clues to the nature of the disease process. Thus delusions (erroneous convictions concerning the nature of the external world maintained 'in the teeth of contrary evidence') and hallucinations (sensory experiences, treated by the patient as such, but arising in the absence of adequate external stimulation) which cannot be accounted for in terms of a primary mood change (as for example can grandiose delusions in states of elation) and occurring in the absence of disorientation (i.e. with intact ability to acquire information concerning temporal and spatial aspects of the immediate environment) are common in schizophrenia. The individual draws erroneous conclusions concerning the external world and special significance and meaning is attached to otherwise unimportant but real events. The mechanisms for distinguishing internal from external stimuli and for attributing appropriate significance to the latter are disturbed. Yet these are not generalised disturbances as may be the case in some organic disorders, e.g. the confusional states. In the latter hallucinations and delusions are often varied and also transient and the mechanisms for acquiring new information are disturbed; in schizophrenia delusions are frequently fixed and sometimes isolated, hallucinations are of particular types and the mechanisms of information acquisition are, at least in major respects, unimpaired.

In an attempt to base diagnosis upon symptoms rather than outcome K. Schneider advanced the concept of the first rank symptoms, that is symptoms whose unequivocal presence indicates with a high probability that the illness is schizophrenic. According to

Schneider's concept these symptoms define a group of schizophrenic illnesses of 'nuclear' type, although illnesses in which these symptoms do not occur may nevertheless be regarded as schizophrenic. Schneider himself regarded the symptoms as a means of arriving at an operational definition of the disease but they may also reveal something of the nature of the process.

The symptoms include:

(1) Auditory hallucinations of certain types — e.g. voices discussing the patient in the third person, conducting a running commentary on the patient's actions, and speaking the patient's thoughts out loud ('gedankenlautwerden').
(2) Delusions concerning the patient's thoughts — for example that thoughts are inserted into or removed from his head (by an agency outside his control).
(3) Delusions concerning the patient's actions or sensations of a similar kind, for example that actions are imposed upon him from outside or that he is 'made to' have certain emotions or sensations.
(4) The phenomenon of 'delusional perception' in which the patient attributes to an otherwise normal sensory experience meaning which cannot be understood either in terms of the experience itself or his previous beliefs, or a combination of the two.

These common but striking phenomena reveal aspects of the disease process which require an explanation, perhaps in physiological terms. Some symptoms, e.g. the auditory hallucinations, might be explained if it be assumed the patient is abnormally aware of some types of neural activity and classifies such activity as arising from the external world. The activity itself might not be abnormal, for example it might represent information processing normally excluded from consciousness. Similarly in the case of the

delusional phenomena it appears that the patient experiences thoughts, sensations and even intentions which he fails to recognise as arising from his own antecedent mental activity and is compelled to attribute to the outside world. The utter unfamiliarity of such experiences to a normal individual and the lack of difficulty which normal individuals have in distinguishing information arising from the external and internal environments reveals an aspect of consciousness which is not self-evident; that consciousness is, as if 'by definition', what is under the individual's own control. The considerable problems of achieving a logical and coherent view of the world when such control is lost are amongst those with which schizophrenic patients are confronted.

Delusions and hallucinations, of which Schneider's first rank symptoms are examples, are referred to as 'positive' symptoms, in the sense that it is the presence of such features which is of pathological significance, and are contrasted with the 'negative' symptoms, which are represented by the loss of some normal function. Negative symptoms are by no means invariable features of the disease, but they are common, probably develop more slowly and may account for some of the more serious long-term disabilities. Thus 'affective flattening', a loss of the ability to experience a range of emotional responses, loss of drive, and poverty of speech, a restriction of the quantity and variety of words used, are classified as negative symptoms. Positive and negative symptoms appear to be independent dimensions of psychopathology and may reflect different aspects or effects of the underlying disease process.

The Nature of the Disease Process

Are there structural changes in the brain?

The corollary of the views of Kraepelin and Bleuler that schizophrenia is a disease which can be clearly distinguished from dementia is that the disease process in the two conditions is quite different. Thus whereas in the dementias (e.g. in Alzheimer's disease) intellectual impairment is associated with structural changes in the brain it has often been assumed (although not by Kraepelin) that such changes are absent in the functional psychoses. This assumption is challenged by findings which suggest that some schizophrenic patients do show intellectual impairments and by evidence, principally radiological, that some have structural changes in the brain. Thus some institutionalised patients have been found to have defects of temporal orientation, often believing themselves to be many years younger than they really are, to have been in hospital a lesser time, and to be mistaken concerning the current year. According to conventional psychiatric criteria such disorientation is characteristic of organic brain disease. These patients have other evidence of intellectual deterioration although they have not suffered from an illness other then schizophrenia (although in most cases this disease has been present for many years) and the cognitive deficit cannot be attributed to the physical treatments they have received. Several radiological studies suggest some patients with chronic schizophrenia also have structural changes in the brain. Such evidence first emerged from air encephalographic studies conducted in the 1930s. This technique involves removal of cerebro-spinal fluid and has some adverse effects. For this reason comparisons with normal subjects were seldom possible and the findings were discounted by some as observer error. The introduction of computerised tomography rekindled interest in this problem. Although the scatter of values is wide it does appear that in the population of patients with chronic schizophrenia mean cerebral ventricular size is larger than in age-matched normal subjects, suggesting that in some schizo-

phrenic patients there is loss of cerebral substance. Within this group of patients increased ventricular size is associated with intellectual impairment. Such changes are more likely to be seen in patients who have been ill for many years. Although the possibility that the ventricular changes may represent a predisposition (i.e. that they may have been present from early in life) to a particularly disabling form of the disease cannot be altogether ruled out it seems likely that in these cases the disease process itself is responsible. Thus some patients with schizophrenia suffer from a disease which more closely resembles dementia than is often thought to be the case.

Neurochemical changes

These findings suggest there is an irreversible component and it might be this which contributes to the poor long-term outcome by which Kraepelin thought schizophrenia could be distinguished from manic-depressive psychosis. On the other hand schizophrenic symptoms can be both improved and exacerbated, and can also be induced in normal subjects, by chemical means. Such observations reinforce the concept of schizophrenia as a functional psychosis the basis of which may be chemical rather than structural. Thus the efficacy of 'neuroleptic' drugs (of which the phenothiazine chlorpromazine is the prototype) both in the treatment of acute episodes and prevention of relapse is well established. Such drugs act as antagonists at dopamine receptors and much evidence supports the view that this pharmacological action is related to their therapeutic effects. Conversely amphetamine-like compounds which can release dopamine from neurones in the brain containing this monoamine (i.e. can potentiate dopaminergic transmission) exacerbate the positive symptoms of the disease and have been shown to induce such symptoms in normal volunteers. On this basis the 'dopamine hypothesis' — that the symptoms of schizophrenia are due to excessive dopaminergic transmission and are reduced by the dopamine receptor blockade brought about by administration of neuroleptic drugs — appears an attractive explanation for at least a part of the disease process. However, neither cerebro-spinal fluid studies nor investigations on post-mortem brain have revealed evidence of increased dopamine turnover. In post-mortem brain increased numbers of dopamine (but not of other neurotransmitter) receptors have been found in some patients. Increases in numbers of receptors can result from neuroleptic drug administration. However these changes are seen in some patients who have not recently received such medication, and the pattern of changes with respect to the different types of dopamine receptor which can now be distinguished does not

appear to be the same in post-mortem schizophrenic brain as seen in animal experiments with neuroleptic drugs. Thus the question of whether the changes seen in post-mortem brain samples from schizophrenic patients are associated with the disease process is of considerable importance.

Two syndromes

The possibility that both structural and neurochemical changes play a role in the pathogenesis of some schizophrenic illnesses suggests there is more than one component of the disease process. Indeed the distinction between positive and negative symptoms may identify two separate syndromes which are associated with different underlying pathological processes. Thus the syndrome of positive symptoms (the type I syndrome — Table 1) responds to neuroleptic drugs and is

Table 1. Two syndromes in schizophrenia

	Type I	Type II
symptoms	positive (delusions, hallucinations, thought disorder)	negative (flattening of affect, loss of drive, poverty of speech)
type of illness in which most commonly seen	acute schizophrenia	chronic schizophrenia (the 'defect state')
intellectual impairment	absent	may be present
response to neuroleptic drugs	good	poor
potential outcome	reversible	irreversible
postulated underlying pathological process	disturbance of dopaminergic transmission (? increased dopamine receptors)	cell loss leading to structural changes in the brain

exacerbated by amphetamine administration. This may be the dopaminergic component. Conversely negative symptoms (the 'type II syndrome') are associated with intellectual impairments, and these features appear to be related to the component of the disease process which leads to structural brain changes. These syndromes are not separate diseases, for both are often seen in the same patient, either at one point in time or sequentially. Thus patients who present with episodes of positive symptoms may later develop the features of the type II syndrome. The syndromes should be seen as overlapping (Fig. 1) and the changes that may occur with time (indicated by arrows) are of particular interest.

The two syndromes may occur together or separately in an individual patient. As indicated in Fig. 1 these combinations correspond to three of the types of schizophrenic illness described by Bleuler (catatonia introduces more complex issues). The apparent irreversibility of the type II syndrome presumably contributes to the poor long-term outcome of schizophrenic illnesses in general and may be attributable to the structural changes postulated as underlying this component of the disease process.

The role of the temporal lobe

For some time it has been recognised that psychoses with symptoms closely resembling those of schizophrenia are occasionally seen in association with temporal lobe epilepsy. Such illnesses occur in patients without a family predisposition and are probably less likely than 'true' schizophrenic illnesses to lead to the type II syndrome (negative symptoms). They may nevertheless manifest typical nuclear symptoms. Presumably in these cases the process which is responsible for the epileptogenic focus in the temporal lobe also causes the confusion between internally and externally-arising stimuli which is so characteristic of schizophrenia.

The functions of the hippocampus are obscure (see Fig. 2). One theory is that it is a device for monitoring discrepancies between the predicted and actual outcome of particular sequences of behaviour. To perform this function the hippocampus would require access to information both from the environment and from the long-term memory store. A confusion between these sources of information is a possible description of the origin of some schizophrenic symptoms. To accommodate the dopamine hypothesis in such a formulation one might suggest that dopamine neurones are involved in one aspect of this process, perhaps in identifying that neural activity which arises from external stimuli. Thus positive schizophrenic symptoms could arise either:— a) by an intrinsic disturbance

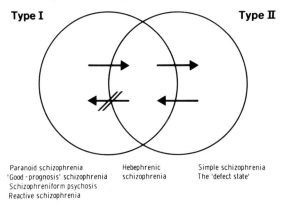

Fig. 1. The postulated inter-relationship between the two syndromes of schizophrenia.
Arrows indicate changes which can take place with the passage of time.

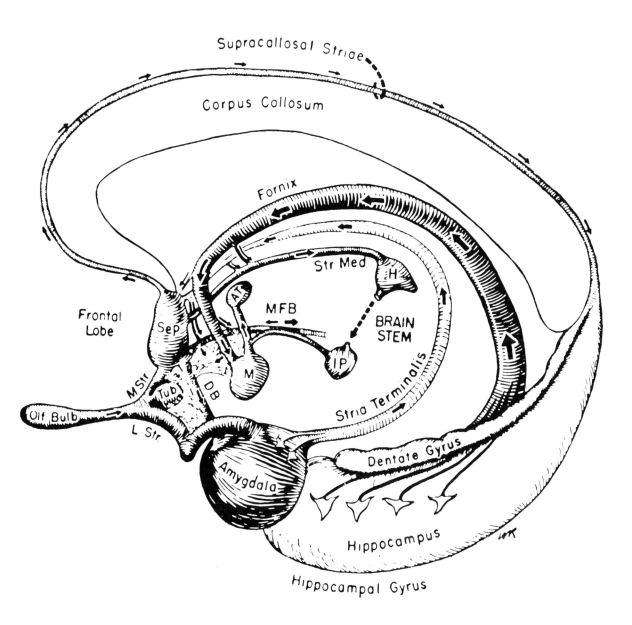

Fig. 2. A schematic representation of the connections of the amygdala and hippocampus. The hippocampus connects through the fornix with the mammillary bodies (M), and these in turn connect with the anterior thalamic nucleus (AT). The amygdala connects via the stria terminalis with the septum (SEP). Other abbreviations: (MFB — medial forebrain bundle; IP — interpeduncular nucleus; H — habenula; STR.MED. — stria medullaris; DB — diagonal band; M.STR. and L.STR. — medial and lateral olfactory striae; OLF.BULB — olfactory bulb; TUB — olfactory tubercle).
Reproduced from Maclean Psychosomatic Medicine, volume 11, 338–353; 1949.

of dopaminergic activity such that dopamine neurones which normally are activated only in response to extrinsic stimuli become excited also by neural activity arising within the organism, or b) by a disturbance in the region of the hippocampus such that incoming activity from two different sources (one of which is related either directly or indirectly to dopaminergic mechanisms) which in the normal subject leads to different consequences within the hippocampus, in the subject experiencing schizophrenic symptoms leads to the same consequence. Thus inputs from the two sources cannot be distinguished.

The temporal lobe has a further possible relevance for schizophrenia. It seems highly likely that the amygdala is concerned with evaluating the biological and adaptive significance of environmental stimuli and elaborating an appropriate emotional and behavioural response. The effects of lesions of the amygdala and its efferent connections in primates have resemblances to the type II syndrome of schizophrenia — such animals show a marked lack of drive and fail to respond appropriately to their peers. Thus it is possible that the type II syndrome is a result of damage to the amygdala and its connections. It is of particular interest that the major efferent pathway, the stria terminalis, travels close to the ventricle and is thus vulnerable to a pathogenic influence approaching from the cerebro-spinal fluid.

What is the cause of schizophrenia?

The genetic contribution to schizophrenia is firmly established by studies on twins of differing zygosities and on children adopted away from families with a predisposition to disease. Both strategies suggest a substantial contribution from the genes. For example the concordance for monozygotic twins is approximately 50% and for dizygotic twins 15%.

However, there are problems for the theory that the genetic components are the only or even the principal factor in aetiology. Firstly the mode of genetic transmission, whether uni- or multi-factorially determined and the 'degree of penetrance', remain obscure. Secondly the prevalence of the disease and its apparent resistance, in spite of the known low fertility of schizophrenic patients, to selective pressure is unexplained. Thirdly there are anomalies in the family data which are not readily explicable along genetic lines. For example it is reported that the concordance in same sex pairs of siblings is higher than for opposite sex pairs, and is also higher for dizygotic twins than for siblings.

A further peculiarity which schizophrenia shares with a number of genetically-influenced psychiatric and neurological diseases is that the onset is often well into adult life. This fact together with the less than 100% concordance in monozygotic twins appears to exclude the possibility that schizophrenia is a simple inherited disorder of metabolism. The evidence points to the genetic component as a predisposition to some other agent rather than as a primary cause.

The possibility that schizophrenia might be a viral disease was first suggested by the appearance of schizophrenic symptoms in some patients who suffered from post-influenzal psychoses following the 1918 epidemic and in patients with sequelae of the encephalitis lethargica epidemic in the early 1920s. Both illnesses were presumably viral although the viruses responsible for these manifestations have either died out or have changed their pathogenicity. But it is still possible that schizophrenia, as it occurs today, is due to an atypical and genetically-determined response to some already identified virus or to some as yet unidentified agent. Host genetic factors are often relevant to viral infections. Such interactions are well studied in the case of the agent which causes the neurological disease scrapie in sheep and may well also occur in human infections such as poliomyelitis. An interesting paradigm for the psychoses as viral diseases of the central nervous system are herpes infections. The herpes viruses have a predilection for certain types of neurone, e.g. sensory ganglia and can become established in a chronic and latent state, with acute exacerbations of symptoms resulting from reactivation.

Some epidemiological observations are consistent with the viral hypothesis. A seasonal trend for the onset of the disease with an excess of cases occurring in the early summer has recently been established. A further tendency for those who later become schizophrenic to have been born in the early months of the year has been reported in a number of countries, and shows a reversal in the southern hemisphere (i.e. the association is with the winter months). Such a phenomenon might be explained if exposure to a virus at the time of birth rendered the individual susceptible (e.g. by the development of tolerance) either to the same or a similar agent on exposure at some later stage of life. Although schizophrenia is not generally thought of as a transmissible disease there is one study that suggests this may be the case. The monozygotic co-twins of a schizophrenic proband are the population known to be at highest risk of the disease. Abe found that the risk to the second twin was greater in the first six months after the onset of the illness in the first twin and that this excess risk was confined to pairs of twins who were together at this time.

The Extent of our Ignorance

It has been argued that a causal agent in schizophrenia remains to be discovered. This is the most important problem. We need to know how it produces the changes which lead to the manifestations of the disease. Is there for example a chronic periventricular encephalitis which damages the stria terminalis, and thus leads to the type II syndrome, as well as to intellectual impairment? Is there a specific neurochemical disturbance that could account for the positive symptoms? What is the relationship between the type I and type II syndromes? Are they chemical (and potentially reversible) and structural (and irreversible) consequences of the same pathological process? What is the nature of the genetic contribution? Is it the possession of some molecular variant (e.g. of a receptor protein) which renders it susceptible to an infective agent? What is the role of the hippocampus in the schizophrenia-like syndromes of temporal lobe epilepsy? Of more general neurophysiological interest what is its role in distinguishing internally from externally-generated stimuli? How is such neural activity normally processed and presented to consciousness? How is the normal person so little aware of the problem of distinguishing neural activity arising from the internal and external environments which so besets the patient suffering from schizophrenia?

References

ABE, K. (1969). The morbidity rate and environmental influence in monozygotic co-twins of schizophrenics. *British Journal of Psychiatry*, **115**, pp. 519–531.

CROW, T.J. (1980). Molecular pathology of schizophrenia: more than one disease process? *British Medical Journal*, **280**, pp. 66–68.

CROW, T.J. (1980). The search for an environmental agent in schizophrenia. *Trends in Neurosciences*, **3**, No. 7, pp. 12–14.

CROW, T.J. and STEVENS, M. (1978). Age disorientation in chronic schizophrenia: the nature of the cognitive deficit. *British Journal of Psychiatry*, **133**, pp. 137–142.

FRITH, C.D. (1979). Consciousness, information-processing and schizophrenia. *British Journal of Psychiatry,* **134**, pp. 225–235.

GOTTESMAN, I. (1978). Schizophrenia and genetics: where are we? Are you sure? In: *The Nature of Schizophrenia.* (Wynne, L.C., Cromwell, R.L. and Matthysse, S., eds.), 59–69. J. Wiley, New York.

JOHNSTONE, E.C., CROW, T.J., FRITH, C.D., STEVENS, M., KREEL, L. and HUSBAND, J. (1978). The dementia of dementia praecox. *Acta Psychiatrica Scandinavica,* **57**, 305–324.

JOHNSTONE, E.C., CROW, T.J., FRITH, C.D., CARNEY, M.W.P. and PRICE, J.S. (1978). Mechanism of the antipsychotic effect in the treatment of acute schizophrenia. *Lancet,* **1**, 848–851.

KETY, S.S., ROSENTHAL, D., WENDER, P.H., SCHULSINGER, F. and JACOBSEN, B. (1978). The biologic and adoptive families of adopted individuals who became schizophrenic. In: *The Nature of Schizophrenia.* (Wynne, L.C., Cromwell, R.L. and Matthysse, S., eds.), 25–37. J. Wiley, New York.

MENNINGER, K.A. (1926). Influenza and schizophrenia. An analysis of post-influenzal dementia praecox as of 1918, and five years later. *American Journal of Psychiatry,* **5**, 469–529.

OWEN, F., CROSS, A.J., CROW, T.J., LOFTHOUSE, R. and POULTER, M. (1978). Increased dopamine receptor sensitivity in schizophrenia. *Lancet,* **2**, 223–225.

DEPRESSION

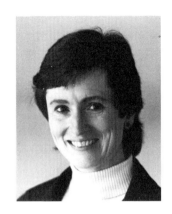

Katherine Noll

Clinical Psychologist, Psychology Department, Elmhurst College, Illinois, USA.

She is also Research Consultant, Illinois State Psychiatric Institute in Chicago, Illinois, USA. Her research has focused on the relationships between alterations in brain chemistry and depression. Her area of special interest is the interface between clinical psychology and neuropsychology, neuropharmacology and psychopharmacology.

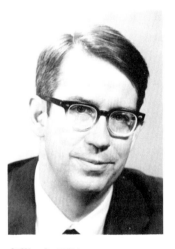

John M. Davis

Gilman Research Professor in Psychiatry, College of Medicine, University of Illinois, USA.

Formerly Professor of Psychiatry, University of Vanderbilt and Director of Research, Illinois State Psychiatric Institute.

Dr. Davis is one of the people who first described the catecholamine theory of depression. He has been active in many studies relating to biological factors of depression and its drug treatment and has also been involved in biological theories of schizophrenia and other mental disorders.

A 40-year old woman is brought to the emergency room of a hospital by her husband who tells the emergency room personnel that he arrived home from work early and found her unconscious. She had apparently taken an overdose of a sleeping medication which a physician had prescribed for her two weeks earlier. After her stomach is pumped and she regains consciousness she appears unable to give a coherent account of what has happened. Her husband reports that she has been acting strangely in the last several weeks, at first seeming withdrawn and uncommunicative and more recently crying frequently for no apparent reason and neglecting her housework and appearance. She is admitted to hospital for observation. The following morning she still appears unwilling or unable to discuss her apparent suicide attempt. She sits staring at the floor much of the day, occasionally crying. When questioned she does not respond directly, but says only, 'Why won't they let me die? I deserve to be dead; I'm already dead inside.' Her husband reports to the staff that as far as he can tell, she seemed to begin acting differently from her normally warm and outgoing self several months earlier. They had recently bought and moved to a new home following his promotion to a better paying position. Shortly after that, their youngest daughter had got married, having a large wedding which had required a great deal of his wife's time and effort. His wife had seemed to take it all in her stride, juggling the wedding arrangements with several projects she was responsible for at work. However, when a more prestigious position had opened in her department, a younger male employee who had been working for her had been promoted over her head. She had seemed to take this hard, feeling on the one hand that she had been passed over because she was middle-aged and a woman and on the other hand that if she had not also been preoccupied with their move and their daughter's wedding she might have done better work which would have

earned the promotion for her. She began to spend long periods of time brooding over the situation, trying to figure out what she should have done differently. She also began to have difficulty sleeping, waking frequently in the night and being unable to go back to sleep again after 3.00 or 4.00 a.m. By the time it was time to get up she felt exhausted. At that point she had seen a physician, who had prescribed barbiturates to help her sleep. However, even after taking this medication and apparently sleeping a normal eight hours, she still had complained of chronic fatigue and her husband's efforts to cheer her up by taking her on weekend excursions seemed only to make her feel worse. She began avoiding their friends and finding excuses not to attend social events. Some days she did not want to get up at all and called in sick to her office. This had been the case on the day she had apparently tried to kill herself, and only the fact that her husband, feeling very worried, had come home early to see if he could do something to help her had prevented her from succeeding in her attempt to die.

What could cause such strange behaviour in someone who appears to have much to enjoy in life? Although she had been disappointed in her desire to be promoted, she seems to have a doting husband who has achieved considerable recognition for his work. They have a beautiful new home which she has decorated exactly to her taste. Although her children have all left home, they do not live far away and call or visit often. Why has she now decided that she wants to die?

This story is fictional, but represents what might be considered a 'typical' case history of a patient suffering from that strange pattern of symptoms and behaviour frequently called simply 'depression'.

The periodic appearance in otherwise normal human beings of severe and abnormal states of sadness, sometimes alternating with periods of excitement and euphoria or aggressive irritability, has been observed throughout recorded history. These periods of altered mood and the behavioural changes which accompany them are often of such severity as to incapacitate the person experiencing them. They are frequently associated with events or transitions in the individual's life which would be expected to cause sadness or excitement in a normal person, but in these people the emotional response is exaggerated and prolonged. Hippocrates, recording symptoms of 'melancholic' patients (whose symptoms were believed to be caused by an excess of black bile), described a pattern of behaviour and mood changes which would be easily recognized today. In addition, there appears to be a group of symptoms which is virtually always present and is relatively invariant not only through time but also in most cultures, even those very different from our own.

There has been a great deal of discussion of which symptoms are essential to the process of depression and which are accidental, but most descriptions of depression start by describing the prolonged experience of sadness and loss of pleasure. This is generally accompanied by loss of appetite (and subsequently of weight), disturbed sleep, particularly waking early and being unable to return to sleep, changes in general activity level, either agitation or retardation, loss of interest in normally pleasurable activities, especially sex, feelings of guilt and worthlessness, reduced ability to think, concentrate, or make decisions, feelings of hopelessness about the future and, frequently, rumination about or actual attempts to commit suicide. These symptoms usually follow an odd daily pattern — they are generally worse in the morning and improve somewhat toward evening. This may last for weeks or months, sometimes even years. If the sufferer receives no treatment, it has been estimated that recovery usually will occur spontaneously in an average of nine months. Once a person has experienced an 'episode' of depression, the probability that this will happen again at some future time in that person's life is high, perhaps as high as 90%. When the person experiences only periods of depression (usually alternating with normal mood), the disorder is considered to be 'unipolar'. If the periods of depression are interspersed with periods during which the person is 'high' (which may become so extreme as to deserve the diagnosis of mania), the disorder is considered to be 'bipolar'.

This suggests significant loss of normal functions in those who are subject to this disorder. The disorder is not limited to persons low in the social hierarchy; it has characterized the lives of some of the most famous and productive of individuals.

Depression is not rare. Estimates of prevalence vary, but some surveys have suggested that as many as one person in five will have this experience at some time in their life, and the odds are higher for women than for men.

It would be possible to write an entire book simply delineating the aspects of depression about which we need to know more. For the purposes of this discussion, however, three primary questions will be posed and will be discussed in terms of what is already known relevant to their answers and what must still be determined.

What is the Nature of the Relationship Between Biological and Psychological Factors in Depression?

Something which has puzzled observers of depressed patients through the ages has been the fluctuating relationship between the occurrence of depression and the experiences the person has had which seem to have 'caused' it. Although almost all depressed patients report some experience, usually of a kind injurious to their security or self-esteem, which caused them to begin to feel depressed, it is not infrequently the case that some of the most severely disturbed patients are unable to identify any specific emotional injuries related to the onset of their symptoms. Theorists have dealt with this in a number of ways. Frequently, especially prior to the discovery of evidence for biological factors in depression, it was thought that experiences early in the individual's life might have produced later depression as a sort of delayed reaction. However, the invariance of the symptoms and particularly the frequent involvement of the physical functioning of the body in the symptoms of depression has indicated that in many, perhaps most, cases there is a biological as well as a psychological component. A number of attempts have been made to distinguish between 'biologically caused' and 'psychologically caused' depressions, but these have been largely unsuccessful. The truth appears to be that in most serious depressions there are both biological and psychological aspects, neither of which can be ignored or rejected. They are almost certainly intricately related and the unsolved question is that of how they are related. Examining the theories and the evidence may show something of the nature of the confusion about this that currently exists.

Factors which predispose to depression

A number of theories deal with the nature of the events or learning which, while not producing immediate depression, 'weaken' the individual in such a way as to make him or her more vulnerable to depression in response to later stresses.

The psychoanalytic viewpoint is probably the best known of these. It has essentially two components: 'anger turned against the self' and the loss of a loved person (sometimes called 'object loss', the term 'object' being an abbreviation of 'love object'). In the former case, fear of losing the love of another person prevents the individual from expressing appropriate anger toward that person, while in the latter case the loved person has either stopped loving the individual or has actually left (perhaps through death). In either case, 'libidinal energy' (the life force which one 'invests' in those one loves) has been withdrawn into the self, leaving the individual unable to form adequate love relationships. In fact, one study reported that 40% of the depressed patients in their sample had suffered significant separations in the year preceding hospitalization.

Recently, there has been an increase in attention to the nature of the thought patterns learned early in life which may make an individual more vulnerable to become depressed later. These are sometimes referred to as 'cognitive' theories of depression. One which has received considerable attention has been Seligman's theory of 'learned helplessness'. This theory argues that depression results from the belief that one cannot control either pleasant or unpleasant events and that this loss of control is due to one's own failing, encompasses all aspects of one's life and is unlikely to change. The early learning which produces the later reaction of helplessness relates to what the child is taught, especially by his or her parents, regarding control of the environment: parents who stress luck as the cause of pleasant or unpleasant events leave the child vulnerable to later helplessness, while parents who teach their child that one can always do something to affect one's fate will have 'immunized' the child against depression. However, while many studies done with both normal and depressed human adults have supported the assertion that depressed individuals feel helpless to control what happens to them, there has been little evidence that depressed adults were taught helplessness as children — in fact, one study suggests that if anything, depressed people learned to believe they were responsible for everything, and it is the contrast of this with their current experience that contributes to their depression.

A number of formulations have been published in the last ten years relating depression to behavior learned by means of rewards and punishments. The main thrust of most of these is that the individual 'extinguishes' behaviours which were maintained by rewards which have now been lost — for example, by the loss of a loved person who supplied the rewards. In addition, the symptoms of depression are also seen as behaviours which are maintained because they are rewarded, as, for example, by sympathy from others. These theorists believe that the depression will be 'cured' by the restoration of the lost rewards or by the withdrawal of rewards for depressed behaviours.

Many of these formulations about the sources of vulnerability to depression seem to make sense. However, evidence has been accumulating that the predisposition to depression may also be transmitted genetically. In the 1960s family studies of depression and mania (often currently called 'the affective disorders') suggested that the pattern of occurrence of these disorders in certain families suggests biologically inherited factors in predisposition as well as environmentally determined learning. The form of affective disorder often considered the most severe, the bipolar form in which the afflicted person has both periods of depression and periods of mania, seems to show the clearest evidence for genetic transmission.

Twins are often studied to try to separate the contributions of genes and environment in producing a disorder. The reasoning behind this is that both identical and fraternal twins grow up in nearly identical environments, but only the identical twins have identical genes. What is then examined is the 'concordance' between the twins for the disorder being studied; that is, the probability that if one twin has the disorder, the other twin will also have it. If it is primarily determined by environmental factors, then the concordance between identical and fraternal twins should be essentially the same. If genetics plays a significant role in generating the disorder, there should be much higher concordance between identical twins than fraternal twins, and fraternal twins should show essentially

the same concordance as that between any siblings. In fact, in almost all studies the concordance for affective disorders is much higher in identical than in fraternal twins, with approximately 40% concordance in identical twins with unipolar depression (vs 11% concordance in fraternal twins) and 72% concordance in bipolar identical twins (compared with 14% concordance in fraternal twins). Obviously, however, there are many cases of identical twins who are discordant (i.e. both do not have depression). The important implication of this is that even though there is good reason to believe that a genetic factor is important in vulnerability to depression, there must clearly be important non-genetic factors involved, since if the disorder were totally determined by heredity, concordance would have to be 100% in identical twins.

Another piece of evidence muddying the relationship between biological and psychological factors in depression is the sex ratio of patients. Virtually all studies have found depression to be more common in women than in men, particularly the unipolar type or types. There have been many explanations posed to account for this, from differential inheritance patterns (one theory has proposed that one form of bipolar illness is transmitted as an X-linked dominant gene, which would give women twice as many opportunities to inherit it) to hormone effects to greater exposure of women to depression-producing experiences. Again, reviews of the evidence suggest that both biological and psychological vulnerability factors are necessary to account for the higher observed rates of depression in women.

An additional method for identifying genetically transmitted characteristics is the study of children adopted at or near birth. Where records are available on both biological and adoptive parents, the children can be observed to see whether they show characteristics of the biological or of the adoptive parents. Again, depression is observed to occur more often in children whose biological parents had it; in one study, 38% of adopted children whose biological mothers had affective disorders later developed it themselves, while only 7% of adopted children whose biological mothers had no history of depression later developed it.

A number of studies have found traits which are almost certainly genetically determined to be found in the same family members who have affective disorders. The 'X-linkage hypothesis' mentioned above has been supported by the evidence that in some families, individuals who have some trait known to be carried on the X chromosome (such as red-green color blindness or a particular blood protein) are also the ones who have the affective disorder. Some families have been found for whom this is not true, however, and in some families there is a relationship between affective disorders and traits believed to be inherited but not on the X chromosome. Some things for which these relationships have been reported are other blood proteins (including the familiar A, B, and O blood types), an unusual brain wave pattern and the combination of low activity of the enzyme monoamine oxidase combined with a tendency of the individual's red blood cells to absorb unusually large amounts of lithium ion.

Thus while we have gained a great deal of knowledge in recent years concerning factors which appear to be related to a predisposition to become depressed, we still do not know conclusively either what produces vulnerability, nor what the exact relationship is between the biological and psychological contributory factors.

Factors which initiate an episode of depression

It is somewhat easier to study the events which immediately preceded the onset of an episode of depression than it is to identify the factors which may have contributed to long-standing vulnerability to depression, but even here the exact triggering factors are unclear and the relationship between biological and psychological-emotional factors is somewhat blurred.

As mentioned above, the majority of depressed patients report that they have experienced stresses of various kinds during the year preceding the beginning of an episode of depression and those events are particularly likely to involve injury to self-esteem or separations from loved ones. A review of such studies concurred with this observation and calculated that depressive risk is increased by a factor of 5–6 during the six months following an extremely stressful life event. This is not true of all cases of depression and the relationship may be somewhat confounded by the fact that the studies were all retrospective – that is, the patient's memory of past events may have been contaminated by his or her current state of mind.

There is considerable evidence that the right kind of physical stress in the right individual can produce the symptoms of depression. It is well known that one of the things that maintains alcohol addiction is the terrible depression that follows alcohol withdrawal. Other physical factors which seem often to precipitate depression are such things as childbirth or even the hormones contained in birth-control pills. Depression arising secondary to some other illness shows some differences from 'primary' depression but still has many of the same characteristics and is often found in patients with other psychiatric disorders as well. Even mania has been observed to result in some cases from such physical stressors as infections, cancer, epilepsy and metabolic disturbances.

Thus there appears to be a great variety of factors, both physical and experiential, which can trigger the onset of an episode of depression or mania, and it is not clear what is necessary, either biologically or psychologically, to bring together predisposing factors and triggering factors to result in depression.

Biological and psychological factors in symptoms and treatment

A number of the most central symptoms of depression were listed at the beginning of this paper. A variety of explanations has been proposed to account for the particular symptoms of depression and again, the issue of the relationship of biology and psychology arises. The level at which one observes the symptoms appears to enter to some extent into what one sees. For the psychoanalyst, the most prominent symptoms are those which relate to the patient's experience of anguish, irrevocable loss, guilt and suppressed rage. The behavioural theorist is interested in the patient's observable behaviour, and from this point of view the most prominent symptoms are the patient's complaints of suffering and the low rate of instrumental behaviours emitted by the patient, which may be due either to the loss of rewards or to punishment-induced suppression of behaviour. The cognitive theorist observes how the patient thinks about the world and his own experience and sees the patient's symptoms in terms of how he processes information and the conclusions he draws from it. The physician is primarily interested in the patient's physical symptoms, as these may provide the clue to what medication to prescribe. The question which arises then seems to be whether these different viewpoints are in conflict.

The first truly medical therapies for depression have come fairly recently. An (incorrect) observation in the 1920s that epilepsy appeared to protect its sufferers against schizophrenia resulted in the treatment of various psychiatric disorders by the induction of seizures. Though this turned out not to be effective in the treatment of true schizophrenia, it did turn out to have striking beneficial effects in treating depression and is even now the most effective single treatment for depression. Until then, the theories developed to try to account for the effects of seizures on depressed patients were directed toward their psychological effects on the patient. One theory held that it was a punishment of such great severity that the patient could then feel that he had atoned for his sins and could now return to normal life; another held that the beneficial effect was derived from the amnesia for the time preceding the treatment in that it allowed the patient to forget the troubles which had led to the depression. Although improvements in method have changed these aspects of convulsive therapy, the beneficial effect of the treatment has not been lost. In addition, the discovery of the antidepressant drugs in the 1950s, both the tricyclic antidepressants and the monoamine oxidase inhibitors, added to the evidence that their therapeutic effect was at least partly derived from the physiological effect of the treatment on the nervous system. Specifically, techniques were being developed for biochemical studies which permitted the study of the chemistry of the brain, and all of the antidepressant treatments were found to have significant effects on the chemistry of the brain.

Observations of the biochemical effects of the antidepressant drugs, particularly their effects on the activity of the chemical messengers of the brain, the neurotransmitters, led in the 1960s to the first neurotransmitter theories of depression. A variety of chemical substances were being identified as being released from nerve cells through electrical stimulation and as having the effect on the cell onto which they were released of either facilitating or impeding electrical activity in that cell. As it began to be apparent that these substances had profound effects on the behaviour of animals, attempts were made to correlate the behaviour of depressed patients with the actions of neurotransmitters known to be functionally altered by antidepressant treatments. In the United States researchers at the National Institute of Mental Health found that drugs such as reserpine and methyldopa, antihypertensive drugs which deplete the neurotransmitter norepinephrine (noradrenaline), produce severe depression in approximately 20% of the patients who take them, while the antidepressant drugs all had the property of facilitating the action of norepinephrine. At the same time, European researchers were studying another neurotransmitter whose action is potentiated by the antidepressant drugs, serotonin (5-hydroxytryptamine). They found that even though this transmitter acts primarily to inhibit electrical activity in nerve cells, there was substantial evidence for the deficit of this transmitter in depressed patients. Another of the neurotransmitters of the same group as norepinephrine (the catecholamines) also seemed to be implicated. This transmitter, dopamine, seemed to be an important factor

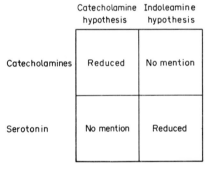

Fig. 1. The catecholamine and indoleamine hypotheses of depression.

in the switch from depression to mania and vice versa in bipolar patients. The relative amounts of the catecholamine neurotransmitters seemed to be elevated in manic patients and reduced in depressed patients. The American theory proposed that depression was caused by a deficiency of brain catecholamines and came to be known as the Catecholamine Hypothesis of depression, while the European emphasis on deficits of serotonin came to be known as the Indoleamine Hypothesis, as serotonin belongs to a family of compounds called indoleamines. The catecholamines and serotonin are often

jointly referred to as the biogenic amines. These two hypotheses are illustrated in Fig. 1. Both theories were supported by significant bodies of research, and in fact deficits of any of these transmitters would account for a number of the common symptoms of depression. Both norepinephrine and dopamine appear to be necessary for the individual to be able to respond to pleasurable events. The catecholamines also seem to control activity level, activity being reduced when these are depleted. They appear to be necessary for the maintenance of normal eating behaviour and normal sexual response. Serotonin, while its primary action is inhibitory, appears to be important in maintaining normal patterns of sleep, pain sensitivity and response to unpleasant experiences. A review of the symptoms of depression listed at the beginning of the paper will indicate that many of the symptoms might well result from deficiencies in these neurotransmitters in the brain. However, the two hypotheses were generally regarded to be in opposition to each other and it was not until 1974 that they were combined. This hypothesis, called the Permissive Hypothesis of Affective Disorders proposed that the predisposition to depression consisted of a chronic deficit in serotonin functions, and that if an alteration of normal catecholamine

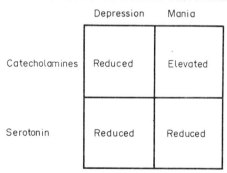

Fig. 2. The 'permissive hypothesis of affective disorders' (after Prange *et al.*, 1974).

activity were superimposed on this serotonin deficit, the symptoms of depression (if catecholamines were reduced) or mania (if catecholamines were elevated) would appear. This is illustrated in Fig. 2. This hypothesis accounted for more of the observed symptomatology than did its predecessors, but there was evidence coming to light implicating another neurotransmitter, acetylcholine. This transmitter appears to be important in the suppression of unrewarded or punished behaviour, and treatments which facilitate this transmitter's action produce symptoms like depression both in normal humans and in patients with mania.

It is apparent that changes in the normal relationships of these neurotransmitters might have a significant effect at a number of levels in humans. A theory which integrates the data on all of these neurotransmitters and integrates the findings concerning the neurotransmitters with the cognitive and behavioural theories of depression has been proposed by the first author of this paper. A relationship between the transmitters and their effects on the individual's experience of rewards (positive reinforcement) and punishment (negative reinforcement) such as that postulated in Fig. 3 could provide an explanation of the

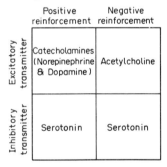

Fig. 3. Neurotransmitter relationships in the brain motivational systems.

effects on behaviour and symptoms of a number of different alterations not only in the absolute amounts of the neurotransmitters but also of perturbations of their relative equilibria. The patterns of altered amounts and relationships of these transmitters suggested in Figs. 4, 5 and 6 to represent several different types of affective disorders would produce not only identifiable

patterns of the symptoms directly related to changes in availability of the transmitters but also predictable effects on learning and thought in the affected individual. For

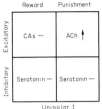

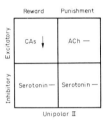

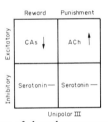

Fig. 4. Three patterns of altered neurotransmitter functioning in unipolar affective disorders. ↑ = functionally elevated; ↓ = functionally reduced; — = functionally unchanged.

example, if the individual had a reduction in the functional availability of the catecholamines and an elevation of the effects of neurotransmission mediated by acetycholine such as that suggested to represent a Unipolar III type of depression, the person would experience little pleasure or reward and the salience of unpleasant events to him would be greatly increased. Thus he would show, over time, the loss of that part of his behaviour motivated by pleasure and he would also experience increasing aversion to various aspects of his life. He would be helpless to exert any control over these and would be correct in interpreting this change in his life to be coming from within himself, affecting all aspects of his life and showing little prospect of improvement in the future. He might feel guilty and ashamed, especially about his inability to feel pleasure with others whom he supposedly loved.

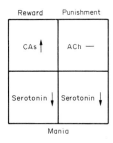

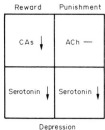

Fig. 5. Patterns of altered transmitter functioning in Bipolar I affective disorder.

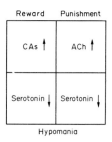

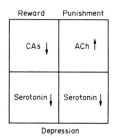

Fig. 6. Patterns of altered transmitter functioning in Bipolar II affective disorder.

While this formulation is undoubtedly an oversimplification of both the physiological and the emotional and experiential aspects of depression, it does suggest some ways in which an attempt can be made to integrate the biological and psychological aspects of depression in such a way as to validate some of the work that has been done in the different fields. It also suggests that these separate ways of looking at depression need not actually conflict with each other.

Seligman and his colleagues have reported some success in treating depressed patients with helplessness-oriented experiences, and Lewinsohn and his co-workers have reported some success in treating depression by reinforcing non-depressed behaviour. Beck and his colleagues have developed a comprehensive treatment for depression using cognitive strategies; they report that in research comparing their treatment to one of the most commonly used of the antidepressant drugs, their cognitive therapy was superior to the drug therapy. Most research comparing drug therapy with psychotherapy has found drug therapy superior in symptom reduction, though both are a significant improvement over no treatment or simply maintaining the patient in a hospital setting. One carefully controlled study showed a reduction in symptoms of depression of approximately 50% with drug treatment or with psychotherapy over a 16-week period; the addition of psychotherapy to drug treatment during the same period resulted in 50% reduction of the remaining symptoms. It was noted that different symptoms were affected by drugs and by psychotherapy. One problem with many studies of this kind has been that little attention has been paid to the quality or even quantity of the psychotherapy to which drug treatment was compared. When the quality of psychotherapy has been carefully controlled, its effects have been more uniformly positive.

Thus the relative contribution of biological and psychological factors to the predisposition to, onset of, symptoms of and treatment of depression is in the early stages of being deciphered, but the relationship is a very close and intricate one and it may never be possible to separate one from the other. Perhaps one of the most effective statements of this relationship still is that of Akiskal and McKinney, who proposed a theory of depression as a 'final common pathway': 'Specifically, we argue that depressive behaviours must be understood as occurring on several levels simultaneously rather than as having a one-to-one direct relationship with a single chemical event in the brain, and that a multiplicity of genetic, developmental, pharmacological, and interpersonal factors converge in the midbrain and lead to a reversible, functional derangement of the mechanisms of reinforcement. According to our hypothesis, then, object losses, interpersonally induced states of frustration and helplessness, and depletion of biogenic amines ultimately result in impairment of the neurophysiological substrates of reinforcement: this impairment is manifested behaviourally as depressive phenomena.'

What Factors are Primary in Depression (either necessary to produce the symptoms or sufficient to diagnose the presence of the syndrome) and Which are Secondary (that is, derived from the primary factors?)

As research on depression has uncovered more and more evidence on the elements of normal functioning that are disordered in the affective disorders, one of the important questions needing to be answered is that of which of the alterations are causal in depression, and which result from other causal factors. Once all of the relevant data on all of the concomitant symptoms of depression have been gathered and when all of the subtypes have been identified and separated, it should theoretically be possible to reach, by combined inductive and deductive reasoning, the point for each where all of the evidence converges on a single or few points from which all of the data can be predicted. Clearly, it is not possible to do this with the data

which we currently have (or if it is, the patterns are not obvious).

The discovery of the antimanic properties of lithium ion by Cade in 1949 eventually led toward the study of alterations in electrolytes in the affective disorders. Patients with affective disorders have been shown to have alterations in the concentration of sodium in their cells and it has also been found that in patients who show an antidepressant response to lithium, the ratio of the concentration of lithium contained in the red blood cell to the concentration of lithium in blood plasma is higher than the ratio found in patients who fail to show a lifting of depressive symptoms when treated with lithium. This relationship suggested that electrolyte transport across the red cell membrane may be related to the vulnerability to affective disorders in an important fashion. Other evidence has been gathered confirming this relationship, including the finding of a manic patient with abnormal lithium-sodium counterflow across the red cell membrane. Other members of this individual's family also have this abnormal transport and it is highly correlated with the occurrence of the affective disorder. Additional evidence of the importance of this abnormality in patients with affective disorder has been gathered; however, what role this plays in the etiology of mania or depression has yet to be determined.

A number of abnormalities of hormone balance and the involvement of the neuroendocrine system in the depressive process have been discovered in recent years. As early as 1969, significantly elevated levels of urinary 17-hydroxycorticosteroids in severely depressed patients were noted and were even proposed to be a predictor of suicide attempts. Since this time a number of studies have shown elevated adrenal-cortical hormones in depressed patients, and a particularly striking finding is the phenomenon of 'escape from dexamethasone suppression'. The secretion of the hormone cortisol, which is usually secreted by the adrenal glands in response to stress, is suppressed by the synthetic hormone dexamethasone in normal individuals. However, not only do depressed patients secrete too much cortisol, they also frequently fail to show cortisol suppression in response to dexamethasone, or if they show some suppression they begin secreting it again after dexamethasone much earlier than do normal persons. In addition, this test seems to identify patients who have classic symptoms of depression and who are more likely to respond favorably to treatment with antidepressant drugs. Other hormones which show abnormalities in depressed patients are prolactin, the hormone which controls the production of milk in women, thyrotropin, the hormone which stimulates normal function of the thyroid gland; human growth hormone (somatotropin), and luteinizing hormone (lutropin) (particularly associated with the menstrual cycle in women). While these hormone abnormalities may have a direct effect on brain function and behaviour, the secretion of these hormones may be controlled by neurotransmitters and therefore be secondary to the neurotransmitter abnormalities discussed earlier. Thus it remains undetermined whether these changes are primary causes of the symptoms of depression or are secondary to other factors.

In the previous section the role of a variety of neurotransmitters and their relationship to each other were discussed. However, the transmitters that have been discussed are only a fraction of the compounds which have modulating effects on nerve cells and the study of the action and importance of various other substances tends to be directly related to the available technology for measuring and observing them. The importance of the role of acetylcholine in depression has been somewhat neglected, largely for the reason that its activity in living humans is very difficult to study. It seems very likely that other substances are also of some significance in depression, either by reason of their presence in excess or their absence. For example, the original mood-altering drugs were discovered accidentally by researchers working on developing new antihistamine drugs for the treatment of allergic conditions. In fact, histamine is now believed to act as a neurotransmitter in the central nervous system and tricyclic antidepressant drugs have been found to be extremely potent antihistamines. Some antihistamine drugs have been shown to act as antidepressants in animal studies, but their effect in humans for depression, and indeed the role of histamine or allergy in depression, has been largely ignored.

The discovery in the last few years of opium-like drugs occurring naturally in the human nervous system (usually called endorphins, a contraction of 'endogenous morphines') has sparked interest in the effects on behavior that might be produced by too much or too little of these in the nervous system. An early uncontrolled study suggested that some of these compounds might offer relief to patients with severe intractable depression, but these results have proved difficult to duplicate. It is relatively difficult to purify this compound for use as a medication and synthetic analogues have also been difficult to produce in the laboratory. This may still prove to be a step forward in the treatment of depression when these compounds can more easily be synthesized or extracted in the laboratory.

As was indicated in the discussion of the symptoms of depression, one of the most frequent symptoms is a disorder of normal sleep patterns. While this sometimes takes the form of hypersomnia — the patient sleeps more than the normal amount — more commonly seen is insomnia, particularly of the type in which the patient sleeps very restlessly, awakens often and finally is unable to return to sleep toward the end of the normal sleep period. Recent research has turned up a sleep characteristic which is peculiar to depressed patients and not only distinguishes them from normal subjects and patients with other disorders or depression secondary to another medical problem, but also from other individuals with insomnia. This is a characteristic called 'shortened REM latency', which means that these patients begin dreaming much earlier after falling asleep than do other individuals. A particularly provocative finding has been that of the antidepressant properties of sleep deprivation. Many depressed patients, when deprived of a night of sleep, show considerable improvement in mood the following day. However, there is a limit to the extent that this treatment can be used as humans cannot tolerate sleep deprivation for long periods, and the benefit from a single lost night of sleep fades rapidly.

A relationship between the abnormalities in sleep patterns and the changes in neurotransmitters observed in depressed patients has been found, in that some of the sleep changes can be produced artificially in animals by drugs that reduce brain serotonin. In addition, administration of drugs that increase the effects of acetylcholine in the brain have been shown to speed up the onset of REM sleep, particularly in people who are currently or who have been depressed.

The observation that sleep cycles are related to the broader concept of circadian rhythms (normal fluctuations in bodily processes over 24 hours) affecting the functioning of the entire nervous system has led to the hypothesis that many of the disturbances seen in depressed patients — possibly even all of the observed symptoms, including disorders of neurotransmitter equilibrium — may be attributed to a disturbance of the normal circadian cycles. Many of the neurotransmitters and hormones would be involved if parts of the circadian rhythm were out of phase with the others. That this factor in depression is primary and that many of the other concomitants are secondary to this is a provocative hypothesis which remains to be tested. How a tendency for circadian rhythms to go out of phase might be genetically transmitted or produced by stressful life circumstances has not yet been spelled out.

The symptom of depression which has always been believed to be the primary, central or defining characteristic of depression is that of the prolonged period of unrelieved sadness from which the disorder gets its name. However, in the last few years there have been several pieces of evidence, generated primarily from research on the antidepressant drugs, which suggest the possiblity that the underlying biological factors which contribute to depression may also be manifested in other forms in which depressed mood is not the most prominent symptom. There appear to be a cluster of symptoms or syndromes which might be considered to be masked forms of depression or depressive equivalents; while this remains controversial, some methods by which they might be identified are that they occur in individuals with a family history of affective disorders, are seen in individuals who later show more classic symptoms of depression, are correlated with high scores on psychological tests of depression, or respond to treatment with antidepressant drugs.

One of the most recent findings has been the response of obsessive-compulsive symptoms to a serotonin-facilitating antidepressant, chlorimipramine. This suggests that some disorders usually believed to be neurotic, other than so-called 'neurotic depression' (this diagnosis has been omitted from the new American classification system, the 3rd edition of the American Psychiatric Association's Diagnostic and Statistical Manual), may actually belong to the family of affective disorders. Other apparently neurotic disorders shown to be responsive to treatment with antidepressants have been a fear of open areas or any area outside the individual's own home, some kinds of anxiety and panic attack, and other phobias, including school phobia. In addition, tricyclic antidepressants have been shown to be nearly as effective or as effective as stimulant drugs in treating childhood hyperactivity and their effectiveness in treating enuresis (bed-wetting) has been noted frequently. Recently there have been some reports of success with antidepressant treatment for some types of chronic or recurrent pain syndromes, such as headache and lower back pain.

Depression has many symptoms and sometimes people who are depressed seek medical help for one of the symptoms other than depressed mood. Whether this is because the individual believes that the emotional symptoms are too shameful to admit openly or whether the other symptom really is more salient than the depression is not clear. Nevertheless, a number of patients seeking treatment for insomnia prove on personality tests to be significantly depressed and follow-up studies on patients hospitalized for anorexia nervosa (self-starvation, most often seen in teenaged girls) have shown that many of these patients later show classical symptoms of depression.

A group of patients who have traditionally been believed to represent a mild form of schizophrenia, as they may at times lapse into periods of psychotic disorganization of thought processes, are now believed by some to represent a form of affective disorder. These patients are currently given a diagnosis of Borderline Personality Disorder in the United States and their disruptive and frequently histrionic behavior has usually been thought to represent a lifelong pattern of maladaptive interpersonal relationships. However, the frequent finding of depression in their parents has suggested treatment for affective disorder and many have been shown to benefit strikingly from treatment with tricyclic antidepressant drugs or with monoamine oxidase inhibitors.

Some of the other psychiatric syndromes traditionally thought to be independent of affective disorders, but now believed by some theorists to be related or alternate forms, are hypochondriasis, neurasthenia and some of the psychosomatic disorders (in which a physical illness is seriously exacerbated by emotional stress).

Thus despite the description of the many symptoms of depression, (including new information being gathered in many laboratories and hospitals around the world), there is still little consensus on which factors are causal in depression or sufficient to produce the other observed symptoms, and which arise only in response to the primary factors. It is to be hoped that further work will soon clarify the nature of these relationships.

Is Depression, or the Predisposition to it, Totally Disadvantageous to the Afflicted Individual, or Might there be Something of Value Associated with it?

There is another interesting aspect of the affective disorders which could be predicted from the transmitter model discussed earlier, which has only occasionally been addressed. Estimates of the predisposition to affective disorder have ranged from a low of 1–4% of the population at large to a high of 20–25%. A recent study of women physicians indicated that over 50% of a sample of 111 had had at least one clinically diagnosable episode of depression; over 30% of a matched sample of women Ph.D.s had also been seriously depressed. This figure is rather similar to that generated from such information as the suicide rate among women physicians. The paper has generated a substantial outcry and a number of letters have been written to the two major American psychiatric journals arguing against these conclusions (women psychiatrists were found to be particualrly susceptible, with nearly 75% of the study sample having been depressed). Few of the writers have seen fit to examine what these data might mean if it is regarded objectively rather than as a slur against women physicians. Some of the effects of the transmitter alterations postulated in this study might be quite beneficial and advantageous to the individual under the right circumstances. One such factor might be improved memory in individuals with elevated acetylcholine function:

facilitating the function of acetylcholine has been found to improve memory in patients showing memory deterioration with age. A recent study has dealt with possible positive effects of affective disorders and found that many bipolar patients, in particular, felt that their disorder had significant positive aspects. This may extend to the children of these patients. Work by Cohler and his colleagues has shown that some of the children of mothers who have had episodes of schizophrenia from which they recovered and were able to return to caring for their children have become unusually creative and productive 'superkids'. The fact that these mothers recovered from their schizophrenic symptoms suggests that they belong to the group of 'good-prognosis' schizophrenics. This group has been shown to be more likely to contain patients with bipolar affective disorders as they tend not only to come from families with more histories of affective disorders than of schizophrenia but also the majority of good-prognosis schizophrenics show a therapeutic response to treatment with lithium, which has little therapeutic value for true schizophrenic patients.

William James, the great American psychologist, is said to have attributed much of his success in his career to the severe depression he experienced at the age of 28, which caused him to re-evaluate his life, its meaning and his goals. Julian Huxley was subject to severe and crippling bouts of depression, as his grandfather Thomas H. Huxley had been. Virginia Woolf died by suicide, as did Ernest Hemmingway. Albert Einstein experienced a nervous breakdown (a colloquial term which frequently means depression) during his final year in secondary school. A recent review of the lives of 400 eminent people living during the twentieth century observed that 'there are many references to periods of acute depression in the biographies and autobiographies of eminent men and women.' Eight of the 400 had already died by suicide even though many were still living at the time of writing — a far higher rate of death by suicide than the rate usually estimated for the general population. The famous Stanford University study of individuals identified as gifted during childhood noted, in the follow-up done when these people averaged 50 years old, that twenty-two of the original 1500 had already died by suicide. This may not be an accident, as it would seem likely that a disorder with effects as devastating as those of the affective disorders would produce selection pressure to reduce its incidence in the general population. That this has not happened suggests that it might be re-evaluated from that standpoint.

The topics discussed here are by no means all of the aspects of depression about which we are still relatively ignorant and need to learn more. It is to be hoped, however, that the excitement that is being felt among researchers working on this new frontier of knowledge will finally generate the answers to these questions. Our ignorance about depression is being chipped away daily.

Further Reading

ABRAMSON, L.Y., SELIGMAN, M.E.P. and TEASDALE, J.D. (1978) Learned helplessness in humans: Critique and reformulation. *Journal of Abnormal Psychology*, **87**, 49–74.

AKISKAL, H.S. and McKINNEY, W.T., Jr. (1973) Depressive disorders: Toward a unified hypothesis. *Science*, **182**, 20–29.

AKISKAL, H.S. and McKINNEY, W.T., Jr. (1975) Overview of recent research in depression. *Archives of General Psychiatry*, **32**, 285–305.

BECK, A.T., RUSH, A.J., SHAW, B.F. and EMERY, G. (1979) *Cognitive Therapy of Depression*. New York The Guilford Press.

BLANEY, P.H. (1977) Contemporary theories of depression: Critique and comparison. *Journal of Abnormal Psychology*, **86**, 203–223.

CADORET, R.J. (1978) Evidence for genetic inheritance of primary affective disorder in adoptees. *American Journal of Psychiatry*, **135**, 463–466.

FIEVE, R.R. (1975) *Moodswing*. William Morrow and Company, New York.

LAPIN, I.P. and OXENKRUG, G.F. (1969) Intensification of the central serotonergic processes as a possible determinant of the thymoleptic effect. *Lancet I*, **6**, 132–136.

RADLOFF, L.S. and RAE, D.S. (1979) Susceptibility and precipitating factors in depression: Sex differences and similarities. *Journal of Abnormal Psychology*, **88**, 174–181.

SCHILDKRAUT, J.J. and KETY, S.S. (1967) Biogenic amines and emotion. *Science*, **156**, 21–30.

WEISSMAN, M.M. (1979) The psychological treatment of depression. *Archives of General Psychiatry*, **36**, 1261–1269.

ZUNG, W.W.K. (1977) Operational diagnosis and diagnostic categories of depressive disorders. In: *Phenomenology and Treatment of Depression* (Fann, W.E., Karakan, I., Pokorny, A.D. and Williams, R.L., eds.), 217–234. Spectrum Publications, New York.

DRUG DEPENDENCE

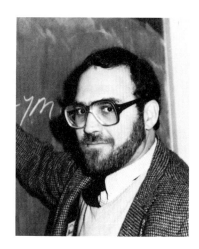

Peter A. Mansky

Associate Professor, Albany Medical College, New York, USA.

He has worked at the N.I.M.H. Addiction Research Center. Has published numerous articles and chapters on drug dependence.

Introduction

The issues and dilemmas in the field of drug dependence are described by several major questions which cover the salient issues. Our ability to answer these questions has improved as more information is gathered and as research is conducted. Some of these dilemmas have been answered more satisfactorily than others and some pose intriguing areas of consideration. The focus of this article will be to describe the major questions, give a brief overview of what is known and to describe some of the most fascinating dilemmas which face us in the field today.

The approach this author uses in thinking about drug dependence is based on a disease model. The first area then, of investigation, would be to consider the natural history of the disease. It must be understood, however, that the natural history may vary with the type of drug, the social setting and the individual using the drug. In general, drug dependence tends to be a chronic recurring disease. This is no more evident than in the folk language of Alcoholics Anonymous when, during a meeting, a member who has not had a drink for fifteen or twenty years, may stand up and say, 'I am an alcoholic', a true statement of the chronicity of the disease and the risk of relapse. Some drug use, however, tends to be self limiting, examples being students using marijuana and hallucinogens, patients with manic depressive illness drinking excessively during a manic phase, or soldiers in Vietnam using opiates while at war but not upon return to the United States. Some of these exceptions will be discussed below and many can be explained by the theories describing the pathogenesis of drug dependence.

In any chronic disease, the first question concerning the natural history would address the initiation of the disorder — that is, how and why it starts. With drug dependence, it would concern the reason a person first uses the drug. Why do some people after they are exposed to the drug go on to use it chronically and, in the case of some drugs, to the point that they become psychologically and physically dependent?

Using the disease model, these two questions involve exposure to the disorder and its pathogenesis. Inherent in this process would be an understanding of the phenomenology of the drug actions, what are its psychological and physical effects on the individual? With each drug, or class of drugs, we would want to know its effects when administered as a single dose and how these effects changed as the drug was chronically administered. During chronic administration of many of the drugs of dependence, individuals often become tolerant to the effects of the drugs and show a physical dependence or withdrawal syndrome when they stop using the drugs. It is interesting to note that although many of the drugs of dependence produce physical dependence, other drugs also produce physical dependence but not drug dependence. Common examples of the latter are anticholinergics such as atropine or the tricyclic antidepressants.

The remaining question related to the natural history of drug dependence would involve the area of relapse. Two of the most interesting concepts in this area are that of conditioned abstinence and protracted abstinence, both of which will be discussed at length in this article.

Areas of Inquiry

Several areas are being and have been investigated to answer the questions raised above. Roughly, these areas concern social factors, factors of the individual or person using the drug (both biological and psychological) and the phenomenology of the drug action both during acute intoxication and with chronic use. Although these areas of inquiry have provided much useful and practical information, they have also generated many questions which are discussed below.

Social factors

Social factors must be considered in drug dependence since drug use appears to follow trends and fads, such that among several drugs with equal pharmacological activity only one may become a popular drug of abuse and although certain people may be more prone to drug use as a drug becomes increasingly popular the type of person using the drug becomes less and less stereotyped.

The questions of legal controls, peer group influence and the setting and social customs will be discussed specifically in this section.

1. *Legal controls.* Legal control has received but little attention in the scientific literature, yet this does represent an interesting approach to drug dependence. The basic premise of legal control is that legal penalties will prevent people from using the drug. It is a fascinating area because legal control should probably effect initial use, continued use and dependence in different ways. Yet we know little of the actual effect. In fact, the most dramatic legal control of an addicting drug, alcohol, in the United States was a dismal failure, at least on the surface. It is still not clear, however, that the cost of the crime enforcement in terms of life, human morbidity and money was greater than the savings in terms of disease, crime and accidents associated with the drug. This would include

cirrhosis of the liver, diseases of the pancreas, other diseases of the gastrointestinal tract, especially the stomach, neurological diseases both of the brain and of the peripheral nervous system, and injuries or deaths as the result of accidents. Crimes such as violent acts especially within families, wife to husband or vice versa and child abuse, are common with alcohol use. Certainly automobile accidents and deaths are an important consequence of alcohol use. All of these areas should be studied to fully ascertain the role of prohibition in limiting alcohol use and its consequences.

Even without this information, we could concede for the moment that alcohol prohibition in the United States during the twentieth century was indeed a failure. If so, are there any other examples of drug prohibition which might be considered a success? Maurice Seevers presented such a case several years ago and it deserves consideration. The use of amphetamines was widespread in Japan after World War II. Strict legal controls were instituted to limit their use. Evidence was presented to show both a decrease in use and a decrease in drug-related diseases such as drug-induced psychosis.

If it is true that prohibition worked for amphetamines in Japan and not for alcohol in the United States, what factors were important in determining this? In this line of thought, one must consider other areas of the world such as the Muslim Countries and their prohibition of alcohol. How successful are they in irradicating use and the negative consequences of use?

2. *Peer group pressure and setting.* Peer group pressure and influence has been a widely discussed topic in drug abuse literature. It is generally conceded that this is a powerful factor in initiating and spreading drug use. Setting, or the factors of the environment may also play a large role in initiating and continuing drug use. Certain people may take drugs to aid them in coping with unpleasant situations. One example might be the soldier in Vietnam who was able to relax and escape the horrors of war and death by using drugs. Peer pressure to take the medications, coupled with easy availability of the drugs, may also have been important factors. To what degree each of these factors determined use is unclear. In any case, the unpleasant feelings associated with the environment may be relieved by the drug. This, in essence, is the negative reinforcement paradigm of behavioral psychology which states that if an action removes or alleviates an unpleasant situation, it is repeated because the removal is reinforcing to the action. Whereas in contrast, the peer approval is directly reinforcing of the drug taking and represents a positive reinforcement paradigm.

An even more intriguing hypothesis states that the environment may be involved in relapse. This involvement may be evident as an essential role in conditioned abstinence and may be one of the explanations of low relapse in Vietnam veterans returning to the United States. This will be discussed as the various abstinent syndromes are described below.

3. *Customs.* In addition to the specific environments discussed here, social customs or membership in cultural or subcultural groups may have an effect on drug self-administration. In investigating pain response and requests for opiate analgesics in patients from different subcultural or ethnic groups, it has been found that some ethnic groups find medications a most acceptable solution whereas others do not. It could be construed that the acceptability is a biological genetic trait but this appears unlikely especially in some of the cultural groups which appear heterogeneous in genetic inheritance but homogeneous in cultural surroundings. Thus, the attitude towards drugs is thought to represent a learned group of responses to various situations. In line with the learned response concept is the factor that some

cultures and subcultures promote a 'safe' medication for relief of dysphoric states such as pain, anxiety and depression. Examples in our culture would be aspirin or mild opiates for pain or an occasional drink for anxiety or mild depression.

Certainly it makes sense to treat dysphoric states in their most severe forms, but it is usually not possible to completely eliminate its occurrence. In the same manner, some degree of dysphoric state is inherent in every day living. In fact, some theories postulate that a certain degree of dysphoria, such as anxiety, provides motivation up to a point but that motivation begins to fall off when anxiety becomes too severe (see Fig. 1). This more sophisticated statement effects both

of these social attitudes will effect the development of drug dependence in cultural groups in different ways.

Thus, we can see that social, environmental and cultural factors play a role in the development of drug dependence, but exactly what these roles are is not clear.

The individual

1. *Psychological and biological.* Just as the social context has been postulated to effect drug use, so have factors of the individual both psychological and biological. These areas include personality type, self-image, the presence or abstinence of biologically determined psychiatric diseases, ordinary psychological

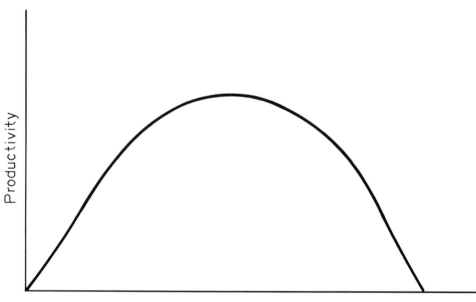

Figure 1.

subculture extremes in that some are so stoic that they will let a dysphoric state become so severe that it limits their productivity, whereas in other subcultures it is treated in its mildest form, so that productivity increased. Each

stresses and experience or learning.

2. *Personality and self image.* Personality types are often discussed using psychoanalytic theories. As such, they represent observable

activity and attitudes as well as assumptions concerning themes of intra-psychic struggle. Personalities described in this way are supposed to represent enduring traits in the individual over time rather than transient attitudes or states. These have then been related to a predominant theme such as obsessive, dependent, hysterical or schizoid.

Studies relating any one of these classical personality types to drug dependence have been disappointing. For example, personalities described as 'dependent' do not generally lead to drug dependence and people who are dependent on drugs of abuse do not necessarily have dependent personalities. Certainly observant clinicians who have worked with drug dependent individuals do often notice some enduring traits. These traits however, are difficult to separate from cause or effect, i.e. are they the result of or the cause of the drug dependence? Furthermore, they usually represent a group of severely impaired drug users who are from socio-economic groups necessitating public rather than private treatment. In this way, one can see that there are additional factors other than drug dependence which may lead to a more uniform selection or a more homogeneous group. As one gains more familiarity with various drug or alcohol treatment programmes the variety of personalities observed among the patients may become increasingly more evident.

Self-concept or self-image although influenced by personality, may be a more essential link to drug dependence. Whether it is indeed, is still open to question. Several observations may help to elucidate this area of investigation. In the early part of this century, several oral opiate preparations were in wide spread use. Their use was legal and people obtained them by prescription, thus behaving as patients or people with an illness. This self-image was fully acceptable. Once the medications were placed under strict control, many people could not give up the self-image of being ill so that they sought treatment for a new disease, drug dependence. Few were able

to see themselves as criminals and obtain the drug through illegal channels. In the same vein, soldiers returning from Vietnam may have discontinued use when returning home because the drugs were available in Vietnam from peers but obtainable at home only through a criminal subculture, a subculture which may have held little attraction for the returning soldier.

3. *Biological factors.* The biological make-up of the individual may also effect drug use. This is a common clinical observation but few systematic studies clearly define the extent of biological diseases in promoting drug use. Among biological diseases it is now clear that depressive illness, both unipolar (repeated depression or lows) and bipolar (repeated depressions and manias or highs and lows) have a strong biological component. Anxiety disorders with panic attacks and agoraphobia tend to occur in families and are considered as hereditary traits and respond to similar medication. Drug use is not uncommon in these disorders but the question remains as to the extent of use and the causal links between the biological disorder and the drug use.

What is of interest is that these disorders are recurring or periodic. As such, an individual may feel and function at a normal level for many years with episodes of mania, depression or anxiety occurring periodically as few as one or two times in twenty years. These episodes may last as long as two to three months. During the time of the episode, the individual may use a drug extensively whereas during the remainder of the twenty years the individual may be completely abstinent or only use the drug occasionally. This is not an uncommon pattern for alcohol use in patients with manic-depressive illness or agoraphobia. In some cases, the drug abuse is limited only to the period of the illness, in others the drug use tends to run a separate course. Much investigation in psychiatry and drug dependence is presently being conducted to investigate the interaction of drug dependence with these psychiatric diseases.

4. *Stress and learning issues.*

(*a*) *Life changes.* Stress may effect a person's biological as well as psychological functioning. Broadly speaking, stress has been related to life changes both positive and negative. The greater the number of changes, the higher the incidence of illness behavior in terms of clinic visits for injury, medical illness, or psychological complaint. Some drug use may occur in order to relieve or mediate the effects of life change stress in the individual. Again, this is an area of much investigative interest.

(*b*) Another area of controversy concerns the role of drugs of dependence in producing a 'high' or a euphoric state. Does the drug stimulate areas of the brain directly that lead to positive reinforcement or do individuals learn to appreciate the high? Opiate euphoria is a good example to explore. Opiate receptor material has been found in the brain gray matter in the diencephalon, an area bordering the inner lining of the third ventricles. This gray matter is part of the central gray system. Electrical stimulation of this area may produce pain or pleasure responses, depending on the particular area stimulated. Furthermore an opiate antagonist, naloxone, may block both responses. It would, therefore, appear that opiate highs are related to direct brain stimulation. Yet, there have been studies which show that many people do not feel a high on first exposure to opiates but may learn this response from repeated exposure in peer groups so the controversy remains unresolved.

The drugs and the phenomenology of dependence

The knowledge of drug dependence has been facilitated by an increased understanding of physical dependence, psychological dependence and the phenomenology of the above with differing groups of drugs. At one time, it was considered that physical dependence, or a well defined withdrawal syndrome upon the discontinuation of chronic administration of the drug, was the key to drug dependence. Drug dependence was at that time thought to involve either addiction or habituation. These were polar concepts. On the one hand, addiction was severe and difficult to change — habituation was mild and easy to change. Addiction at first did not require the presence of physical dependence but as it spread into wider use as a concept, most people took it to imply the presence of physical dependence. Thus, with the use of the terms addiction and habituation, physical dependence was thought to be the key differentiating the two polar concepts.

These terms were widely used in the 1950s but several observations contradicted the explanatory model of addiction–habituation with its implications of physical dependence as a key to drug dependence. The first observation concerned dependence on central nervous system (CNS) stimulants such as amphetamines, methamphetamine, methylphenidate (Ritalin), phenmetrazine (Preludin) and cocaine. In the 1950s the CNS stimulants were observed to produce prominent and devastating drug dependence without physical dependence. Today it is felt that these particular drugs may have a well defined withdrawal syndrome but historically they represented an example of drug dependence without physical dependence. Less well known, outside of professionals dedicated to studying drug dependence, was the observation that other drugs such as narcotic agonist–antagonists, produced physical dependence but no drug dependence. For example, two drugs, cyclazocine and nalorphine, were observed to show a withdrawal syndrome after chronic administration. What was even more surprising was that this withdrawal syndrome was similar to morphine withdrawal and at least as unpleasant, yet, unlike morphine withdrawal, it was not a negative re-inforcer of continued drug use. Thus, there was an example of physical dependence without drug dependence.

without drug dependence.

Putting the two observations together: (1) drug dependence without physical dependence and (2) physical dependence without drug dependence changed peoples' concepts in this field. Physical dependence could no longer be considered the *sine qua non* of drug dependence. It could still, however, be a powerful negative reinforcer of drug dependence but only if an unknown ingredient were present. This unknown ingredient was identified as psychological dependence.

dependence to former drug users in an experiment they will report that they like the drug and that it makes them feel good. Furthermore, this can be demonstrated to have a dose-related score on several sophisticated tests measuring drug effects. Thus, the higher the dose, the more the drug is enjoyed or appreciated by the former drug user. An example may be useful in illustrating this concept. If morphine is given intramuscularly in doses of 10, 20 and 30 milligrams, former users will report a dose-related response on a

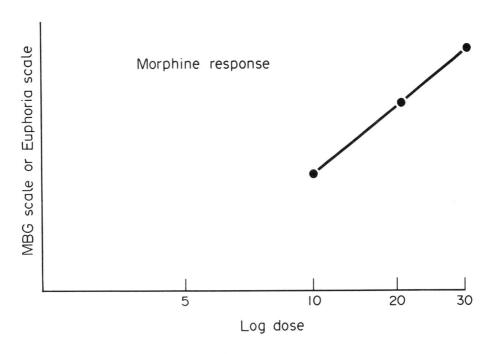

Figure 2.

At first, examining psychological dependence as a concept appears fuzzy. It is easy to let the mind wander and talk of psychological dependence on food, sex, gambling and other positive reinforcers as well as on drugs of dependence. Yet, psychological dependence as it applies to drug use cannot only be defined as taking a drug to get high but also in an operational manner. If one gives a drug of

euphoria scale (Fig. 2). If morphine is then given chronically several times a day for three to four weeks, the subjects will become physically dependent, i.e. they will experience a well-defined physical withdrawal syndrome when administration of the drug ceases and seek the drug for relief of the syndrome.

In contrast, if the opiate agonist-antagonist nalorphine were given to former users, they

Table 1.

Classification	Drugs	Physical dependence	Psychological dependence
Agonist	morphine codeine	yes	yes
Agonist—antagonist	nalorphine cyclazozine	yes	no
Pure antagonist	naloxone naltrexone	no	no

would not experience any euphoria or pleasure from the drug. They would generally report that they did not like the drug. If this drug were then given chronically, the former user would also develop physical dependence. In contrast to morphine withdrawal, the former user would not request nalorphine to relieve their physical symptoms of withdrawal. They would just appear pleased to be off the chronic administration schedule of this opiate agonist—antagonist (Table 1).

It is, therefore, concluded by many investigators in the field of drug dependence that psychological dependence measured by how much one enjoys the drug, or gets high on the drug, is necessary for physical dependence to promote continuing drug use. Psychological dependence is then like an all or nothing switch, an on-off switch, which when on, allows physical dependence to be a powerful negative reinforcer, but when off, negates the reinforcing properties of physical dependence. This conclusion seems obvious and well documented when looking at the examples of opiates and opiate agonist—antagonists. It still remains to be established with such diverse drugs of abuse as phencyclidine, atropine, glue sniffing and nicotine inhalation.

We have just discussed physical dependence as of secondary importance, psychological dependence being the primary or necessary ingredient. When psychological dependence is present however, physical dependence can be very important in drug dependence, the presence of psychological dependence is still needed to reveal its very important role.

The phenomenology of physical dependence.

Physical dependence is a term used to indicate that a well-defined physiological and behavioural syndrome will occur when chronic administration of a drug is discontinued. Physical dependence occurs with a variety of different types of drugs, including opiates; opiate agonist—antagonists, sedative hypnotics such as secobarbital, pentabarbital and alcohol, CNS stimulants such as the amphetamines, and atropine-like drugs. On the other hand, controversy still surrounds the presence of physical dependence in the case of marihuana, cocaine and other drugs.

The most thoroughly studied drug dependence or withdrawal syndromes have been described with opiate-like drugs and they will be discussed as a prototypal example. Three major types of withdrawal syndromes have been described with opiates (see Table 2). The first is called acute or primary abstinence. This syndrome occurs within hours of discontinuing the drug, reaches its peak within one or two days and lasts for about one to three weeks. With opiates, this is a rather dramatic

Table 2. Physical dependence syndromes

The Syndrome	Time Course	
	start	duration
primary or acute abstinence	hours	days
secondary or protracted abstinence	weeks	months
conditioned abstinence	variable	

syndrome resembling a bad case of the flu. The patient has nausea, vomiting, diarrhea, running nose, watering eyes, goose flesh ('cold turkey'), involuntary muscular contractions ('kicking the habit'), restlessness, insomnia and anorexia. Along with this are well-defined changes in vital signs such as body temperature, pulse rate, blood pressure, pupil size and respiratory rate. This is accompanied by drug craving and prominent drug-seeking behavior.

In addition to this acute or primary abstinence syndrome, two additional syndromes have been described with opiates, secondary or protracted abstinence and conditioned abstinence. These two syndromes are far more subtle in intensity than primary abstinence but may play a prominent role in relapse to drug use. These two syndromes have not been well described with other classes of drugs but may well exist with sedatives such as alcohol and with other classes of drugs. Even with opiates, these two syndromes are accepted by many investigators as established fact but since they are on the frontiers of recent research, others still ponder their importance if not their existence. These two concepts of protracted abstinence and conditioned abstinence raise more questions than they

answer and they are rightfully discussed as not only showing our knowledge but also our ignorance.

Protracted abstinence, as described after opiate use, starts several weeks after the primary withdrawal syndrome has subsided and lasts about six months. It is very mild in intensity and physiologically represents many changes that are opposite in direction to the changes seen with acute withdrawal or primary abstinence. For example, in primary abstinence pupils in the eye tend to dilate and become larger. In protracted abstinence, they constrict or become smaller. As alluded to above, the intensity of the change is so small and slight, one wonders what it might have to do with continuing drug use.

The final answers are far from established but several observations do allude to the importance of secondary abstinence. First, it has been observed that during the six-month duration of protracted abstinence the former opiate users are more sensitive to physiological stress. Secondly, it appears that those former users who have been drug free for about six months, have a greater chance of staying drug free in the long run.

Conditioned abstinence as a concept is even

less well established than protracted abstinence in its role in promoting drug dependence. It originates as a concept from clinical and experimental observations. This syndrome has been observed for some time in former opiate users when they visit neighborhoods, areas, or even rooms where they had formerly used drugs. At this time they would experience mild opiate withdrawal or mild primary abstinence. This would even occur if they made their visits years after they had been drug free. Animal experimenters noted that dogs who had been dependent on opiates would exhibit withdrawal long after their drug use when faced with the person who formerly injected them with the drug.

It was postulated that in both animals and humans, there would be a slight withdrawal just prior to each injection. Furthermore, this withdrawal would be conditioned to environmental factors by classical or Pavolovian conditioning. Abraham Wikler devised elaborate experiments in the rat to show conditioned abstinence and Charles O'Brien has shown this in former opiate users. Still, the question remains as to the importance of conditioned abstinence in relapse. Here one can speculate freely and here investigators are presently looking for answers. The conditioned abstinence may be experienced by the former drug user as either mild withdrawal or simply as anxiety. In either case, it is accompanied by craving for the drug and drug seeking behavior. If an individual mysteriously feels anxious or drug craving, they may cognitively label this experience as a defect in their psychological and physical makeup. Thus, they may become demoralized and discouraged, turning to their former drug for solace. However, if they are warned they will experience anxiety, drug craving and even mild withdrawal in certain

situations or places, they may not be discouraged but at least on guard for just this feeling. They would not have to see this as a defect in their makeup but as a conditioned feeling they can overcome by extinction. Indeed, this labeling of the experience has been useful to this author in treatment.

This may also explain the practical statement alluded to earlier and made by alcoholics in Alcoholics Anonymous stating 'I am an alcoholic', even if they have been drug-free for years. It has been assumed that this statement refers to an inherent psychological or personality defect. Some have postulated that the tendency to relapse may not be psychological but secondary to a genetic defect. It could also be simply a statement reflecting the experience of conditioned abstinence in alcoholics. It must be remembered that this latter explanation is rather tenuous but our ignorance only begins to dissolve as such speculations are formed into hypotheses and tested experimentally.

Another use of the conditioned abstinence hypothesis would be to test it in groups of drug users who have a low relapse rate. Several explanations have been offered for the low relapse rate among Vietnam veterans living in the United States. Most if not all of their opiate use was confined to Southeast Asia. Certainly they are no longer faced with the positive reinforcement of peer pressure or the negative reinforcement of the war. But they are also no longer in an environment which is conditioned to elicit an abstinent syndrome. This too, may lead to a low, long-term relapse rate.

In this chapter we have reviewed the field of drug dependence, highlighting the areas which represent the frontier of our knowledge and clearly illustrating our ignorance.

Further Reading

GUNDERSON, E.K.E. and RAHE, R.H. (eds.) (1974) *Life Stress and Illness.* Charles C. Thomas.

JAFFE, J.H. (1980) Drug Addiction and Drug Abuse. In: *The Pharmacological Basis of Therapeutics.* Gilman, A.G., Goodman, L.S. and Gilman, A., eds.) Macmillan, pp. 494—534.

JAFFE, J.H. and MARTIN, W.R. (1980) Opioid Analgesics and Antagonists. In: *The Pharmacological Basis of Therapeutics.* (Gilman, A.G., Goodman, L.S. and Gilman, A., eds.) Macmillan, pp. 494—534.

JASINSKI, D.R. (1977) Assessment of the abuse potentiality of morphine-like drugs (methods in man). In: *Drug Addiction I: Morphine, Sedative/Hypnotic and Alcohol Dependence.* (Martin, W.R., ed.) Handbuch der Experimentellen Pharmakologie, **Vol. 45**, Pt. I. Springer-Verlag, Berlin, pp. 179—258.

MANSKY, P.A. (1978) Opiates: Human Psychopharmacology. In: *Handbook of Psychopharmacology,* **Vol. 12** (Iversen, L.L., Iversen, S.D. and Snyder, S.H., eds.) Plenum.

MANSKY, P.A. and ALTMAN, J.A. (1977) A Conceptual Model of Drug Dependence. In: *Renewal in Psychiatry: A Critical Rational Perspective.* (Manschreck, T.C. and Kleinman, A.M., eds.) Hemisphere.

MARTIN, W.R. (1967) Opioid antagonists. *Pharmacology Reveiws,* **19**, 463—521 (373 references).

McLELLAN, A.T., WOODY, G.E. and O'BRIEN, C.P. (1979) Development of Psychiatric Illness in Drug Abusers. *New England Journal of Medicine,* **301**, pp. 1310—1314.

O'BRIEN, C.P., TESTA, T., O'BRIEN, T.J., BRADY, J.P. and WELLS, B. (1977) Conditioned narcotic withdrawal in humans. *Science,* **195**, pp. 1000—1002.

WIKLER, A. (1973) Dynamics of drug dependence. Implications of a conditioning theory for research and treatment. *Archives General Psychiatry,* **28**, pp. 611—616.

WINKLER, A. and PESCOR, F.T. (1967) Classical conditioning of a morphine abstinence phenomenon, reinforcement of opioid-drinking behavior and "relapse" in morphine-addicted rats, *Psychopharmacologia,* **10**, pp. 255—284.

CHEMICAL COMMUNICATIONS IN THE BRAIN AND MECHANISMS OF ACTION OF PSYCHOTROPIC DRUGS

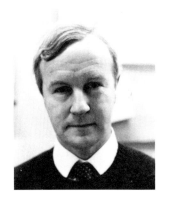

Leslie Lars Iversen, F.R.S.

Executive Director of the Neuroscience Research Centre, Merck Sharp and Dohme Ltd.

Formerly Director of the MRC Neurochemical Pharmacology Unit, Cambridge. Associate of the Neurosciences Research Program, M.I.T., USA. His main research interest has been chemical transmitter substances of the central nervous system in health and disease.

Chemical Messengers in the Brain

In broad terms we understand the function of the brain as a highly sophisticated computer-controlled telephone exchange, perceiving and analysing the environment through myriads of sensory inputs and generating thought and action, but we know little of the detailed cellular and chemical mechanisms involved. The billions of brain cells signal to one another by means of minute electrical impulses that travel along the often extended nerve fibres connecting cells to each other. At the junctions between cells, however, the transmission of information takes place not by direct electrical contacts but by means of chemical relays. At synapses, the tiny regions of close proximity between the terminal of one neurone and the receiving surface of another, the arrival of a nerve impulse causes a sudden release of molecules of chemical neurotransmitter from the nerve terminal. The transmitter then diffuses across the fluid-filled gap between the two cells and acts at specific receptor sites on the post-synaptic target cell membrane, thereby altering the electrical activity of the receiving neurone.

Some thirty different substances (Table 1) are known or thought to act in this way as transmitters in the brain and each has a characteristic excitatory or inhibitory effect on target neurones. These chemicals are not

Table 1. Known and possible candidates (?) for neurotransmitter function in mammalian brain

Monoamines	Amino Acids
Acetylcholine	GABA (gamma-aminobutyric acid)
Noradrenaline	Glutamic acid
Dopamine	Glycine
Adrenaline	Aspartic acid (?)
Serotonin (?) (5-hydroxytryptamine)	Taurine (?)
Histamine (?)	

Peptides	
Angiotensin (?)	Insulin (?)
Avian pancreatic polypeptide (?)	β-Lipotropin (?)
Bombesin (?)	LHRH (luteinising hormone releasing hormone or luliberin)
Bradykinin (?)	Neurotensin (?)
Carnosine (?)	Oxytocin (?)
Pancreozymin (?)	Prolactin (?)
Endorphin (?)	Somatostatin (?)
Leu-enkephalin	Substance P
Met-enkephalin	TRH (thyrotropin releasing hormone or thyroliberin) (?)
Growth Hormone (somatotropin) (?)	Vasopressin (?)
Glucagon (?)	VIP (vasoactive intestinal polypeptide) (?)

uniformly distributed throughout the brain, but are localized in specific groups of nerve cells, whose fibres project specifically to certain other regions. Some of these substances, such as acetylcholine and noradrenaline, have been known for many years to exist in the peripheral nervous system, where they are released as neurotransmitters from nerve terminals and control the activity of muscles and visceral organs. Many of the peptides recently discovered in the brain are known also to exist in the peripheral system, where they function as local hormones in the gut, or as blood-born hormones co-ordinating the activity of various body organs.

In terms of brain function, the biological significance of the existence of such a large number of different chemical messengers remains unknown. Models of neuronal circuits can be constructed in which not more than one or two chemical messengers (one excitatory and one inhibitory) are needed. Whatever the explanation, it seems certain that yet more chemical transmitters remain to be discovered in mammalian brain. For example, the millions of fibres in the optic nerve almost certainly transmit information from the eye to the brain by means of a release of chemical transmitter in the brain, yet the identity of this transmitter remains unknown. Many other similar gaps in our knowledge of chemical circuitry in the brain exist, and it would no longer be surprising to contemplate the existence of as many as one hundred different chemical messengers in the brain.

Thus, complex chemical coding is superimposed on the already stupendous anatomical complexity of neuronal circuitry within the brain. The importance of such chemical coding is obvious from the dramatic effects that small amounts of certain foreign chemicals (psychotropic drugs) can have on brain function. Thus, stimulant drugs such as amphetamine heighten arousal and excitement, sedatives cause sleep, anaesthetics dull all sensation and hallucinogens, such as lysergic acid diethylamide (d-LSD), vividly distort perception. Although such drugs are thought to act by interfering with the normal processes of chemical transmission of information within the brain, in most cases their detailed mechanisms of action are not yet understood.

Studies of the function of chemical transmitters in the brain remains technically exceedingly difficult. They are present in vanishingly small quantities, and the brain is structurally and chemically so complex that it is not easy to isolate a particular transmitter system for examination. Future progress will depend heavily on the development of new techniques to surmount these difficulties. Major advances have already been made in the development of selective staining techniques that allow visualization of neurones containing a particular transmitter, and this has provided a flood of information about the detailed anatomical distribution of individual transmitters in the brain.

Monoamines and Drug Mechanisms

The most thoroughly studied brain transmitters are the monoamines, noradrenaline, dopamine and serotonin. Neurones containing these substances will fluoresce green or yellow if the transmitters are converted into fluorescent derivatives by reacting them with formaldehyde or glyoxylic acid. Extensive mapping studies have revealed that many of the noradrenaline-containing cells in the brain are concentrated in small clusters at the base of the brain, in the brain stem. From these clusters of cells highly branched fibres project to many brain regions, particularly the hypothalamus, cerebellum and forebrain. The noradrenaline system has been implicated in the maintenance of arousal, in the brain system of reward, in dreaming sleep and in the regulation of mood. Other groups of neurones containing the related monoamine transmitter dopamine are concentrated in the upper brain stem, and their fibres terminate in particularly high density in a region near the centre of the brain known as the basal ganglia. In this region dopamine appears to play a crucial role in the control of complex voluntary movements. The degeneration of the dopamine fibres in this region gives rise to the muscular rigidity, lack of voluntary movement and tremors of Parkinson's disease. Other dopamine-containing fibres project to the forebrain, where they are thought to be involved in regulating emotional responses. A third amine transmitter, serotonin, is concentrated in a cluster of neurones in the brain stem raphe nuclei. As with the noradrenaline and dopamine cells, serotonin-containing fibres are highly branched and project to many regions of the forebrain, including the hypothalamus and cerebral cortex. Serotonin is thought to be involved in temperature regulation, sensory perception and the onset of sleep.

Although the precise function of these amine-containing neuronal systems is far from clear, they appear to represent key targets for the actions of several types of psychotropic drugs. Thus, the stimulant and appetite-suppressant effects of amphetamine and related drugs are due to their ability to release dopamine, and to a lesser extent noradrenaline, from nerve terminals in brain. Excessive use of amphetamine by addicts can lead to disruption of thought processes, hallucinations, and delusions of persecution, symptoms which closely mimic those found in some forms of schizophrenia. This and other evidence had lead to the hypothesis that an overactivity in the brain dopamine system may underly the symptoms of schizophrenia.

Another important finding is that the various antischizophrenic drugs (major tranquillizers) that have been developed, such as chlorpromazine and haloperidol, all share the common property of acting as antagonists of dopamine at its receptor sites on target neurones in the brain. This discovery has proved to be one of the most promising leads in modern schizophrenia research, and studies

on human post-mortem brain tend to confirm the idea that excessive amounts of dopamine and abnormally large numbers of dopamine receptors exist in the brains of patients dying with schizophrenic illness. Such findings have encouraged further research which may lead to the development of more selective dopamine-blocking drugs that might avoid some of the undesirable side effects associated with those currently available.

Other psychoactive drugs may also act by mimicking or blocking the effects of monoamine transmitters at their post-synaptic receptors. Many hallucinogenic drugs, such as LSD and psilocybin are related structurally to serotonin, although their precise modes of action are still not known. Drugs used in the treatment of depression seem to act by potentiating the effects of amine transmitters such as noradrenaline and serotonin. One such group of drugs is represented by iproniazid, and other drugs that inhibit the enzyme monoamine oxidase, which degrades noradrenaline, dopamine and serotonin in the brain. As a result, the arousing effects of these monoamines are enhanced, perhaps accounting for the anti-depressant actions of such drugs. A second group of anti-depressants, the tricyclics, also enhance the effects of noradrenaline and serotonin in the brain. These drugs, such as imipramine and amitriptyline, block the re-uptake of noradrenaline and serotonin after their release from nerve terminals, thus prolonging their effects at the synapse. The stimulant drug cocaine appears to work by the same mechanism. These findings have led to the suggestion that depression may be associated with low levels of amine transmitters at brain synapses, whereas mania may be associated with excessively high levels of such transmitters. Despite these modest successes however, a great deal remains to be learned about the chemical basis of schizophrenia and depression, the most common major mental illnesses. Not all patients with schizophrenia or depression respond favourably to treatment with currently available drugs, and it seems likely that the mental symptoms of schizophrenia or depression can arise from a number of different underlying chemical imbalances in the brain, only some of which are corrected by presently available psychotropic drugs.

GABA and Minor Tranquillizers

The most widely prescribed psychotropic drugs are the minor tranquillizers, such as diazepam (Valium), which are used to treat neuroses and other anxiety states and as 'sleeping pills'. Such drugs belong to a chemical class known as benzodiazepines, and their unique anti-anxiety effects were first discovered in the early 1960s. Until recently their mechanism of action was unknown, but new evidence suggests that these drugs may act by increasing the effectiveness of the amino acid GABA (gamma-aminobutyric acid) at its receptor sites in the brain. GABA is the commonest inhibitory transmitter in the brain, and is unique among amino acids in that it is manufactured almost exclusively in the central nervous system and is not incorporated into larger molecules such as peptides or proteins. It has been estimated that as many as one third of the synapses in the brain may use GABA as their transmitter. It has also been discovered that a specific deficit in brain GABA occurs in Huntington's chorea, which is an inherited neurological disease. The uncontrolled movements of Huntington's chorea are caused by progressive deterioration of the basal ganglia in middle age. Post-mortem analysis has revealed that the brain damage involves a major loss of inhibitory neurones that normally contain GABA, suggesting that a deficit in this transmitter might be responsible for some of the symptoms of the disease. Attempts to treat patients by replacing the missing brain GABA is currently not possible since GABA-like drugs that are capable of penetrating the brain from the blood stream have not yet been developed. The nature of the interaction of minor tranquillizers such as diazepam with the GABA system also remains obscure. Although specific diazepam receptor sites have been identified in the brain, by virtue of their ability to bind the radioactively labelled drug with high affinity and specificity, these sites are clearly distinguishable from the GABA receptors, although the two types of receptor appear to interact. The intriguing possibility exists that the brain contains some undiscovered substance that normally acts on the diazepam receptors, perhaps a natural anxiety-producing or anti-anxiety compound?

The Chemistry of Pain

Another success story for brain chemistry research has been the dramatic improvement in our understanding of the mode of action of pain-relieving drugs (analgesics) in recent years. The most important of these is morphine, a complex natural organic chemical derived from the opium poppy. Despite the widespread abuse of morphine and related substances (collectively known as the opiates) by addicts, they continue to play a crucial medical role in the treatment of severe and chronic pain. During the 1970s it was discovered that morphine and related opiates are recognised by specific receptors present in certain regions of the brain. These were identified by their ability to bind radioactively labelled opiate drugs with high affinity. The opiate receptors did not recognize any of the known transmitter chemicals and an intensive search was started to discover what naturally occurring chemical might exist in brain that might mimic the effects of morphine on opiate receptors. This led, in 1975, to the discovery of a wholly new series of brain chemicals, the enkephalins and endorphins. The enkephalins, leu- and met-enkephalin, are small peptides consisting of chains of five amino acids. They are identical in amino acid sequence except for the terminal amino acid, which in one is methionine and in the other is leucine. Other morphine-like peptides, named endorphins, were subsequently isolated from the pituitary gland. The enkephalins and endorphins seem to represent chemical transmitters, synthesized and released normally by neurones in certain regions of the brain and spinal cord, with an important role in modulating the input of pain stimuli to the higher brain centres. It seems likely that several procedures used to treat chronic pain, including acupuncture, and direct electrical stimulation of the brain, and even hypnosis, may act by causing a release of enkephalins or endorphins in the brain and spinal cord. The effectiveness of all these procedures can be largely blocked by administration of naloxone, a drug that specifically blocks the effects of morphine and enkephalins on opiate receptors. As research proceeds in this area, however, it seems likely that the enkephalins and endorphins will be shown to have other roles to play within the brain apart from the modulation of pain inputs. Enkephalin-containing neurones and opiate receptors exist in abundance in regions of the brain, and even in the retina of the eye, where they have no obvious relation to pain pathways. Detailed pharmacological analysis also suggests that more than one subcategory of receptor may exist capable of recognizing morphine and enkephalins. The possibility thus exists that more selective pain-killing drugs can be developed, and entirely novel psychotropic agents may emerge, as drugs are selectively designed to act on these sub-varieties of opiate receptor. Only one of the receptor types appears to be critically involved in mediating the pain-relieving properties of the opiates. A selective agonist for the other receptor sub-type would have a hitherto unknown pharmacological profile. Perhaps a pure euphoriant? Despite this rapid progress, however, we are still no closer to understanding the problems of tolerance and addiction associated with morphine and related drugs. With repeated use progressively larger doses are needed for them to be effective (tolerance), and after long-term use physical dependence (addiction) develops, manifested by an unpleasant collection of mental and physical withdrawal symptoms if the drug is abruptly stopped. The challenge of developing a safe analgesic drug, perhaps based on the enkephalin structures rather than on morphine, which would not suffer from the disadvantages of tolerance and addiction liability remains an important challenge for future research. The possibility that such research might also lead to the emergence of 'safe' euphoriant drugs is an intriguing and alarming possibility. Western societies have strict laws to discourage trafficking and use of opiates, to protect people against the medical dangers of their abuse. What would our attitude be if these dangers were removed? Are we ready to tolerate the 'Soma' of Aldous Huxley's 'Brave New World'?

Peptide Hormones in the Brain

The enkephalins and endorphins represent only one example of the newly discovered brain peptides. More than twenty other peptides are now known to exist in mammalian brain. Some of these have been known for many years to exist as local hormones in the gut (pancreozymin, gastrin, vasoactive intestinal peptide) or secreted as hormones into the blood from specialized glandular tissues (insulin, glucagon, corticotropin). The discovery that they also exist within the brain has been highly unexpected, and perhaps suggests that during evolution these molecules have been adapted to serve a variety of different functions within the body. In most cases, their function within the brain is totally unknown. Perhaps the strongest candidate among the neuropeptides for neurotransmitter status is substance P, a peptide consisting of a chain of eleven amino acids. As with many of the other peptides, it was first discovered in the gut and later found to be present in the nervous system. It is present in a number of specific neuronal pathways in the brain and also in some of the primary sensory fibres in peripheral nerves. Substance P is released from the terminals of sensory nerves in the spinal cord, where it is known to be able to excite relay neurones. This suggests that it may function as one of the sensory transmitters. Because substance P excites those spinal neurones that respond most readily to painful stimuli, it has further been suggested that it may be associated specific-ally with the transmission of information from peripheral pain receptors into the central nervous system.

Such specific functions have not yet been proposed for most of the other peptides known to exist in the brain. One remarkable feature of the neuropeptides is that many of them are able to elicit remarkably specific behavioural responses when administered in very small amounts directly into the brain. For example, injection of nanogram (one thousand millionth of a gramme) amounts of the neuropeptide angiotensin II elicits intense and prolonged drinking behaviour in animals that were not previously thirsty. Another peptide, luteinizing hormone releas-ing hormone (luliberin), induces characteristic sexual behaviour when it is injected into the brain of a female rat. Even more remarkable, the administration of small amounts of the neuropeptide vasopressin appears to improve markedly the memory of learned tasks in laboratory animals. The peptides may repre-sent a means of chemical coding for patterns of brain activity associated with particular functions, such as body-fluid balance, sexual behaviour, pain or pleasure, and learning and memory. If this were true, it suggests the possibility of developing wholly novel categories of psychotropic drugs that might specifically affect intellectual performance, memory, libido, and other appetites. The possibility of developing drugs that would improve intellectual function and memory

would be of enormous significance, not only to undergraduates, but also to the increasing numbers of people in our ageing population who suffer from the intellectual impairment and memory defects associated with various forms of 'senile dementia'. As many as one in ten in the over sixty five years age group, and up to one in five in the over eighty age group may expect to suffer some form of dementia, making this a medical problem of epidemic proportions for the twenty first century. So far we have little or no under-standing of the cellular and chemical mecha-nisms underlying such senile deterioration.

Some Outstanding Areas of Ignorance

We do not know how several major classes of psychotropic drugs act, and we know little of the cellular and chemical basis of several important brain disorders. For example, the most widely used of all psychotropic drugs are alcohol and nicotine, yet we have very little knowledge of their actions in the brain, or of the mechanisms that lead many people to become dependent upon them, often in a life-threatening manner. Nor do we really understand how anaesthetics act to deaden sensation without significantly impairing the life supporting functions of the brain, or why caffeine is a stimulant and wards off sleep, or why cannabis is pleasurable. One of the commonest brain disorders is epilepsy, in which at intervals, regions of the brain be-come vastly over-active, leading to the seizures (fits) characteristic of this illness. The uncontrolled neural discharges of an epileptic seizure strongly suggest an underlying chemical imbalance, with some failure in the normal inhibitory chemical systems in the brain. But the precise chemical nature of this imbalance remains completely obscure, and the drugs used, often very effective in pre-venting seizures in epileptic patients, have a completely unknown mode of action.

The phenomenon of mental retardation

also presents an enormous challenge to re-search, and represents a terrible burden in terms of human suffering. In England about four per thousand of the people who survive to the age of 15–19 years are likely to be severely retarded (with I.Q. values of less than 50). As many as twenty per thousand of the population will suffer from milder forms of mental retardation. There is no common cause of such conditions, which arise instead for a multitude of different reasons. In a few cases specific biochemical abnormalities have been detected, often involving the lack of one of the enzymes needed for the normal meta-bolism of amino acids, sugars, or lipids in the brain. Although only a few per cent of mentally retarded children suffer from con-ditions in which a specific biochemical cause can be established, the importance of such understanding is emphasized by the dramatic improvements in treatment now possible for some such conditions. For example, phenyl-ketonuria is a very rare metabolic disorder in which the amino acid, phenylalanine, can-not be metabolized normally. Soon after birth, blood phenylalanine concentrations begin to rise and as a consequence an excess of phenylalanine metabolites accumulates in blood and urine. If the condition is left un-diagnosed and untreated, severe mental retardation invariably ensues. However, treat-ment by phenylalanine-restricted diets is successful in preventing such retardation, and is now a practical proposition and the disease can be diagnosed by a simple blood test routinely applied to newborn babies.

Clues are beginning to emerge from basic research about the nature of the chemical factors that guide nerve cells and allow them to make suitable connections during develop-ment. It seems likely that a series of 'nerve growth factors' will be discovered in coming years, and our increased understanding of the specialized chemistry that underlies normal brain development may help us to devise means of controlling abnormal develop-ment, and even to persuade nerve cells in the adult brain to regenerate after damage.

In conclusion, it is clear that ignorance greatly outweighs knowledge in the field of brain chemistry and understanding psycho-tropic drug actions. Further knowledge of the basic mechanisms involved is needed to help us unravel the nature of the abnormalities that underly mental illness and to improve the possibilities for developing rational drug treatments of such illnesses. To the research worker lucky enough to be involved in this area, the study of brain chemistry retains the excitement and adventure of a scientific frontier.

Further Reading

BURGEN, A.S.V., KOSTERLITZ, H.J. and IVERSEN, L.L. (eds.) (1981) *Neuroactive Peptides*. The Royal Society, London.

COOPER, J.R., BLOOM, F.E. and ROTH, R.H. (1978) *The Biochemical Basis of Neuropharmacology*, 3rd Edition. Oxford University Press, New York.

IVERSEN, L.L. and IVERSEN, S.D. (1981) *Behavioural Pharmacology*, 2nd Edition. Oxford University Press, New York.

'The Brain' *Scientific American*, September, 1979.

MULTIPLE SCLEROSIS

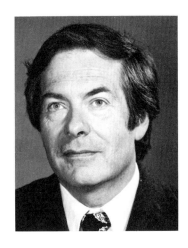

Alan N. Davison

Professor of Neurochemistry, Institute of Neurology, University of London.

Formerly Professor of Biochemistry, Charing Cross Hospital Medical School, London. His recent interests include the biochemistry of brain degenerative disorders, including multiple sclerosis and dementia, central nervous system development and mental retardation, and muscular dystrophy.

With a few exceptions such as infectious disease (e.g. poliomyelitis) or deficiency states (c.g. lack of vitamin B group), the causes of most brain disease are completely unknown. For example, there is no satisfactory explanation of the selective damage to nerve cells found in the basal ganglia region of the brain in the movement disorder known as Parkinson's disease. Equally baffling are the presumably subtle metabolic factors producing psychiatric conditions such as schizophrenia or certain behavioural disorders. At first sight, the same applies to multiple sclerosis (sclerosis is thickened scar tissue), for the cause of this relatively common neurological disease remains an enigma and effective treatment is lacking. However, there are clues which, as we shall see, have led to considerable speculation on the aetiology and pathogenesis of the demyelinating disorder.

The Problem with Multiple Sclerosis

Multiple sclerosis (MS) is a disease affecting the central nervous system (CNS), but not the peripheral nervous system. Since various sites in the brain and spinal cord are affected, MS may first appear in a number of clinical forms, for example there may be transient impairment of vision or perhaps unsteadiness of gait.

Not until there is more than one lesion disseminated in both time and space can MS be safely diagnosed. In areas of damage, the insulating myelin sheath is primarily attacked, leaving the conducting axons of the nerve fibre intact. In this process of demyelination, certain parts of the central nervous system are affected more than others. One site of predilication is the optic tract and indeed blurred vision is a frequent symptom of MS. Since demyelination is commonly found in the optic nerve and the ventricles (the cavities in the brain filled with cerebrospinal fluid), it has been suggested that these sites are exposed to the action of a soluble taxic factor possibly emanating from the circulation. Another feature of multiple sclerosis is that it has a relapsing—remitting pattern. Although the exact cause of a relapse is not known, stress and intercurrent infections are associated with attacks. Some periods of remission may extend for many years, or the disease may be slowly progressive. Less commonly there is a rapid downhill course. It may be, therefore, that these conditions represent a broad spectrum of a single disease, or alternatively that there are distinct diseases in which the benign condition differs from the fulminating type.

Clues to Multiple Sclerosis

Epidemiology

Although MS is not thought to be infective in the same way as well-defined diseases such as measles or rubella, it is slightly more common amongst close relatives. There is a characteristic geographical distribution of MS, just as was found when paralytic poliomyelitis was endemic. The disease is much commoner in colder Northern climates. More cases are found in the Northern States of the USA than in the South, and a high proportion in the Hebrides (1 in 800) compared with the rest of the United Kingdom (1 in 2000). MS appears to be virtually absent amongst the Bantu of

South Africa or amongst native-born Israelis. In some parts of the world there have been restricted outbreaks of MS. For example, in the Faroes the disease was rare from 1929 to 1943, but then an outbreak occurred terminating in 1960. It was suggested that this restricted cluster of MS was related to an epidemic of canine distemper which occurred on the islands during the second World War. Similar outbreaks have been found in Iceland and in Alaska and again canine distemper has been implicated. This has led to a trial of a distemper vaccination programme, to see if this prevents incidence of new cases. Unfortunately, other evidence for the incrimination of the distemper virus is not as convincing.

An infective agent

There is little evidence that MS is transmitted to relatives or those in contact with patients. Neither has it proved possible to infect experimental animals nor nervous tissue in culture. Nevertheless, a number of viruses have been considered as possible infective agents. So far, it has not proved possible to isolate any one, but recovery experiments of this type are notoriously difficult. With the development of improved tissue culture procedures, there is a better chance that renewed attempts to recover and identify one or more viruses will succeed. Occasionally, virus-like bodies have been recovered from MS tissue, but this has usually proved to be either artifact or contaminant. It has been claimed that a para-influenza virus can be identified in replicate cultures obtained from bone marrow samples obtained from MS sufferers. Serological studies indicate a slight increase in measles antibodies in MS, and there is immunological data to suggest an abnormal response to this virus. It does not necessarily follow that any such virus persists in the CNS throughout the illness, or indeed that the same infective agent is associated with renewed relapses. In the cerebral spinal fluid, increased antibody titres to several different viruses have been reported. One explanation of these findings is that MS sufferers may be more vulnerable to infection, so that the disease may be initiated by one of a number of viruses. Alternatively, the disease may stimulate recall of antibody directed against past infection, and viruses may have only a secondary role in the pathogenesis.

Pathology

Although in the brain and spinal cord some disseminated plaques (thickened scar tissue) may be large enough to see, it is evident from microscopic examination that there is much more extensive damage to white matter than is apparent to the naked eye. Using a combined histological and biochemical study of apparently unaffected MS white matter, Allen and McKeown (1979) in Belfast found that 72% of samples were abnormal. There was evidence of cellular proliferation (gliosis due to fibrous astrocytes) away from plaques, suggesting some localised pathological process, as may be associated with a chronic viral infection of glial cells. This could be the key factor initiating demyelination, for the oligodendroglial cells are connected with and sustain the myelin sheath (see Fig. 1).

Areas of demyelinated tissue are frequently close to blood vessels in whose endothelial cells there are often cuffs of inflammatory cells. The acute type of perivascular cuffs contain lymphocytes (a type of white blood cell or leucocyte), whereas the older chronic lesions contain mainly macrophages and plasma cells (see Figs. 1 and 2). It is suspected that the macrophages release lipolytic and proteolytic enzymes (Table 1), which are responsible for digestion of the fatty and protein components of the myelin sheath, although peeling or stripping of myelin sheaths is not usually observed. In the plaques basic protein of the myelin sheath disappears at an early stage. However, loss of a myelin-associated glycoprotein is even more widespread, extending around the lesion into the apparently normal areas of white matter. The

digestion of these proteins appears to be due to the action of acid and neutral proteinases. Proteolytic enzyme activity is increased close to fresh lesions, and is thought to be due to infiltrating cells – macrophages and polymorphonuclear leucocytes. Some proteolytic activity may also come from astrocytes. It has been proposed by Cammer and her colleagues at the Albert Einstein, New York, that stimulated macrophages in the CNS release plasminogen activator and so form plasmin, a potent proteolytic enzyme. The result of the proteolytic attack on the myelin is to release fragments of myelin and low molecular weight peptide fragments. Fragments of myelin and encephalitogenic peptides have been identified in the spinal fluid during a relapse. It is known that myelin basic protein and some peptides derived from it, are powerfully encephalitogenic. Thus, it has been postulated that an autoimmune response to these myelin degradation products contributes to the pathogenesis. There is evidence that other hydrolytic enzymes – such as phospholipases – facilitate the proteolytic destruction of myelin. Dr Banik and I showed that, while added trypsin readily removed basic protein from myelin preparations, the membrane ultrastructure remained intact. However, in the presence of phospholipase there was extensive splitting of myelin lamellae and numerous free strands of dissociated single lamellae were observed. Elevated phospholipase activities have been demonstrated in tissues from patients with MS and in animals with encephalitis.

Experimental Allergic Encephalomyelitis (EAE)

Inflammation of the brain (encephalomyelitis) sometimes occurs in individuals following rabies vaccination, where the vaccine was prepared from infective brain tissue. This has led workers to attempt to reproduce the encephalomyelitis by repeated

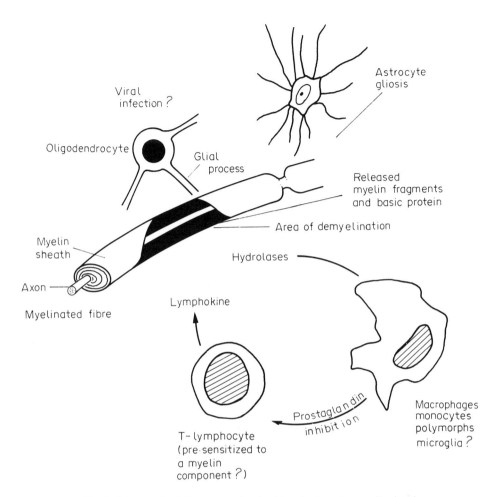

Fig. 1. Scheme of cellular changes involved in attack on the myelin sheath.
Lymphokine is a soluble factor released from T-cells. It is a chemotactic factor,
attracting lymphocytes and polymorphs to the inflammatory site. The macrophage is a phagocyte, which helps digest damaged myelin.

injection of nervous tissue into animals. When the central nervous tissue was combined with an oily preparation (Freund's adjuvant), paralysis developed one to two weeks after injection. The animals usually showed signs of hind-limb paralysis, loss of weight and very often incontinence (see Plate 1). Although inflammatory changes occur in the CNS, in rodents the degree of demyelination is slight. A condition with relapses and remissions can be produced by injection of young sensitive strains of animals. This is a closer model of

MS, for in this case there is demyelination and plaques of scar tissue form in the CNS.

Experimental allergic encephalomyelitis is an example of a delayed hypersensitivity reaction in which the neuroantigen (basic protein) activates lymphoid tissue (see Fig. 1). With the first sign of paralysis, circulating 'early' or 'avid' T-lymphocytes (detected by a rosetting test in which rabbit red cells stick in a rosette arrangement to the sensitized lymphocyte) decrease in number. There is evidence that some of these cells appear to

Table 1. Some biological effects of lymphocytic activation products

Released Factor	Target Cell	Effect
Blastogenic factor	Lymphocytes	Provokes transformation, including B-cell to plasma cells
Antigen-specific and non-specific helper and suppressor factors	Lymphocytes	Help or suppress activation or differentiation of B- or T-lymphocytes
Chemotactic and leucocyte inhibitory factors	Neutrophil Polymorphs	Affect movement of polymorphs
Migration-inhibitory factor	Macrophages	Inhibits macrophage migration

(modified from *Immunology* (Ed. by J—F Bach) 1978)

When lymphocytes are cultured in the presence of a specific antigen, the supernatant from the culture contains factors which act on different types of target cell. The term 'lymphocyte activation product' or lymphokine refers to all such factors.

enter the CNS where they may release soluble products (lymphokines) and so initiate the inflammatory reaction. In acutely paralysed animals, about 65% of the infiltrating cells are lymphocytes, 25% are mononuclear phagocytes, and a small proportion neutrophils (polymorphs). Of the lymphocytes recovered from the CNS, about half have been identified as T-cells, some of which are sensitized to myelin basic protein. Development of encephalitis can be partially suppressed by administration of excess myelin basic protein and by immunosuppressant drugs, if they are given before the onset of paralysis. Inhibitors of proteolytic enzyme activity (particularly plasminogen inhibitors) also delay the onset of paralysis and reduce the histological damage to the brain and spinal cord. The protective effect is exerted up to seven days after sensitization with white matter or myelin basic protein. Thus, these enzyme inhibitors probably prevent some of the localized damage resulting from release of proteinases by infiltrating macrophages.

Some years ago it was shown that animals deficient in essential fatty acids were particularly vulnerable to EAE. Conversely, treatment with essential fatty acid such as linoleic acid reduces the severity of EAE. The effect is thought to be related to the concentration of the biologically highly active prostaglandins which are derived from long chain polyunsaturated fatty acids. Prostaglandins of the E type are implicated in regulation of the immune response. Of particular interest is the claim that prostaglandins activate suppressor T-cells. The likely involvement of the prostaglandin E series has been supported by experiments showing modification of EAE when synthesis inhibitors (e.g. indomethacin), antibodies to prostaglandins and prostaglandin analogues, are given. As a result of

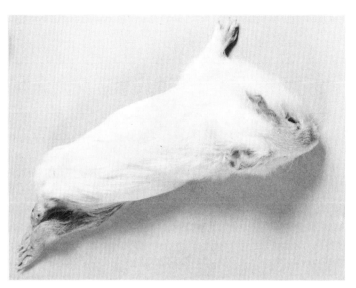

Plate 1. Guinea-pig showing signs of experimental allergic encephalomyelitis. The first signs of the disease are loss of weight, hind-leg paralysis and incontinence.

Table 2. Some secretory products of mononuclear phagocytes

Enzymes:	neutral proteinases (e.g. plasminogen activator), acid hydrolases (proteases, lipases, etc.)
Complement components	
Enzyme inhibitors:	plasmin inhibitors, α_2-macroglobulin
Biologically active lipids:	prostaglandin E_2, thromboxane, leucotriene, platelet-activating factors
Neutrophil chemotactic factors	
Lymphocyte activating factors	
Lymphocyte replication inhibition	

(after Nathan, Murray and Cohn, 1980).

this research, there is renewed attention to the validity of EAE as a model of the auto-immune reaction in MS. There have been several trials investigating the potential value of dietary supplementation with polyun-saturated fatty acids in treatment of patients with MS, but the results so far are not striking.

Immunology of Multiple Sclerosis

Some diseases (e.g. rheumatoid arthritis and myasthenia gravis) tend to be associated with a certain kind of inherited genetic pattern found on chromosome six within cell nuclei. The mapping or expression of these genes is easily identified by characteristic markers of the human leucocyte antigens (HLA) pre-sent on the human lymphocyte. This method had led to the important discovery that many MS sufferers have a characteristic HLA pattern. Since similar genes in mice control immunological reactivity, the changed HLA type in MS suggests that there is some defect in their body defence mechanisms. There are indications of a defect in immuno-regulation in MS sufferers, not only in the raised cerebrospinal fluid antibody, but also in changes found in circulating lymphocytes during the course of the disease. A defect in cell-mediated immunity is indicated by aberrant response to viral antigens and the altered leucocyte migration to antigens (measles or myelin basic protein).

The cerebrospinal fluid

On electrophoresis of the cerebrospinal fluid from MS cases, discrete bands of anti-body separate. These so-called oligoclonal bands of restricted heterogeneity presumably originate from a limited number of B-cell clones. Oligoclonal antibodies can also be detected in the cerebrospinal fluid of patients suffering from viral encephalitis and other conditions where there is a known infectious aetiology. In the case of a rare measles in-fection of the brain (subacute sclerosing panencephalitis), it has proved possible to show that some of the cerebrospinal fluid antibody combines with measles antigen. However, in MS all attempts to identify antigens to which most of the antibody might be directed, have failed. Indeed, it has been suggested that the oligoclonal bands are 'nonsense' antibodies derived from aberrant clones of B-lymphocytes. Data of Arnason and his group from Chicago shows that different patterns of oligoclonal antibody can be recovered from individual plaques in the same patient. This is interpreted as being due to the involvement of different antigens in each separate plaque or to the synthesis in each plaque of antibodies, irrelevant to the pathogenesis of the disease. In contrast, identical antibody patters are seen in the antibody recovered from different areas of brain from a patient with subacute sclerosing panencephalitis.

In a relapse, cells are detectable in the cerebrospinal fluid. Frequently macrophages (histiocytes), lymphocytes and occasional polymorphs are seen. A decrease has been observed in a subpopulation of immuno-logically active T-cells corresponding to clinical disease activity. These T-cells possess immunosuppressor potential and the cells appearing in the CSF presumably are derived from peripheral blood, where similar de-creases occur during a relapse. Although immune complexes are generally absent from the cerebrospinal fluid in remission and in other neurological diseases, low concentra-tions of immune complexes are detectable in about half of MS patients during exacerba-tion. Since immune complexes are digested (phagocytosed) by polymorphs, these may correlate with the reported appearance of these cells, and for the increase in cell-bound proteinase activity found during a relapse in both the cerebrospinal fluid and the blood.

The blood

With the help of our neurological col-leagues, Dr Louise Cuzner and I began a syste-

70 A.N. Davison

matic study of the properties of circulating leucocytes (white cells) in the hope of finding changes which could be related to the inflammatory cells appearing in the CNS during a relapse. We first found that there were increases in blood polymorph neutral proteinase activity in association with an exacerbation.

Up to a few years ago there were conflicting reports of changes of circulating lymphocytes (T- and B-cells) in relationship to the progress of the disease. While it is now generally agreed that there is little alteration in the proportion of B-lymphocytes, well documented differences in T-cell subsets have been reported. T-lymphocytes have both effector and regulator immunological roles. The effector T-cell functions include release of lymphokines and direct cytotoxic effects

on target cells. Regulator cells may either amplify or suppress the immune response by both B- and T-cell effectors. Those T-cells which reduce the immune response are designated suppressor cells. It is the suppressor cell population which appears to be significantly depleted in a relapse. It has now been found that patients with clinically definite MS have a reduced lymphocyte suppressor activity in response to added measles virus, compared with control individuals and others with strokes. Normally, suppressor cells moderate the lymphocyte response to infectious disease, so that the reduction in suppressor cells in MS patients may also indicate a defect in immunoregulation. The results of Neighbour and Bloom (1979) show a failure of MS-lymphocytes to produce significant amounts of a soluble

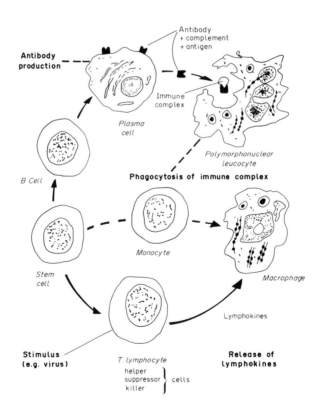

Fig. 2. Diagram of cell types involved in immunological reactions.

immunosuppressive and antiviral factor (possibly interferon). Attempts have been made to restore this function by use of an immunopotentiating agent -- transfer factor -- derived from lymphocytes of non-affected volunteers. Such attempts have generally not been successful, but some modest improvement has been claimed by an Australian group when transfer factor was prepared from relatives and given for a 2-year trial period. During a remission, a clone of T-cells can be detected which are sensitized to a factor present in aqueous extracts prepared from the brain of MS sufferers. So far, this factor has not been identified — it may be a degradation product of myelin or the oligodendroglial cell, or even an antigen derived from the causative agent. As an attack of MS develops, circulating sensitized cells are no longer detectable and there is a decrease in the proportion of 'early' T-cells. By analogy with EAE, it could be that the sensitized T-lymphocytes are attracted into the CNS by lymphokines at a site of damage, together with other cells (polymorphs, macrophages, monocytes) also involved in the inflammatory reaction. It is of considerable interest that Dore-Duffy and her colleagues have found that a small proportion of lymphocytes from the blood of established MS sufferers binds preferentially with the myelin-containing white matter of cerebellum sections. Clearly, it is important to demonstrate that the lymphocytes which stick to the white matter include those sensitized to myelin components, and that the same lymphocytes disappear from the circulation during a relapse. It seems possible that chemotactic factors at the site of a new lesion are responsible for attracting lymphocytes into the white matter from both blood and cerebrospinal fluid. It would be of further interest to see if drug therapy could prevent sensitization and possibly thereby remove one of the factors contributing to the pathology of MS.

Major questions remaining unanswered

Is there an infective agent? Is there continuous antigenic stimulus from an on-going degenerative process in the central nervous system? How is an exacerbation initiated, and could the cycle of relapses and remissions be suppressed? What is the role of the suppressor cell in a relapse? These basic questions indicate the depth and extent of our ignorance in understanding multiple sclerosis.

References and Further Reading

ALLEN, I.V. and McKEOWN, S.R. (1979) A histological, histochemical and biochemical study of the macroscopically normal white matter in multiple sclerosis. *Journal of Neurological Science*, **41**, 81−91.

BACH, J.−F. (1978) *Immunology*. J. Wiley & Sons, New York.

BLOOM, B.R. (1980) Immunological changes in multiple sclerosis. *Nature*, **287**, 275−276.

CUZNER, M.L. and DAVISON, A.N. (1979) The scientific bases of multiple sclerosis. *Molecular Aspects of Medicine*, **2**, 147−248.

DAVISON, A.N. and CUZNER, M.L. (1980) *The suppression of experimental allergic encephalomyelitis and multiple sclerosis*. Academic Press, London.

DORE-DUFFY, P., GOERTZ, V. and ROTHMAN, B.L. (1980) Lymphocyte adherence to myelinated tissue in multiple sclerosis. *Journal of Clinical Investigation*, **66**, 843−846.

KURTZKE, J.F. (1980) Epidemiologic contributions to multiple sclerosis: an overview. *Neurology*, **30**, 61−79.

MATTSON, D.H., ROOS, R.P. and ARNASON, B.G.W. (1980) Isoelectric focusing of IgG eluted from multiple sclerosis and subacute sclerosing panencephalitis brain. *Nature*, **287**, 335−337.

NATHAN, C.F., MURRAY, H.W. and COHN, A. (1980) The macrophage as an effector cell. *New England Journal of Medicine*, **303**, 622−626.

NEIGHBOUR, P.A. and BLOOM, B.R. (1979) Absence of virus-induced lymphocyte suppression and interferon production in multiple sclerosis. *Proceedings of the National Academy of Science*, **76**, 476−480.

THE HYPOTHALAMUS AS AN AGING CLOCK

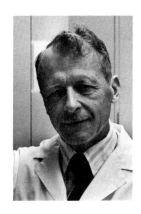

T. Samorajski

Director of the Neurobiology Section of the Texas Research Institute of Mental Sciences.

He is also Professor of Biology, Texas Woman's University and Adjunct Professor, Department of Neurobiology and Anatomy, University of Texas Medical School of Houston. Early in his career, he turned his attention to the nervous system and the changes associated with its aging. He is a charter member of the American Aging Association and currently its president.

The rate at which a human being ages may be controlled by hypothalamic neurotransmitter substances and hormones. By stimulating the nervous and endocrine systems the neurotransmitters and hormones are believed to regulate cellular events connected to aging and age-related illnesses.

Not so long ago, the study of aging was seen as either a mystical search for the fountain of perpetual youth, or heretical tampering with a process that only God could control. And yet, today's rapid advances in cell biology make it possible to investigate the underlying mechanisms of physiological aging. If these processes could be identified and their actions understood, perhaps some measure of control might be imposed on them and the debility of advanced old age postponed to the final moments.

Various theories have been proposed in an effort to identify the underlying cellular and molecular mechanisms of aging. Some hypotheses focus attention on changes in the DNA molecule. Alterations in DNA may result from a variety of sources including radiation effects and free radicals. Free radicals are highly reactive molecules resulting from biochemical oxidation that, like irradiation may damage DNA and other cell structures. Another possibility involves changes in DNA-directed protein synthesis, called the DNA error (somatic mutation) hypothesis. Of the many variants of DNA theories, the DNA error hypothesis is a particularly attractive one. It introduces the possibility that errors in transfer of information from the DNA to the final protein product may be a more likely basis for aging than changes in the DNA molecule itself. A related theory involves the formation of cross-links of specific proteins. Both the protein error and the cross-link theories assume that a typical protein may be detrimental to cell function. Another theory with popular appeal is the 'wear-and-tear' hypothesis. This theory assumes that an organism wears out much as a machine might under operational conditions. Adherents of this theory claim that excessive stress contributes to aging causing small damages which accumulate with time and accelerate the degenerative process.

It has also been proposed that a combination of protein misspecification at the cellular level and changes in the immune system may be the cause of aging (error-autoimmune theory). While thymic and immunologic involution are a characteristic feature of aging, their relation to the aging process in organs like the brain, which has non-dividing cells, remains unexplained. For completeness, the hypoxia theory of aging should be mentioned. This theory suggests that aging is primarily the result of lowered oxygen tension in critical areas such as the brain. There is little experimental evidence, however, of any significant decline in oxygen intake when it is calculated on the basis of cell numbers. With the possible exception of the error-autoimmune theory, none of these hypotheses deal with possible interactions among cells or control mechanisms that maintain the integrity of the total animal.

From a physiological standpoint it now seems that aging might be regarded as a breakdown or impairment of endocrine and neuronal control mechanisms which together function as pacemakers for the aging process. Unfortunately investigators trying to sort out the causes of senescence have found it difficult to determine whether changes associated with old age cause the disturbances or whether the reverse is true. Equally problematic is the question of which organ or organs are most critical for aging and the susceptibility of older persons to disease.

Age-associated changes in the brain, particularly loss of memory and confusion, are of greatest concern to most people. Loss of nerve cells and vascular alterations may be inevitable, but the rate at which these changes occur may be influenced by environmental factors to a far greater degree than has been suspected. Because of the brain's key role in regulating physiological processes, even a small change in some critical areas of the aging brain may precipitate a cascade of events that alters the rate of aging, hastening the onset of age-associated diseases that diminish the quality of late life.

In a multicellular organism, cells have two major pathways of communication: the nervous system and the endocrine system. Neurons communicate with each other by releasing neurotransmitter substances into synaptic clefts, tiny spaces between adjacent nerve cells, which change the electrical activity of the receiving cells. In the endocrine system, specialized cells release hormones which are carried by the blood throughout the body and influence the activity of responsive target cells. If a complex organism is to function well, its cells must operate in a coordinated fashion. Like an orchestra, the system needs a conductor.

Located between the pituitary gland and the base of the brain, the hypothalamus (see Fig. 1) is uniquely suited to coordinating the metabolic and physiologic activities of several organ systems. More specifically, assigning the role of an 'aging clock' (or clocks) to the hypothalamus is based on location and on the possibility that age-associated changes in neurons and their responses to neurotransmitters, hormones, and other regulatory substances may alter homeostatic systems in such a way that a pathological condition may develop.

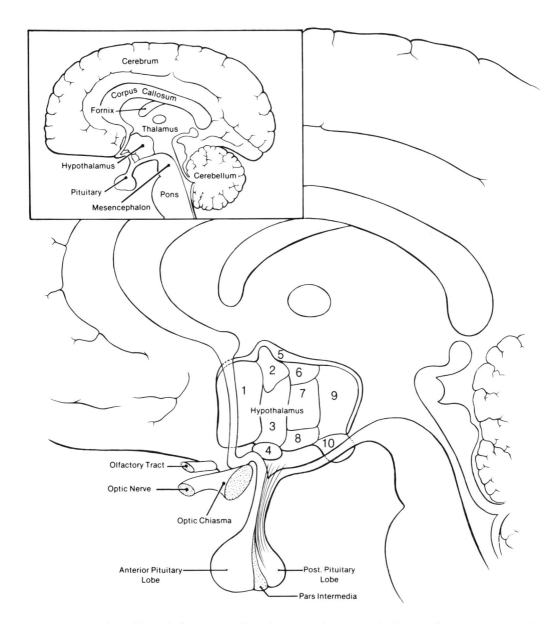

Fig. 1. Schematic illustration of interrelation between hypothalamus and pituitary gland. Ten cell groups or areas are found in the hypothalamus (preoptic nucleus — 1, paraventricular nucleus — 2, anterior hypothalamic area — 3, supraoptic nucleus — 4, lateral hypothalamic area —5, dorsal hypothalamic area — 6, dorsomedial nucleus — 7, ventromedial nucleus — 8, posterior hypothalamic area — 9, and mammillary body — 10).

Let us review some current concepts of the hypothalamus as an aging clock. As presently conceived, an organism ages in two ways: systems deteriorate from predetermined genetic causes with the passage of time (chronological aging) and as a result of neuro-endocrine responses to environmental conditions (physiological aging). Thus, differences in the rate of aging and duration of life among individuals are evidence of an interaction between a genetic programme and external conditions that may modulate the rate at which the timing mechanism runs. The central role of the hypothalamus (see Fig. 2) in the adaptation of the organism to environmental influences and the diversity and importance to its regulatory function led A.V. Everett of the University of Sydney to propose that the hypothalamus may be the central site for regulating aging. Abundant experimental evidence in animals documents the fact that lifespan may be altered by extrinsic conditions, but little is known about the underlying mechanisms.

Some scientists believe that changes in the hypothalamus may result in oversecretion of 'aging hormones' from the anterior lobe of the pituitary gland; this accelerates aging throughout the body. Physiological studies by V.V. Frolkis and his colleagues at the Institute of Gerontology in Kiev reveal that different hypothalamic areas age in different ways and at varying rates. These researchers suggest that non-uniform aging in the hypothalamus may cause hypothalamic disregulation, followed by changes in the release of hypothalamic hormones. V.M. Dilman of the Research Institute of Experimental Medicine at Leningrad proposes another theory. He believes that age-associated intrinsic changes may produce an elevation of the hypothalamic threshold to circulating hormones. In the reproductive system, for example, this change may be reflected in an age-associated decrease in sensitivity of the hypothalamic-gonadotropic system to the inhibitory action of oestrogens. We need to examine the aging mechanism in more detail to understand how a limited population of cells in the hypothalamus might control the course of aging throughout the body.

The nerve cell, or neuron, is the basic structural and functional unit of the nervous system. Information in the form of an electrical signal is conveyed along elongated fibres of a neuron (axons), triggering the release of a chemical (neurotransmitter) into the gap, the synaptic cleft, that separates the fibre terminal from the receiving neuron. The neurotransmitter travels across the gap and, as it interacts with receptors on the outside of the neuronal membrane, causes a change in electrical potential across the membrane and a subsequent discharge of the neuron. Neurotransmitters that have been identified in the central nervous system with some degree of certainty include acetylcholine (ACh), dopamine (DA), norepinephrine (NE) (also known as noradrenalin) and 5-hydroxytryptamine (5-HT). In addition, several amino acids have recently been recognized as possible

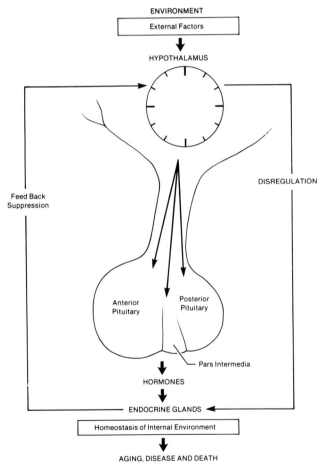

Fig. 2. Diagram illustrating the interaction between external environmental and internal homeostatic factors on aging, disease and death mediated by the hypothalamus and the pituitary gland.

neurotransmitters in the brain. These actions may be sufficient to account for the chemical controls normally operating in the brain. There are, however, certain neurons located primarily in the hypothalamus that perform an additional function, the production and release of peptide hormones in response to conventional signals relayed across synapses. Because of the dual role of these cells, they are frequently referred to as 'neuroendocrine transducer ceels' or 'peptidergic neurons'.

Many peptide-secreting cells in the hypothalamus and adjacent areas secrete their hormones into the pituitary-portal system to

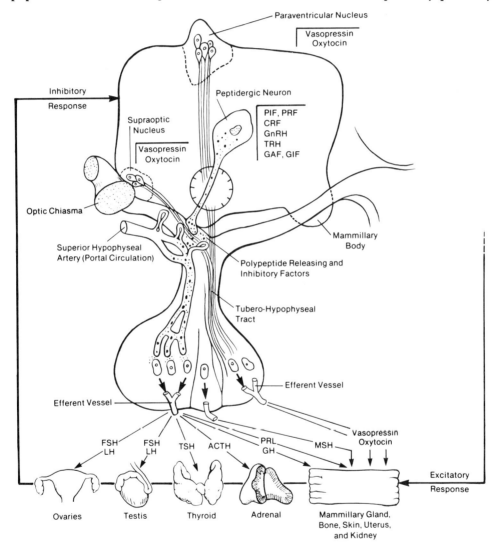

Fig. 3. Possible actions of hypothalamic releasing and inhibitory factors and neurosecretory substances on release of pituitary hormones. Abbreviations: PIF = prolactin inhibitory factor (prolactostatin), PRF = prolactin releasing factor (prolactoliberin), CRF = corticotropin releasing factor (corticoliberin), GnRH = gonadotropin releasing factor (gonadoliberin), TRH = thyrotropin releasing factor (thyroliberin), GRF = growth hormone releasing factor (somatoliberin), GIF = growth hormone inhibitory factor (somatostatin), FSH = follicle stimulating hormone, LH = luteinizing hormone (lutropin), TSH = thyroid stimulating hormone (thyrotropin), ACTH = adrenocorticotropin, PRL = prolactin, GH = growth hormone (somatotropin) and MSH = melanotropin.

be carried to the anterior pituitary. At present there is evidence for the existence of at least five 'releasing' factors and two 'inhibitory' factors in the hypothalamus which control the release of six different hormones from the anterior pituitary gland (see Fig. 3). With the development of radioimmunoassay techniques it is now possible to measure circulating levels of pituitary hormones. Apart from some increase with age in follitropin and lutropin, there are surprisingly few changes with age in basal plasma levels of pituitary hormones. It is possible, however, that dramatic environmental circumstances such as chronic stress, long-term drug administration, or exposure to toxic and noxious substances might lead to an overproduction of hormones. This would accelerate aging processes by producing permanent damage in tissues.

The posterior lobe of the pituitary also secretes some powerful hormones. Two similar neuropeptides, oxytocin and vasopressin, are synthesized in neurons of the supraoptic and paraventricular nuclei (see Fig. 4) and stored in axons that terminate in the posterior pituitary. With the appropriate stimulus they also are released into the blood stream. In human beings, the neurons in the supraoptic and paraventricular nuclei enlarge with age, but the significance of this change for oxytocin and vasopressin release and aging is not clear.

The spatial and temporal domain of these neuropeptides suggests that their principal

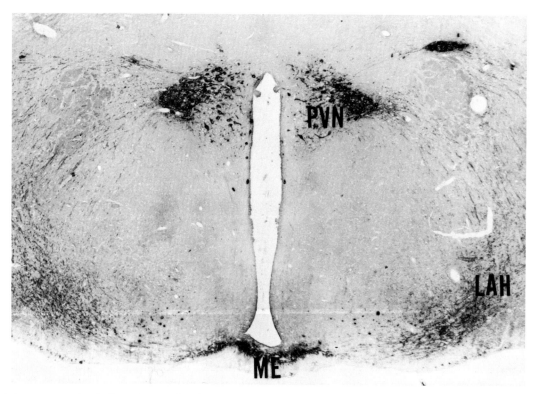

Fig. 4. Immunocytochemical reaction product in oxytocin containing cell bodies in the paraventricular nucleus (PVN) and axons in the lateral hypothalamic area (LHA) and zone interna of median eminence (ME) of the rat. Magnification X 24 (Courtesy of Dr. Gerald Kozlowski, University of Texas Medical School, Houston, Texas).

action is that of 'modulators' or 'regulators'. As R. North of the Loyola University School of Medicine points out, stimulation produced by a peptide develops slowly and is of long duration. In contrast, excitation or inhibition by neurotransmitters occurs rapidly and is short-lived. The action of a neurotransmitter at the synapse has been likened to a telephone conversation between two people — private and instantaneous. The response of a neuron to a neuromodulator may be more like a radio broadcast which can be picked up by any properly sensitized receiver within range of the signal. In addition, a peptide or other agent released by the neuron could affect neuronal activity by altering the synthesis or metabolism of a neurotransmitter, neuromodulator or neurohormone. Extensive efforts to identify the neuropeptides, establish their mode of action and map the neurons that produce them are currently under way.

How might the peptidergic neurons be regulated by influences from the internal and external environment? We have already learned that feedback control from circulating hormones within the hypothalamus might activate the release of appropriate activating or inhibitory factors for the maintenance of internal homeostasis. This does not mean that the anterior pituitary is completely under hypothalamic control. In all probability, a number of pituitary functions are controlled directly by changes in the concentration of various hormones in the blood.

The biogenic amine neurotransmitters (NE, ACh, DA, 5-HT and GABA) also have a major role in regulating pituitary function. Evidence has accumulated from fluorescent histochemical studies that peptidergic neurons are widely innervated by afferent connections from cholinergic, noradrenergic, dopaminergic, serotonergic and GABAminergic fibre systems. There is as yet only limited evidence as to which neurotransmitter(s) is involved in the release of a particular excitatory or inhibitory factor from the hypothalamus. Other work on the localization of neurotransmitter substances has demonstrated that their concentration and turnover, particularly in the hypothalamus, can change in response to various external stimuli reaching the brain, as well as stimuli from within the body. It appears, therefore, that internal and external stimuli alter anterior pituitary release by some kind of competition between the number of available hormone molecules in the pituitary and concentration and turnover of one or more biogenic amines in the hypothalamus (see Fig. 5).

Of all the substances measured in the brain, the NE- and DA-containing systems seem to be most vulnerable to aging and age-related brain diseases. An examination by us and others of life-span changes in brain biogenic amines of mice, rhesus monkeys and humans has shown a significant decline of norepinephrine in the hypothalamus and dopamine in the basal ganglia. This finding seemingly fits one of the requirements of mammalian aging, namely that of species universality. Some interesting inferences may also be drawn from changes in neurotransmitter substances in the brain of patients with age-related brain diseases. The major neurochemical finding in Alzheimer's type of dementia, Parkinsonism, and Huntington's chorea is a significant decline, compared to age-matched controls, of one or more neurotransmitter substance(s) in the basal ganglia, cortex and other regions of the brain, most with afferent projections to the hypothalamus.

Is it possible, then, that subtle neuronal changes, progressing at a rate determined by environmental conditions and genetic programme, eventually result in a critical shortage of one or more neurotransmitter substance(s)? Might the loss of these chemicals

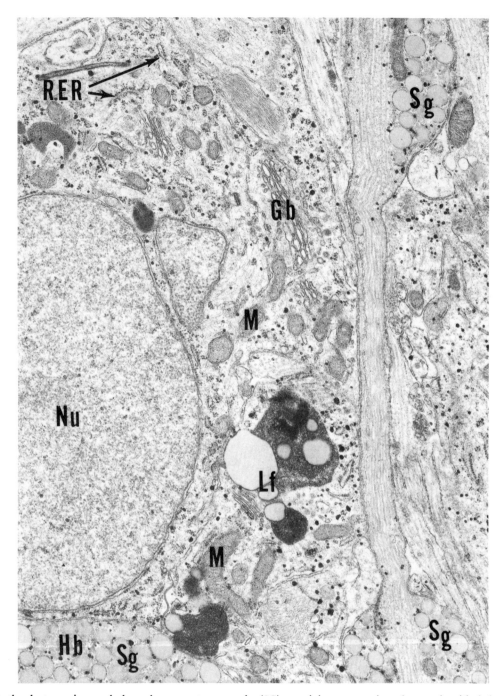

Fig. 5. In the electron micrograph shown here, secretory granules (SG) containing vasopressin and oxytocin with their respective carrier proteins (neurophysins) are localized in a granule aggregate (Herring body: Hb) and in two locations within an axon. Translation of messenger RNA occurs on the rough endoplasmic reticulum (RER) of the neuronal cell body yielding a precursor (propeptide) molecule. Packing into secretory granules occurs in the Golgi body (Gb). Lipofuscin (age) pigments (Lf), mitochondria (M), and two portions of a nucleus (Nu) are identified. Magnification, ✕ 8000.

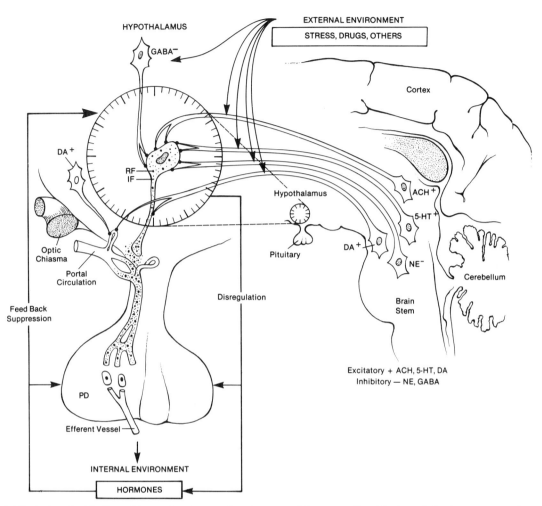

Fig. 6. The 'aging clock' effect of internal and external environmental factors mediated by hypothalamic neurotransmitters. Releasing and inhibitory factors (RF, IF) from neuropeptidergic neurons reach the pars distalis (PD) of the pituitary gland through the pituitary portal circulation. Other abbreviations: dopamine (DA), gamma-amino butyric acid (GABA), acetylcholine (ACh), 5-hydroxytryptamine (5-HT), norepinephrine (NE).

be prevented by favorable environmental conditions or, if lost, might they be replaced by the administration of a drug, hormone or precursor? If so, would the neuropeptidergic neurons respond favorably or are they also victims of their own degenerative process? These are some of the questions behind the mystery of the hypothalamic aging clock (see Fig. 6).

The strongest support for the hypothesis that hypothalamic neurotransmitter substances function as regulators of the aging process has been provided by studies of senescence in male and female rodents. Data from several laboratories have shown that depressed levels of catecholamine (norepinephrine and dopamine) and enhanced serotonin metabolism in the hypothalamus may underly the cessation of cyclic gonadotropin production in female rats. Administrations of L-dopa, epinephrine, or iproniazide (a monoamine oxidase inhibitor), all of which increase brain catecholamine, were able to reinitiate oestrous cycles in female senescent rats. Further, the atrophied ovaries of old rats could be made functional again with appropriate stimulation by gonadotropic hormone. In aging humans, as in the aging rat, deficiencies begin to occur in each of the reproductive organs, but the primary fault seems to lie in the hypothalamus. It becomes less responsive to stimuli that control the release of lutropin, follitropin and prolactin.

In view of the belief that increasing old age seemingly involves a progressive imbalance between various neurotransmitters in the hypothalamus and other areas of the brain, the question whether changes might be imposed on the rate of aging through nutrition, drug administration or other means of intervention is interesting. Unfortunately, data from research with human beings are too scarce to have any bearing on this proposition. What then is the evidence from animal models in which the role of neurotransmitters in the aging process can be studied?

Investigators have begun to develop more precise techniques to explore the role of neurotransmitters in the aging process. P.S. Timiras and associates of the University of California at Berkeley have shown that tryptophan deficiency causes delayed growth, development and maturation of the central nervous system of female rats. In parallel experiments, these investigators also demonstrated that chronic treatment with dl-para-chlorophenylalanine, an inhibitor of serotonin synthesis, inhibited growth and delayed sexual maturation. G.C. Cotzias and colleagues at the Brookhaven National Laboratories have shown that long-term addition of a high concentration of L-dopa to the diet of mice enhanced the animals' fertility and increased their mean life span by about 50%. These findings support the hypothesis that neurotransmitter substances influence growth, maturation, and aging. We further believe that the component of senescence referred to as physiological aging is largely determined by extrinsic or environmental factors and the rate at which the biogenic amine transmitters of the hypothalamus are synthesized and eventually broken down to metabolic end products. Under this concept, age-related diseases and their related syndromes may result from the tendency of the mammalian brain to lose its stores of neurotransmitter substances during aging. Such changes could lead to hypothalamic deregulation and/or feedback suppression as proposed by V.V. Frolkis and V.M. Dilman. Thus, the hypothalamus becomes the clock that does the aging.

Perhaps the most interesting evidence concerning environmental influences on the rate of aging comes from recent work by C.L. Goodrick at the Gerontology Research Center in Baltimore. He found that voluntary wheel exercise significantly increased the longevity of both male and female rats compared with that of control rats. The influence of exercise on growth duration was suggested as a possible explanation for the increase in longevity.

The physiological influence of exercise on the circulatory system and skeletal muscle is, of course, well known. Studies of animal and human subjects have shown that physical exercise can reduce fat, cholesterol, triglycerides, and phospholipids in blood serum, in addition to lowering blood pressure and heart rate. Some investigators believe that exercise in combination with dietary adjustments may act in a prophylactic way and delay or halt vascular disease in adult human beings. How might our model of the aging clock be involved in such a process? U.S. von Euhler of the Karolinska Institute in Sweden has stated that 'physical exercise represents a kind of stress in the organism in which hemodynamic as well as biochemical functions are exclusively involved'. It seems likely, therefore, that the hypothalamus, which plays an important part in regulating autonomic, metabolic, hormonal, and circulatory systems, should be affected. Whether changes in brain neurotransmitters occur as a direct or indirect consequence in relation to prolonged motor activity is an open question. Exercise and nutrition appear to be the most obvious means of altering mammalian life span. Both are important in terms of ultimate applicability to humans.

In addition to alterations in neurotransmitters, neuromodulators, hormones and neuropeptidergic substances, other aspects of cell function must be considered. The 'second messenger' system of transmitting hormonal signals to the interior of the cell (for functional regulation) is only now beginning to be understood. So many steps influence the final result that it is impossible to conceive how so complicated a process actually reads out an aging programme directed by the genetic material.

Nevertheless, old age is a period of the life span that has its own physiological characteristics. Depending on many factors that remain to be discovered, growing old may bring fulfilment of personal goals and ambitions to some individuals and frustration, maladjustment and increasing isolation to others. If the usefulness of human beings is to be extended along with their longevity, understanding the process of aging becomes a central issue. Only when all of the findings already discussed and yet to be discovered are put into proper perspective will we begin to understand the aging clock and the region of the brain most concerned with its regulation.

Further Reading

MERVIS, R. (1981) Cytomorphological alterations in the aging animal brain with emphasis on Golgi studies. In: *Aging and Cell Structure*, Vol. 1 (Johnson, J.E., Jr., ed.), 143–186. Plenum.

ORDY, J.M. (1975) Principles of mammalian aging. In: *Neurobiology of Aging*, Vol. 16, (Ordy, J.M. and Brizzee, K.R., eds.), 1–22. Plenum, New York.

SAMORAJSKI, T. How the human brain responds to aging. *Journal of the American Geriatrics Society*, **23**, 4–11.

SAMORAJSKI, T. (1981) An introduction to normal and pathologic aging of the brain. In: *Brain Neurotransmitters and Receptors in Aging and Age-related Disorders*, (Enna, S.J., Samorajski, T. and Beer, B., eds.), 1–12. Raven Press, New York.

SAMORAJSKI, T. and HARTFORD, J. (1979) Brain physiology of aging. In: *Handbook of Geriatric Psychiatry*, (Busse, E.W. and Blazer, D., eds.), Van Nostrand and Reinhold Co., New York.

SENILE DEMENTIA

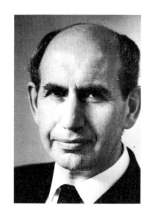

Sir Martin Roth

Professor of Psychiatry, University of Cambridge.

Formerly Professor of Psychological Medicine, University of Newcastle-upon-Tyne and Honorary Director at the MRC Group for the study of relationships between functional and organic metal disorders. He serves in an advisory capacity on many other committees on mental health and problems of the aged. He has published papers on psychiatric aspects of ageing, depressive illness and schizophrenia in various psychiatric and mental journals.

The Nature and Dimension of the Problem

The mental diseases to which old people are liable constitute one of the most urgent medical problems faced by contemporary society. They are causing growing hardship to families, communities and social and medical services as well as the individuals affected. Whereas illnesses such as cardiac or respiratory disease impose mainly physical restraints and limitations upon the manner in which old people live, the progressive forms of mental decline undermine their autonomy and cause them to become dependent upon others.

Epidemiological studies in different parts of the world have shown that between four and six per cent of those aged sixty-five and over are affected by dementia, that is, a progressive global decline of the individual's intellectual and emotional faculties which ultimately destroys the distinctive features of his personality. A further proportion suffers from milder degrees of impairment. According to one estimate, approximately 400,000 aged people in England alone suffer from one or other form of this disorder. More than four-fifths of those affected suffer from one of two main diseases. The first is the form of progressive mental deterioration in which the brain shows the distinctive pathological changes first described by the psychiatrist and

neuropathologist, Alzheimer. This is responsible for some two-thirds of the cases affected.
In a further 25% the presence of multiple
occlusions in a number of cerebral arteries
leading to a patchy destruction of the tissues
of the brain is the cause of the mental decline.
This second type of disease is known as
'multi-infarct dementia'.

The numbers of the aged in highly developed and in underdeveloped countries are
steadily increasing, both proportionately and
in absolute terms because of declining birth
rates, improved social conditions and advances in the science and practice of medicine.
In consequence, the most common forms of
dementia are undergoing a parallel increase.
It has been estimated that if present trends
continue, people of pensionable age will
account for 10% of the world's population
before the year 2000. On the basis of prevalence rates recorded in Newcastle-upon-
Tyne, this would mean that approximately
one-half per cent of the world's population
will then be suffering from dementia.

Social, Biological and Medical Approaches

Social and medical services in many
countries are already straining at the seams
with the growing dimensions of the problem.
However, the families of the aged and the
communities in which they live are bound to
be even more heavily taxed in the future.
Although dementia shortens life considerably, the period of survival of those with the
disease may be increasing. Until quite recently, only about 1—2% of those affected were
being cared for in hospitals or institutions, the
majority have continued to live within the
community. With the increasing employment
of women and the growing mobility of young
people, however, the means by which families
have cared for many disabled aged people
is being slowly but surely eroded. A measure
of the urgency of the problem is reflected in
the fact that within the age group of those

aged 80 years and over, the prevalence of
dementia climbs to approximately 20%. In
consequence, enquiries into the medical,
biological and social aspects of dementia
have all been intensified in the last few
decades.

The proportion of old people in gainful
employment has been declining steeply for
some decades and they constitute in most
societies an impoverished leisured class. The
status and dignity of old people tends to decrease after retirement, and this is particularly true of the underprivileged sections of
the community. Such deprivations cause
great unhappiness and the poor, isolated and
childless are also more likely to be admitted
to hospitals and institutions. There is no
evidence, however, that dementing illnesses
affect certain classes preferentially. The most
common forms of disorder respect neither
wealth nor social prestige. No class or segment of society is immune.

As far as biological factors are concerned,
the first degree relatives of patients with
senile dementia have been shown to be four
times as liable to the disease as corresponding
age groups in the general population. Heredity
therefore contributes to causation, and it
has been estimated that the single dominant
gene responsible might be present in some
12% of the population. As penetrance increases with age, by the age of 90 some 40%
of carriers of the gene would be affected.
From the point of view of natural selection,
old age may be regarded as a backwater —
a repository for many kinds of genes with
harmful effects which may initially have been
manifest at an earlier age. Older people are
bound to be less numerous than the young,
having been more often exposed to the hazard
of extinction by diseases and injuries that
occur at random. Consequently, genes that
favour the more potent and numerous young
at the expense of the aged will tend to be
more rapidly disseminated than those with a
reverse effect. Moreover, the effects of harmful genetic mutations tend to be progressively

postponed to a later age until they are manifest after the end of the reproductive period. Thereafter no selection for or against them can occur since they no longer exert any effect upon 'fitness'.

This theory, which derives from ideas advanced by Haldane and Medawar, has interesting implications. As the reproductive life of men is longer, one might expect them to be less liable to ageing than women. In fact, the life span of men is substantially shorter and their mortality from many diseases in middle and late life is significantly greater. However, the evidence regarding the origin and significance of such sex differences is scanty. The explanation may be that cardiovascular and respiratory disease, disorders of the liver and many forms of cancer are due in large measure to noxious exogenous agents such as smoking and alcohol to which men have until quite recently been far more exposed than women. The effects of such environmental influences might to some extent override and mask those due to inherent genetic factors. On the other hand, the most common form of mental deterioration, the dementia of Alzheimer's type, occurs more often in women than in men. Although the disorder generally begins two decades or more after the menopause, a proportion of the most severe and rapidly progressive forms of the disease commence in middle life.

Medical hypotheses of dementia regard it as a disease *sui generis*, caused by biochemical infectious or other exogenous or endogenous factors exerting their effects in middle or late life. Such a view is not in conflict with but rather complementary to the biological theories previously considered. For example, genes must ultimately exert their influence through biochemical effects. Although there is some reason for regarding senile dementia of Alzheimer's type as arising from an accelerated ageing of the central nervous system, such extreme deviations from the norm are very liable to runaway effects culminating in

qualitatively distinct pathological processes. As we shall see, there is reason to believe that something of this nature may be occurring in the case of 'senile' and some other forms of dementia in middle or late life. Hence, when the most common form of dementia (that named after Alzheimer) was delineated as a specific disease instead of being regarded as merely due to old age, an important advance was made, for the disease model focuses on the difference between the normal aged and the severely demented, the individuals robust and intellectually productive in their eighties compared with those in a state of total oblivion at the age of 50 or 60 years. Currently the central purpose of research is to diminish, postpone or eliminate the decay of intellect and personality. This battle is being fought on a number of fronts.

The Starting Points of Contemporary Research

The modern era in the scientific study of dementia probably began with clinical observations which established that the mental disorders of old age were not varying expressions of cerebral degeneration, but comprised a number of different illnesses each with a distinctive presentation, course and outcome. Two main groups were defined. The first were the depressions, manias, neuroses and paranoid illnesses of old age and the second comprised the pre-senile and senile dementias and those forms of intellectual and personality decline due to strokes. Although there was some measure of overlap between the groups, emphasis in clinical practice and scientific work had to be laid on the differences between them. The expectation of life of those in the first group proved to be identical with or similar to that of individuals of comparable age in the general population. Also, their intellectual functions and personalities were found over a number of years of observation to remain intact. In the second group the life expectation was found to be only 20—25% of the normal. In general, these patients entered a course of progressive decline. The exceptions were the small minority in whom specific and remediable causes for the dementia such as pernicious anaemia or hypothyroidism came to light and required treatment. Individuals in the first group were found to possess brains whose structural characteristics did not differ from those in mentally healthy old people in old age. However, in the second group distinctive pathological changes were almost invariably found. Although such changes in the brain were not exclusively confined to those with senile and multi-infarct dementias, their constancy and intensity enabled a close link to be established between the mental changes observed during life and the pathological alterations evident in the brain after death. Because the changes found in the brains of the second (demented) group were qualitatively similar to those found in the brains of well-preserved people of advanced age, their true significance had been obscured for some decades. It was not until quantitative measurements were applied that the situation was seen in its true light.

Although the basic causes of the main forms of dementia have not yet been established, some progress has been made in recent years. The Alzheimer type of dementias, for example, is believed to be in some way connected with changes known as plaques, neurofibrillary tangles, granulovacuolar degeneration in certain specific cells and some other less conspicuous pathology. Plaques are amorphous argyrophilic (i.e. they are shown up by silver stains) masses 40—80 μm in diameter found in the cortex and grey matter of the elderly brain. Neurofibrillary tangles are aggregations of filamentous material that accumulate in the nerve cell bodies. Both are found in the aged and in the demented but to a far greater extent in the latter. There are also some differences in distribution. Under the electron microscope plaques have been shown by the work of Terry and his colleagues to be made up of three main components: swollen and degenerate nerve terminals, amyloid and glial cells (macrophages, microglia and astrocytes). The neurofibrillary tangles appear as sheaves of fibrillar elements measuring 22 nm and constricted to about 10 nm at internals of 80 nm. They were originally regarded as 'twisted tubules', but later enquiries by Kidd showed them to be composed of bundles of paired helical filaments. The neurofibrillary tangle is very rarely found outside the hippocampus (within the temporal lobe) in well preserved old people, and abundance of tangles in the cerebral cortex is found only in indubitably demented subjects. Some of the changes have been described in other conditions, such as Down's syndrome and amyotrophic lateral sclerosis. However, there is not the same intensity of proliferation as in senile dementia nor the same clear quantitative relationship between the clinical findings and pathological changes.

In dementia due to multiple infarcts the aggregation of strokes could be held responsible for the mental disorder, for although the first one to three strokes is often associated with no impairment or transient impairment, a succession of strokes or one or two exceptionally large ones will cause progressive deterioration.

It is the Alzheimer type of dementias that pose the most interesting questions because the pathological changes here appear to be the same changes as those of old age but in an accelerated or intensified form. Can any hypothesis accommodate both the similarities between the cerebral changes and clinical status of normal and demented subjects?

The 'threshold' concept

One possibility is that senile dementia falls into the group of disorders that includes late onset diabetes and essential hypertension, in which a threshold effect is observed. No disability is demonstrated until the underlying changes brought on by ageing develop beyond a certain critical point.

Among normal people who die accidentally, the proportion of those in whose brains plaques and tangles are found increases with advancing age. This may reflect the extent to which a destructive process associated with ageing has been encroaching upon their reserves of cerebral neurones. Were this the case, one would expect that the effects of other forms of brain damage would be additive to those manifest in plaques or tangles and other forms of so-called 'senile' change. This proves to be so. Equally, the effects of a small amount of damage arising from strokes can in rare instances be combined with this senile change and result in a swiftly-evolving dementia that would not have appeared in the event of either kind of change in isolation.

In addition, above the age of 75 the prevalence of plaques and tangles in the brain of normal people has been shown to rise sharply. Also, above this age there is a parallel increase in the prevalence of the Alzheimer type of dementia, affecting a substantial minority of 12.5%.

The concept of a 'threshold' would explain why dementia develops so rapidly after the first symptoms and signs have made their appearance. Dementia is not a solitary phenomenon in which a qualitatively distinct process appears to evolve following the aggregation of a quantitatively graded pathological change or of a large number of genes, each with a small affect. Arterial hypertension and epilepsy are among the more common examples of this group of phenomena.

Since the brain cell population is post-mitotic and fixed at birth, the threshold concept has important practical implications. It suggests that damage to cerebral neurones at any stage of the life span is likely to increase the chances that dementia will develop as the individual reaches an age when the concomitants of normal ageing begin to make

their appearance. Something of this nature appears to occur in boxers who have suffered a large number of cerebral injuries. The onset of dementia may be deferred until a decade or more has elapsed since the last encounter in the boxing ring.

Biochemical theories

The biochemical abnormalities found in the brains of those with senile dementia of the Alzheimer type have attracted increasing attention in recent years and the activity of numerous transmitters and enzymes has been investigated. A powerful impetus was given to such studies by the successes achieved in the case of Parkinson's disease. Here the administration of the drug *L*-dopa can bring considerable relief to many patients who in the past were seriously and progressively incapacitated. Investigators in a variety of centres in a number of countries have demonstrated a widespread deficit in the enzymes concerned with the synthesis and breakdown of acetylcholine in the brains of people who suffered from Alzheimer's disease of the presenile and senile types. Acetylcholine is a neurotransmitter in certain specific parts of the brain.

It is of interest that the cerebral cortex contains very few intrinsic cholinergic neurones (Emson and Lindwall, 1979). The observed decline in the activity of choline acetyltransferase must therefore reflect a decrease or impaired function of cholinergic projections to the neocortex from the substantia innominata. The finding carries high promise: the deficiency is specific to Alzheimer's disease, being absent in the depressions and neuroses of old age and in the dementias due to multiple strokes and other causes. The severity of the defect appears to correlate well with the measured number of plaques found in those parts of the brain which show the most intense pathological changes. Moreover drugs such as hyoscine (which antagonizes the action of acetylcholine on muscarinic receptors) produce in human subjects a form of memory impairment similar to that prominent in the early stages of dementia, although cognitive impairment is rarely confined to memory, even in early Alzheimer's disease. Hence chemical treatments which might remedy these deficiencies are now the subject of intensive investigations in different parts of the world. For the present attempts to remedy the cholinergic deficit with the aid of drugs have not succeeded. There are, however, indications that the deficiency relating to acetylcholine may be one of a number of interacting biochemical abnormalities. Loss of cortical and subcortical noradrenaline and of cortical dopamine β-hydroxylase activity have been reported. In the hippocampus noradrenaline, 5-hydroxytryptamine, and 5-hydroxyindole acetic acid are diminished as well as choline acetyltransferase. In consequence, pharmacological treatments may have to incorporate a 'cocktail' to compensate for all the defects identified.

Dementia due to an infective process

The discovery in recent decades of the infective nature of the precocious forms of dementia, kuru and Creuzfeldt-Jacob's disease, has led to the theory that other forms of dementia might be caused by infective agents.

Kuru, which was until recently endemic amongst the cannibalistic Fore tribe of New Guinea, was shown by Carleton Gadjusek to be passed on to women and children of both sexes in the tribe by rituals associated with the practice of devouring the brains of the recently deceased. The precise mode of transmission is unknown, but the disease has vanished since cannibalistic practices were eradicated. Gadjusek also demonstrated that Creuzfeldt-Jacob disease, previously attributed to brain degeneration, was transmissible to chimpanzees and New World monkeys by the inoculation of brain tissue from infected patients. Accidental transmission has also

taken place from one human brain to others. Both diseases are now suspected to be caused by a virus or minute virus-like particle, a 'slow' virus which resists destruction by the usual antiviral agents and does not generate the usual inflammatory reaction or neutralizing antibodies. It is possible that a 'viroid' organism such as that found in some infections of plants may be responsible, but there is no known example of such a disease in man.

Carleton Gadjusek was awarded a Nobel Prize in 1977 for his pioneering work. His laboratory and many others in different parts of the world aim at uncovering the underlying organisms in kuru and Creutzfeldt-Jacob disease, and it is not impossible that infectious micro-organisms will be exposed at the root of some cases of Alzheimer's disease. Were this to be the case it would not become a treatable disorder overnight, but in preliminary experiments in the treatment of Creuzfeldt-Jacob disease with the antiviral agent Amantadine encouraging results have been obtained in a few cases.

Treatable dementias

Gradually, then, the progress of knowledge is encroaching upon this group of disorders, which was regarded a few years ago as uniformly hopeless in outcome. The number of treatable cases is slowly but surely increasing as the sphere of scientific comprehension expands.

A minority of patients suffers from dementias that can already be treated. The disorder may arise from hypothyroidism, vitamin B12 deficiency, tumours in certain parts of the brain, intestinal malabsorption, chronic subdural haematoma or alcoholism. Prompt and appropriate treatment may bring about complete recovery in such cases. The picture of dementia may also arise in immunologically incompetent individuals suffering from Hodgkin's disease or chronic leukaemia. Here the dementia may be due to invasion by a Papova-like virus of those parts of the brain concerned with memory. There are also rare forms of brain infection due to viruses such as the Herpes simplex virus or the measles virus. The encephalitis caused by these viruses frequently proves fatal. The prospects for such patients would be transformed by any advance in the treatment of viral infections.

Dementia can also be caused by a form of hydrocephalus. Here it begins with a characteristic disorder of gait and impaired control of the sphincters, followed by a slowly developing mental impairment heralded by apathy and inattention. Relief of the obstruction may sometimes mitigate or cure the condition, particularly in younger patients who have sustained a head injury or subarachnoid haemorrhage.

A rare form of dementia — Guam-Parkinsonism-dementia

Occasionally the investigation of rare disorders provides unexpected insights into the causes of other related but more common diseases. It is possible that this may prove to be so in the case of Guam-Parkinsonism-dementia. The disease is endemic among the Chamorro peoples of the island of Guam in the Philippine Sea. It gives rise either to a combination of mental deterioration with Parkinsonism or to a characteristic type of progressive muscular wasting, which occurs in an identical form in many parts of the world. It causes premature death in a relatively high proportion of men in the island — one in five over the age of 25. One of the most interesting features of the disorder is that two of the pathological changes found in the brains of its victims after death appear to be identical to two of the characteristic lesions in Alzheimer's disease of the pre-senile and senile type: neurofibrillary tangles and granulo-vacuolar degeneration. Furthermore, a substantial minority of well-preserved and mentally fit Chamorros proves to have had similar changes in their brains in an attenuated form, a phenomenon which provides a striking parallel with the distribution of neuritic plaques between the well-preserved

aged Caucasian and those with Alzheimer's disease. The neuritic plaque itself is not found in the Chamorros. In contrast, neurofibrillary tangles are exhibited in a substantial minority of normal middle-aged and elderly subjects from the island of Guam and also in some Japanese: in the West they are virtually never found in any number in the aged cerebral cortex except in Alzheimer's disease.

Clearly, as far as the most conspicuous structural changes found in the ageing brain are concerned, there is no one type of alteration that proves to hold for all members of the human species. There is, however, enough overlap between Guam Parkinsonism dementia and Alzheimer's disease to make it likely that any advances in knowledge in respect of the former would also shed light on the most widely prevalent forms of dementia in the world.

Future Perspectives

The prospects for clinical and scientific work on the subject of dementia have been greatly enhanced by a number of important technical advances. Among them, the CAT (computerised axial tomography) scan provides a picture of the detailed regional structure of the human brain by a technique a hundred times more sensitive than the conventional X-ray. Moreover, unlike the methods available in the past, this new type of X-ray examination is simple and entirely safe and can be undertaken without anaesthesia or invasive procedures.

The pioneering studies of Lassen and Ingvar in the investigation of the blood flow of the brain have been further developed by the recently introduced techniques of Sokoloff and his colleagues in Bethesda. It is now possible to study the metabolism of the human brain in detail following an intravenous injection of a radioactive analogue of glucose. In positron emission tomography the rate at which this substance is taken up by nerve cells provides an accurate index of their functional activity. Information about oxygen and glucose consumption as well as cerebral blood flow are provided and modifications of the technique can shed light on other metabolic processes.

Until less than a decade ago it was assumed that brain chemistry could not be studied because of the artefacts created by autolysis post-mortem. The demonstration that such an assumption was in error has made it possible not only to investigate the chemistry of neurotransmitters and other substances in the brain, but also to correlate these findings with structural changes in the brain and with psychological observations and diagnoses recorded during life. A relatively new science has been born. It tries to shed light on the clinical phenomena recorded during life with the aid of investigation of the regional neurochemistry and pathology of the human brain after death.

The results accruing recently have led workers on ageing to revise some firmly ingrained ideas. In the past it has been assumed that the intellectual deterioration manifest in dementia stemmed from the progressive and generalized death and outfall of brain cells. However, it is no longer certain that the earliest mental changes are caused by irreversible cellular destruction. When neurones do die, the fall-out may be highly selective, affecting cells in which impulses are mediated by one kind of transmitter, while leaving others intact.

The concentration in the brain of many chemical substances concerned with neuronal activity has been investigated. This includes a number of neuropeptides within the cell bodies of neurones intrinsic to the cerebral cortex such as vasointestinal polypeptide, pancreozymin, vasopressin and somatostatin. Estimations of these substances in certain areas suggest normal concentrations of the first two and a 50% decrease in somatostatin in senile dementia patients relative to control subjects. One possible explanation is that

there is a corresponding selective fall-out of somatostatin-containing neurones. Quite recently, investigations in Cambridge and Newcastle demonstrated that one group of cells, the nucleus coeruleus, suffers a loss of as much as 70–80% of its cell population in forms of dementia that commence at a relatively early age. This nucleus provides the cells of origin for the noradrenergic innervation of the cerebrum.

The complete picture remains to be unravelled. It is possible that the situation could turn out to be basically similar to that obtaining in Parkinsonism where there was both a fall-out of cells in the nigrostriatal system and a biochemical deficit which proved to be correctible up to a point. This is the highest promise that has been opened up in relation to dementia by the enquiries of the last half century.

Down the ages men have cherished dreams of being able to overcome the toll of the years. Although this has not yet been accomplished, those working in the field hope that eventually this aspiration will not prove to be completely without substance. Senile dementia is in many respects a parody of old age and the brain with its fixed cell population would be particularly susceptible to the effects of ageing. Any advances in the knowledge of causation of dementia in old age would very likely shed light on the general problems of senescence.

Although this paper has been largely devoted to the subject of dementia, it should be added for the purpose of perspective that advances have also been made in the mitigation of many other forms of mental suffering in the aged. The distress of large numbers of old people affected by paranoid psychoses, severe depression and anxiety, obsessions and phobias, who suffered for years without hope of relief, can now be alleviated and sometimes banished. These conditions are merely coloured by the qualities of old age, not determined by the process of ageing as such. There is however, one fact about dementia that particularly spurs on those involved in its investigation. This is the enormous disparity between those who go into their eighties and nineties with minds undimmed and those who in their seventies or even earlier are already incapable of independent existence. How are we to account for the gap between Pablo Picasso and Bertrand Russell, who displayed vitality and creative genius into their nineties (but were merely outstanding examples of the majority who die with minds intact) and that relatively small proportion which becomes demented and have to end their lives in mental hospitals or other institutions after years of oblivion?

Although he may hope that one large leap will achieve this aim, the psychiatrist working with the aged must meanwhile adopt a strategy that has little sanction from stringent evidence. He works on the assumption that stimulus and challenge preserve the mind and that human relationships keep the emotions alive. This is a hypothesis less easy to test than those stemming from virology, genetics, immunology, neurochemistry or neuropathology. We cannot be at all certain that those who continue to be vital and mentally active into advanced age owe their happy state to their manner of life rather than their genetic predisposition. Yet this view is not without some basis in fact, and it provides some validation for attitudes towards the care of those in middle and late life that draw their main sanction from humane concern and common sense.

References

ANDERSON, F.H., RICHARDSON, E.P., OKAZAKI, H. and BRODY, J.A. (1979) Neurofibrillary degeneration in Guam. *Brain,* 102, pp. 65–77.

BONDAREFF, W., MOUNTJOY, C.Q. and ROTH, M. (1981) Selective loss of neurones of origin of adrenergic projection to cerebral cortex (nucleus locus coeruleus) in senile dementia. *The Lancet,* April 4, pp. 783–784.

CROSS, A.J., CROW, T.J., PERRY, E.K., PERRY, R.H., BLESSED, G. and TOMLINSON, B.E. (1981) Reduced dopamine-β-hydroxylase activity in Alzheimer's disease. *British Medical Journal,* 1, pp. 93–95.

GAJDUSEK, D.C. and GIBBS, C.J., Jr. (1975) Slow virus infections of the nervous system and the laboratories of slow, latent and temperate virus infections. In: *The Nervous System,* Vol. 2, Tower, D.B., ed., pp. 113–135.

KAY, D.W.K., BEAMISH, P. and ROTH, M. (1964) Old age mental disorders in Newcastle-upon-Tyne. Part I. A study of prevalence. *British Journal of Psychiatry,* 110, pp. 146–158. Part II: A study of possible social and medical causes. *British Journal of Psychiatry,* 110, pp. 668–682.

PERRY, E.K., TOMLINSON, B.E., BLESSED, G., BERGMAN, K., GIBSON, P.H. and PERRY, R.H. (1978) Correlation of cholinergic abnormalities with senile plaques and mental test scores in senile dementia. *British Medical Journal,* 25, pp. 1457–1459.

ROSSOR, M.N., EMSON, P.C., MOUNTJOY, C.Q., ROTH, M. and IVERSEN, L.L. (1980) Reduced amounts of immunoreactive somatostatin in the temporal cortex in senile dementia of Alzheimer type. *Neuroscience Letters,* 20, pp. 373–377.

ROTH, M. (1955) The natural history of mental disorders arising in the senium. *Journal of Mental Science,* pp. 281–301.

ROTH, M., TOMLINSON, B.E. and BLESSED, G. (1966) Correlation between scores for dementia and counts of 'senile plaques' in cerebral grey matter of elderly subjects. *Nature,* 209, p. 109.

ROTH, M. (1971) Classification and aetiology in mental disorders of 'old age'. Some recent developments. In: *Recent Developments in Psychogeriatrics* (Kay and Walk, eds.), pp. 1–18. (Special publication of the *British Journal of Psychiatry*, No. 6). Headley Brothers Ltd.

TERRY, R.D. and WISNIEWSKI, H. (1970) The ultrastructure of the neurofibrillary tangle and the senile plaque. In: *Alzheimer's Disease and Related Conditions* (Ciba Foundation Symposium) (Wolstenholme, G.E.W. and O'Connor, M., eds.), pp. 145–168. Churchill, London.

TOMLINSON, B.E., BLESSED, G. and ROTH, M. (1968) Observations on the brain in non-demented old people. *J. Neurol. Science,* **7**, pp. 331–607.

EPIDEMIOLOGY OF CORONARY HEART DISEASE

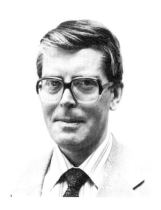

Hugh Tunstall Pedoe

Professor and Director of the Cardiovascular Epidemiology Unit, Dundee.

He has held clinical training posts at several London teaching hospitals. At St. Mary's Hospital, London he worked on the United Kingdom Heart Disease Prevention Project.

Introduction

Most doctors are in the front-line of the battle against disease. They wrestle with individual cases, diagnosing, investigating and treating them. Behind the lines however are the epidemiologists, the intelligence corps of the army, sifting through the routinely collected data, collating and analysing it and attempting to build up an overall picture of the battle, the size and disposition of the enemy, and whether the local tactics or even the overall strategies are likely to succeed. A lot of this is armchair work with routine reports (Fig. 1), but their reliability has to be assessed and periodic sorties are made not only to the front but into no-mans land and beyond to answer the basic questions of epidemiology:

Who gets the disease?
When?
Where?
How do they get it?
How many of them get it?
Why do they get it?
What happens to those who get it?
What can we do about it?
So what?

As much epidemiological research effort has been expended on coronary heart disease

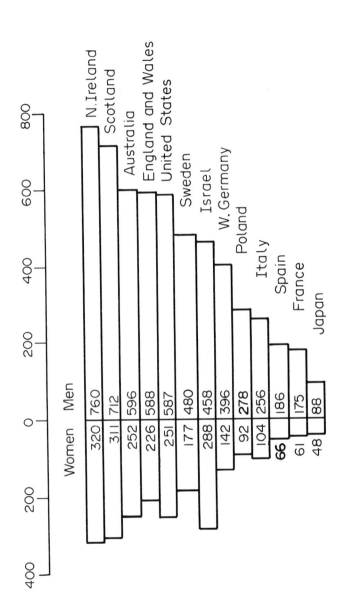

Figure 1. Mortality rates from coronary heart disease in men and women aged 35–74 in selected countries in 1977 (age standardised, based on World Health Organisation data).

as on all other human diseases put together and therefore I shall discuss epidemiology in relation to this disease. The present confusion and lack of acceptance of the conventional answers to the above questions, is related to a number of conceptual problems and areas of ignorance which may not be solved simply by a glib prescription of more research. An understanding of these may lead to a more balanced appreciation of what is known and what more might be found out.

Definitions of the Disease and the Clinical Problem

Coronary heart disease is synonymous with ischaemic heart disease, defined by the World Health Organisation as 'the cardiac disability, acute or chronic arising from reduction or arrest of blood supply to the myocardium (i.e. the heart muscle) in association with disease processes in the coronary arterial system'. Unfortunately this definition can only be used indirectly to recognise the disease in life because the heart muscle, its blood supply and the coronary artery system are buried in the centre of the chest. The diagnosis must therefore be made either by recognising the association of patients' complaints (the symptoms) and the external evidence of disordered function (the physical signs) that occur with the disease, or by specialised investigations, or by examination of the heart at necropsy, a procedure reserved for fatal cases.

Manifestations of Coronary Heart Disease

There are three major manifestations:
(a) When the blood supply to part of the heart is interrupted the muscle concerned may die, undergoing immediate loss of function followed by breakdown of structure and replacement with scar tissue. This phenomenon of cardiac (or myocardial) infarction

was described by pathologists many years before the condition was recognised in life (which occurred in the first two decades of this century). The episode is associated with severe chest pain in most cases and is confirmed by a typical series of changes in the electrical record made of the activation of the heart beat (the electrocardiogram) and by the release of intracellular heart muscle enzymes into the blood. Death of heart muscle, changes in the electrocardiogram and release of enzymes all take minutes to hours to take place. If the subject survives long enough to be seen by a doctor and to have the relevant tests performed then the diagnosis of cardiac infarction may be made. If however, the patient dies, as often happens, from a breakdown of the electrical activation of the heart causing a disorganised writhing motion (ventricular fibrillation) rather than a rhythmic pumping, then the evidence of infarction may never appear. When it was first described cardiac infarction was attributed to coronary thrombosis, blockage of the relevant artery by a clot at a point of narrowing from fatty deposits called atheroma. There has been recent doubt as to which is the cause and which effect i.e. whether:

Atheroma → Thrombosis → Cardiac infarction
(Old theory)

or whether:

Atheromatous Narrowing → Cardiac
                infarction → Thrombosis

In addition, while some pathologists blame the thrombosis on breakdown of the arterial lining over a fatty atheromatous deposit, others claim that atheroma, the fatty deposit itself, is a residue from recurrent episodes of localised thrombosis. To complicate explanations even further, it is now known that an old and thoroughly discredited idea, that coronary arteries can go into spasm, is in fact true, so that it is possible to postulate that both infarction and coronary thrombosis and even atheroma, are precipitated by spasm in the artery wall.

It might be thought that our ignorance of mechanisms is compensated for by our ability to diagnose the condition accurately once it occurs. There is, however, a complete spectrum of severity of attacks. There is a poor correlation between a clinical history of chest pain, the development of electrocardiographic changes, and necropsy findings of infarction or scars in the heart muscle. All these phenomena frequently do occur together but many subjects who are found to have electrocardiographic (ECG) evidence of an episode have no history of chest pain and the same is true of those with necropsy evidence of old infarction. Moreover the correlation between necropsy scars and prior ECG abnormalities is also poor. On the other hand severe chest pain is more common than cardiac infarction. About half of the patients sent into hospital as cases of cardiac infarction do not have it confirmed. In a middle-aged population of men about 7% will remember having had an episode of severe chest pain at some time but only 1% will have unequivocal ECG evidence of infarction.

This major manifestation of coronary heart disease, cardiac infarction, may therefore be missed or the diagnosis may be in doubt in investigated cases.

(b) The oldest manifestation of coronary heart disease is angina pectoris of effort (chest pain or discomfort brought on regularly by effort and relieved within a few minutes by rest) described by Heberden two hundred years ago. While cardiac infarction is virtually a specific indication of coronary disease, angina pectoris can occur in other heart diseases and its course and manifestations are very variable. It can be of any degree of severity and is mimicked by some other complaints. Again, the classical case is easily recognised but there may be argument about the others.

(c) The third manifestation of coronary heart disease, which again is not specific, is sudden death. This may occur during the course of cardiac infarction or as the result of electrical instability in the heart caused by local differences in blood supply leading to ventricular fibrillation. The subject may literally drop dead or become dead whilst about his or her everyday affairs, e.g. hanging curtains, while asleep, reading, eating, in the bathroom or toilet. Because coronary disease is the leading cause of sudden unheralded death it may be a diagnosis of convenience. In some countries routine necropsies are not done on subjects found dead and in others they may not be done very carefully, with additional microscopic examination of the heart. Patients with other diseases or after big operations may die unexpectedly and be given a coronary label as may deaths from overdose of drugs or alcohol or even the odd murder.

Methods of Investigation

The electrocardiogram

The secret electrical messages transmitted by the heart have fascinated electrocardiographers for 70 years. Researchers in the 1940s and 1950s showed however that cardiologists were highly idiosyncratic in their interpretation of these messages, often basing it on text-book dogma rather than scientific validation. Not only did different observers vary but one observer would be inconsistent given the same ECG to re-read in a proportion of cases. This discovery prompted the design of a standardised coding system, the Minnesota code in 1960, for use in epidemiological research, but even with this results are only 70–80% repeatable and attempts to reproduce it by computer have not been so successful that manual coding of ECG records for large surveys could be abandoned.

Enzyme tests

Ideally a blood test for cardiac infarction should be sensitive (positive in all cases) and specific (positive only in cases). Many tests launched with these claims have proved to be disappointing in practice. Criteria cannot be generalised in quantitative terms because of differences between laboratories. Even if tests were standardised the timing of them is critical; many subjects reach medical care rather late.

Symptom assessment

Many patients have difficulty in describing a pain that is unlike any previous experience. Doctors can influence them so that after several interviews the description fits the classical picture. What appears to be chest pain to one doctor seems to be in the upper abdomen to another. Interpretation of angina is very variable. If one physician thinks a patient has angina, there may be only a 50% chance that a second physician would agree. A special symptom questionnaire designed to detect angina-like pain was found to be repeatable, but two thirds of cases found to be positive in a population study had never complained to their doctors. When reviewed a year later a substantial proportion of cases denied that they had the symptom or had ever had it. Those positive to the questionnaire had a high subsequent mortality from coronary heart disease giving it some validity, but this was not true for young people. It has also been used in the West Indies where coronary disease is rare but the prevalence of positives was high (as are ECG findings which would indicate old infarction in a Western community). The questionnaire is therefore sensitive but not specific for coronary disease.

Necropsy

Most necropsies are done for medico-legal reasons and once an 'unnatural' cause such as violence, poisoning, alcohol, old war wounds or industrial causes is excluded coronary disease of some degree is often found. Pathologists have to produce a label. Careful microscopy or serial sectioning of the heart might reveal another pathology such as a viral inflammation or scarring of the specialised conducting tissue of the heart but this is seldom done.

Other newer tests

It is now possible to take cine-X-ray pictures of the coronary arteries while they are injected with liquids opaque to X-rays. This technique silhouettes the healthy artery and any narrowing or obstruction. Results are valuable but errors in interpretation can result from differential streaming of the liquid or bends concealing blockages. Radio-isotope techniques are under investigation for showing up damaged heart muscle. Neither of these techniques is suitable for epidemiological use because even if they are perfected they are too 'invasive' for population surveys.

Natural History of Coronary Heart Disease

There is no such thing as an unbiased picture of the effect of coronary heart disease. The viewpoint and set of criteria used influence the results (Table 1).

The hospital specialist sees only the cases severe enough to warrant his attention and who live long enough to reach hospital. The general practitioner sees milder cases but his experience is restricted to about six cases of infarction or death a year. The really mild cases of angina pectoris and the so-called 'silent' cases of cardiac infarction will not present for medical attention. Sudden death cases concern the coroner and the police surgeon rather than ordinary medical services. The coroner's pathologist sees fatal cases but no survivors.

One way of obtaining a more comprehensive picture is to follow-up a group of subjects over many years with repeated questionnaires and diagnostic tests, picking up mild angina and silent infarction. This can only be done with willing volunteers who may not be representative of the general population in all respects. Volunteers tend to be

Table 1. How defining a heart attack affects differently
apparent frequency and fatality

	Number of events qualifying	% fatal within 28 days
Definite post mortem evidence	157	100
Definite or possible post-mortem evidence	205	100
Typical chest pain	508	23
Definite electrocardiogram evidence	277	8
Raised enzymes in blood	351	9
Definite cases (all criteria)	534	35
Definite and possible cases	707	38

Table 2. Relationship of early behaviour in attack and method
of reaching hospital to fatality

	% fatal within 28 days
Patient went direct to hospital	25
Seen at home by general practitioner	26
Seen in surgery (office) by general practitioner	15
Hospital by ambulance (dead or alive)	47
Hospital by car (passenger)	14
Hospital by taxi, bus, on foot or driving self	1

healthier than 'non-responders' who have been shown in many studies to have an excessive death rate.

The apparent behaviour of the disease is strongly dependent on diagnostic criteria. The evidence of coronary thrombosis or visible cardiac infarction can only be obtained at necropsy. Conversely patients with raised cardiac enzyme levels in their blood or who have diagnostic ECG findings must have lived long enough to have the tests done. Their death rate is low. Each method of diagnosis picks out a specific sub-group of cases, a different section of the spectrum of disease.

Not only do the tests and the medical source of cases reflect different sorts of cases but so does the behaviour of the patient in the attack. On grounds of common sense it is suggested that someone having an attack should stop and rest and summon a doctor or an ambulance. In a community survey I discovered that patients who did this had a higher death rate than those who waited and went to the general practitioner's surgery (office). Those who walked to hospital had a very low mortality. The explanation seems to be that the behaviour in the attack did not influence the outcome so much as reflecting the severity of the illness (Table 2).

Community studies allow estimates to be made of the apparent length of survival of a patient in an attack. Unfortunately eye-witness evidence is frequently missing or unobtainable. Subjects who last an hour or so are more likely to involve others, whereas instantaneous death can occur when the subject is alone. By insisting on well described witnessed events the investigator seriously biases the result towards long survival. By including all cases he or she must decide what to do with those on whom no information is available so mixing good data with poor.

Mortality from Coronary Heart Disease

As has been described death certification is not always accurate, but almost always the subject himself is dead so that mistaken diagnoses must be allocated to or from another cause of death. Although diseases genuinely come and go, fashions occur in diagnosis and new diagnostic terms appear. It is therefore possible to argue that coronary deaths have always occurred, buried under such diagnoses as 'fatty heart' or 'sudden indigestion' until the modern terminology came in (most authorities however do agree that there has been a real increase). The most recent terminological change was when 'arteriosclerotic and degenerative heart disease' was renamed 'ischaemic (or coronary) heart disease'. Coronary heart disease was known originally as the 'executive disease' and it was first described in Britain among wealthier patients. However such descriptions tend to be self-fulfilling and there is a suggestion that what was called 'coronary thrombosis' in the rich was called 'myocardial degenerative disease' in the poor for rather longer. Now the difference is the other way round with more coronary death in the lower social classes. The diagnostic terminology and classification used in death certificate analysis undergoes a necessary revision once every ten years or so. However this creates problems in assessing long term trends in disease.

For most countries in the world, however, the problem is not one of interpreting published mortality statistics, there are none. Much of what is reported on coronary disease in the Afro-Asian countries is no better than travellers' tales, whether or not it is seen in the big city hospitals.

One method of assessing whether differences in mortality rates between countries are genuine would be to subject all deaths in defined areas to the same set of diagnostic criteria used by a central team of assessors. The logistic problems of such a study are so formidable that it has never been done on a large scale. Central criteria have been applied by peripheral teams and specimen case histories have been interpreted in different countries. The latter exercise demonstrated that even between English speaking countries there are considerable differences in diagnostic practice.

Epidemiological Studies of Risk Factors and Causation

The best known epidemiological studies of coronary heart disease have involved the standardised examination of large numbers of subjects by questionnaire and clinical tests (employing obsessional quality control) who are then followed for a number of years and possibly re-examined periodically. Success depends on a high response rate to the original recruitment, minimal losses to follow-up, a good number of disease cases occurring in the study group and good luck in the choice of factors to be studied. Such studies can only demonstrate the relevance to the risk of developing the disease of the factors that were measured. They cannot confirm or deny the importance of anything else. Thus for example, serum cholesterol and serum triglycerides have both been claimed to be useful as predictors of coronary risk. Whether they are independent can only be demonstrated by measuring both in the same large study. Obesity appears to be a risk factor when measured by itself. When included with blood pressure and serum cholesterol its effects seem to be explained away. Thus it is always possible to argue that what is being measured is not the primary causal factor but a by-product. The argument is only of scientific value if the postulated primary factor can be defined and measured, when it is possible to test it against the established conventional factors. A factor that appears to relate to risk on its own has therefore to undergo a sort of mediaeval trial by tournament when it is measured at the same time as the old guard and its independence and power are compared with them. Such studies have to be large and factors that appear frequently together may be dissociated only with difficulty. This

problem is also true of international correlations. Thus both animal fat and sugar have been postulated as causes of coronary disease. Countries that consume a lot of animal fat also consume a lot of sugar so the two cannot be easily separated and both correlate with coronary disease mortality. Conversely the countries that eat less animal fat and sugar tend to eat more cheese and wine so these come out of such studies as protective (as do garlic and onions). The mass of correlations do not reveal the underlying factor or factors.

Another problem with risk factors is their variability. Height would be an ideal subject for study as it is reasonably constant so that tall, medium and short people can be distinguished by a quick single test. Some of the chief coronary risk factors vary within individuals so that subjects whose serum cholesterol (or nowadays their lipoproteins) or blood pressure place them in one category on one occasion, may appear quite different on another. A whole series of measurements may be necessary to classify one subject reasonably accurately within his group. This is particularly true of diet where one day's consumption of food may be totally unrepresentative, both in quantity and in its detailed breakdown, of the long-term average characteristics of that individual. Despite this variability, factors such as lipoproteins, cholesterol and blood pressure do predict coronary risk. If we could measure their true average values rather than taking only sample readings, we should be able to predict coronary disease more accurately.

When large scale studies are analysed they are subjected to powerful statistical tests employing mathematical models that assume the relationship of increasing levels of each risk factor to risk is simple, e.g. that it is linear or follows a simple curve. Such an assumption may be the simplest to make for purposes of analysis but it may be misleading if the smoothed curve is used, rather than the original data, for purposes of proposing an ideal level of the risk factor. Even if the original data are used, different effects may occur at different ages and the pooled simplified curve may conceal these differences.

Trials of Coronary Disease Prevention

It might be thought that the definitive proof that current theories of coronary disease causation are correct could be tested by trials of prevention. This is true but the problems are formidable. It is only practicable to do such trials over 5—7 years. If the risk of developing the disease is say 1% per year then 95% of participants will be subjected to the regime unnecessarily as this proportion of the untreated control group will emerge unscathed. In order to demonstrate benefit to the 5% a vast army of participants must be recruited. Interventions that are practical in small studies are seriously weakened in studies on this scale. As many preventive measures involve behavioural change such as stopping smoking, diet change, weight loss, increase in exercise, the dangers are that not only will many 'treated cases' fail but that a lot of the control group may follow the regime, so that the two groups are little different. For this reason most preventive trials run the risk of being too small in numbers because the change in risk factors is too little and sustained too temporarily for the causal relationship to be seriously tested. A so called 'negative' trial result is often an inconclusive one in which a worthwhile benefit may have occurred but the trial was too small to demonstrate it. The first generation of trials which were successful included two in which diet was manipulated in closed institutions. Massive current trials on several risk factors at once in free-living subjects may be successful. If not, it may be because risk factor changes are too small, because changing risk factors in middle-

age is too late or even dangerous, or because theories of causation are wrong. Unfortunately the interpretation of trial results is as difficult as their design and execution.

Mortality Trends

Recently the world of coronary disease epidemiology has been excited by the discovery that coronary disease rates in the USA and some other countries such as Australia and Belgium are declining while those of Britain appear stable (Fig. 2). Despite the volume of research done in the United States the explanation is not clear. Changes in certifying practice and the effects of other diseases have been discounted. The effect seems real and substantial. In the USA there has probably been some decline in blood lipid levels but methods of measurement have changed since 1960, blood pressure is being treated more and more people take exercise and have stopped smoking, but none of these effects fit the decline well in terms of timing and size. There may be some correlation with a change to vegetable fats but this has also happened in Sweden where coronary rates are rising. There is some doubt as to whether the decline in mortality is because fewer people get the disease (a fall in incidence) or whether fewer people with the disease die from it (a fall in fatality). Large scale studies are now being planned in many countries in which all coronary events, fatal and non-fatal, over ten or more years will be monitored using defined criteria in communities of 300, 000 population and the trends in these event rates will be correlated with trends in coronary risk factors. Epidemiologists, like nuclear physicists have reached the stage of having to build bigger and bigger investigative machines to answer topical questions.

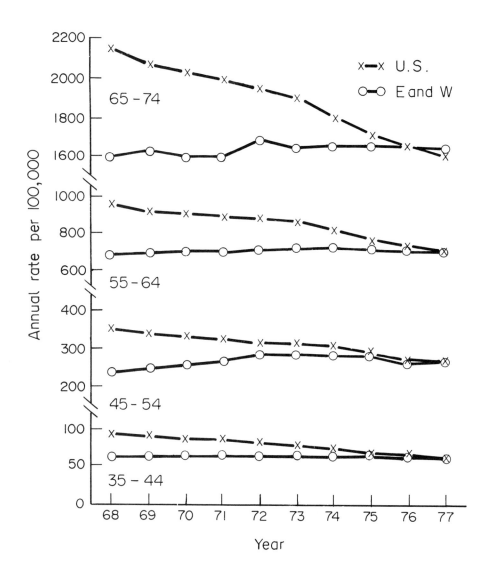

Figure 2. Mortality rates for men in different age groups in England (E) and Wales (W) and in America, 1968–77.

Further Reading

DAWBER, T.R. (1980) *The Framingham Study — The epidemiology of atherosclerotic disease.* Harvard University Press, Cambridge.
HAVLIK, R.J., FEINLEIB, M. (eds.) (1979). Proceedings of the Conference on the Decline in Coronary Heart Disease Mortality. U.S. Dept. of Health Education and Welfare, Washington.
TUNSTALL PEDOE, H. (1982) Coronary Heart Disease. In: *Epidemiology of Disease* (Miller, D. and Farmer, R.L. (eds.).) Blackwells, Oxford.

CARDIOVASCULAR SYSTEM

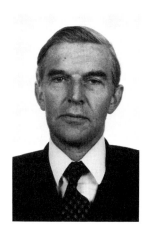

John Dickinson

Professor of Medicine and Chairman of the Department of Medicine, St. Bartholomew's Hospital Medical College, London.

He has held academic appointments at University College Hospital, London and was formerly visiting Professor in the Department of Medicine, McMaster University, Canada. He is a general physician with a special interest in applied physiology and in hypertension.

Autoregulation — How do Body Tissues get the Right Amount of Blood?

Suppose a cancer begins to grow in a woman's breast. In most cases a tumour begins from unrestrained proliferation of one type of cell which goes on multiplying, apparently lacking normal restraints. Think what would happen if the cells simply divided and the tumour comprised a mass of cancer cells with no blood supply. If we look at the rate of diffusion of, say, a glucose molecule in water, we find that although this can diffuse on average ten micrometres (the diameter of a red blood cell) in one-tenth of a second, it will take 16 minutes to move 1 mm and more than a day to move, on average, 1 cm. Thus a tumour without a blood supply and dependent on diffusion of nutrients would soon die. However it is common knowledge that such tumours can, if left untreated, grow to a large size. I have seen a neglected breast cancer the size of an orange. It would obviously be impossible for nutrients to be supplied fast enough to such a malignant tumour by a simple process of diffusion from surrounding healthy tissue. As the surgeon who excises it knows very well, the tumour mass includes extensive blood vessels which have emerged from the surrounding tissues and permeate its substance. Only rarely we find such a process going wrong, with the rate of growth of new blood vessels being inadequate to nourish the tumour. When that does happen the central part of the tumour dies. Unfortunately it is exceedingly uncommon, if indeed it ever happens, that a tumour chokes itself to death by outstripping its blood supply. If a tumour grows to an enormous size it will be supplied with arteries, veins and lymph vessels of comparable size.

Normal tissues exhibit exactly the same behaviour. In the months after the loss of a leg the artery which supplied the leg gets much smaller, because it does not need to carry so much blood. When a baby grows in a mother's womb, the womb itself develops a very extensive blood supply to nourish the baby, but after birth the blood vessels shrink down. After the menopause, when the womb may get quite small, the size of the blood vessels gets smaller still. In fact it seems that the body is so constructed that the blood supply (i.e. the size and number of blood vessels) is automatically adjusted to meet the needs of the tissues.

This is one aspect of what is called 'autoregulation', which is a term used to describe the phenomenon by which tissues regulate their own blood supply to get just the right amount. When the system breaks down and the blood supply becomes inadequate we are usually made aware of the fact by feeling pain in the affected part. The best known example is, of course, angina pectoris (literally pain in the chest). When a man takes exercise and the heart has to perform more work than is possible within the limits of narrowed coronary arteries, he feels a heavy tightness in the chest. If the exercise is prolonged pain becomes sufficiently intolerable to force him to stop and rest. A similar pain may be felt in the leg muscles of people whose main leg arteries are partially or completely blocked. This condition is known as intermittent claudication (literally 'limping') because it interferes with the subject's ability to walk.

Just about the only time when we see actual death of tissues from an obstructed blood supply is when this has been very sudden, as in the case of coronary artery thrombosis (suddenly causing a heart attack through death of some portion of the heart muscle) or a clot in a brain artery (producing a stroke because of death of a small piece of tissue in the brain). On the other hand, when restriction of blood supply occurs because of gradual blockage of one major artery, the healthy body reacts by enlarging other arteries.

Long term autoregulation is extremely efficient, but even in short time scales, tissues can respond in a remarkable manner. For example, it is possible to measure the total amount of blood flowing into the leg by the simple device of measuring the volume of the limb in the few seconds after suddenly damming back the return of blood to the heart. The rate of increase of limb volume equals the rate of blood inflow. If the main femoral artery is tied, there will of course be a very sharp fall in blood flow through the leg, but within about half an hour the total flow of blood to the leg will be back to normal. A man would, of course, be disadvantaged and would doubtless suffer pain on exercising later, but the blood supply of the limb at rest is usually enough to prevent any death of tissues, even though the main artery, prior to being tied, had been supplying 95% of all the blood going through the limb.

How does this happen? In most cases the phenomenon most certainly does not involve the brain, since parts of the body to which all nerves have been cut can still 'autoregulate' their blood supply, both over short and long periods of time. Obviously body tissues generally have some 'in-built' negative feedback system by which the tissue itself can detect a discrepancy between the blood supply required and the blood supply currently available, and so alter the calibre of the arteries so that the situation is corrected. Undoubtedly the most critical nutrient is oxygen. It is possible to do experiments in which the blood supply to some part of the body is gradually reduced and the amount of oxygen taken up continuously measured. When this is done it is usually found that the blood supply can be reduced to about one-third of normal before any measurable reduction in the up-take of oxygen occurs. If we take other nutrients such as glucose or fatty acids, which are metabolic fuels of the body, we find that if oxygen is available in adequate amounts, the blood supply can be reduced to about one-tenth of the normal before consumption of the fuel begins to diminish. Because of this many people have suggested that tissues have some means of detecting a fall in oxygen supply (probably by a reduction of the partial pressure of oxygen in the tissue concerned) and that the reduction in this partial pressure is the immediate stimulus for growth of blood vessels. There are several other possiblities. For example, to burn up metabolic fuels, like glucose and fatty acids, tissues use up oxygen and evolve carbon dioxide, which is passed by the blood supply to the lungs and excreted in the air we breathe out. As the blood supply to a tissue is progressively reduced, the partial pressure of carbon dioxide gas in the tissue will rise roughly in proportion to the amount that the oxygen tension falls, though the rate of rise is not relatively as fast because of the very big stores of carbon dioxide in the tissues. Again, when many tissues run short of oxygen, metabolic acids (particularly lactic acid), are produced in excess so that the tissues them-selves and the blood draining them becomes more acidic. Various highly potent substances such as kinins may be released from tissues which are inadequately supplied with blood and some of these have been shown to be capable of making arteries enlarge.

There is at present no unanimity amongst physiologists as to the factor which controls the blood supply and makes it increase when a tissue becomes 'ischaemic', i.e. short of blood. There is absolutely nothing known about the reverse mechanism, which shuts down the blood supply to a tissue whose needs for blood have gone down. One big problem which has not so far received the attention it deserves is the mystery of how the message is passed 'upstream', i.e. up the artery (towards the heart) instructing that artery to change its calibre. Diffusion is a very slow process over distances greater than 1 mm or so, but blood passes through most arteries quite rapidly. It is quite impossible that some chemical change in the blood works its way upstream against the flow of blood. It has been suggested that the reason why arteries and veins to many organs run close to each other is to allow a message of some sort to be passed from the vein across to the adjacent artery telling it, in effect, that the current blood supply is either too big or too small and that the artery calibre needs to be adjusted. Teleologically I find this conclusion almost irresistible, but as far as I know it is unproven and the nature of the chemical or nervous signals passed from vein to artery is likewise unknown.

I regard autoregulation as one of the major and absolutely crucial mysteries of the circu-lation. An analogy might be to challenge an engineer to design pipework to supply an enormous building with centrally heated water for its radiators but to specify, for economy in pipe size and bulk of water re-quired for the system, that the calibre of all the pipes should be self-adjusting so that when a radiator was turned on the supply pipe would automatically increase in calibre.

I have just one personal observation which makes me inclined to think that in most cases the tissue tension of oxygen is the controlling factor. Some years ago I examined the main arteries supplying the brain of a man who had died at the age of twenty-five from Fallot's tetralogy — a congenital deformity of the heart in which a high proportion of the blood by-passes the lungs altogether. He had been born a 'blue baby' and had remained blue all his life so that from birth onwards all his tissues had been supplied with blood at a very low oxygen tension. Not only were the brain arteries about twice as large in diameter as normal brain arteries but in addition the whole of the base of the skull was penetrated by many large arterial channels. These are unnoticeable in normal people but in this man's case had clearly been carrying large amounts of blood to the brain. Judging by the size of the arteries I would guess that brain blood flow must have been at least twice or perhaps three times normal. We know that in such individuals the partial pressure of carbon dioxide in the blood does not rise in proportion to the fall of oxygen, because breathing is stimulated by rising carbon dioxide levels and carbon dioxide is blown off. The tremendous growth of this man's brain arteries must therefore have been a consequence either of the very low oxygen level in the blood supplying the brain or (just conceivably) of the presence of some very subtle chemical which normally is inactivated in the lungs but which was present in the arterial blood in this case because a substantial amount of the blood coming to the heart by-passed the lungs and entered the arteries directly. I can see no reasonable alternatives; and although it is certain that the lungs have various metabolic functions in addition to the well known ones of exchanging blood gases with the surrounding air, we do not (yet) know of any material which has an artery-dilating effect and which is inactivated by the lungs. It would be easy to multiply such hypotheses, but plausible hypotheses which take no account of oxygen tension changes are very difficult to construct.

The Regulation of Arterial Blood Pressure

In the previous section I described the way in which any organ or tissue of the body seems to be able to acquire arteries and veins of a calibre appropriate to its needs. The intrinsic regulation of the blood supply to organs clearly presupposes that blood is supplied at a pressure sufficient to overcome the resistance of the many small blood vessels, which ramify into a network whose capillaries are only some 1/100th of a millimeter in diameter. It is approximately correct to say that the flow of the blood through tubes is something like the flow of electricity through a resistance. The rate of blood flow (current) is proportional to the pressure (voltage) divided by the flow resistance (electrical resistance). It immediately becomes obvious that tissues and organs of the body could obtain the same amount of blood flow by having a twice normal driving blood pressure together with a twice normal intrinsic resistance, or for that matter, a half normal pressure together with a half normal resistance. Since it is abundantly clear that organs and tissues can adapt themselves to any reasonably adequate prevailing arterial blood pressure, the next problem which raises its head is 'What determines the arterial blood pressure?'.

We can say straight away that there is a certain minimum pressure. In the capillaries it has been known for a hundred years or so that the hydrostatic pressure tending to drive fluid out of the bloodstream into the surrounding tissues is matched by a contrary suction pressure provided by large molecules, particularly of albumin, which circulate in the bloodstream but are only to a small extent permeable through the lining capillary membrane. Thus they exert a colloid osmotic pressure which balances the hydrostatic pressure tending to extrude fluid. The capillary pressure is of the order of 15 mmHg (1/50th of an atmosphere) and the difference between colloid osmotic pressure inside the bloodstream and immediately outside it is approximately 22 mmHg (though it varies a lot in different places and at different times). The apparently anomalous 7 mmHg difference reflects the pressure in the tissues being this amount negative to atmospheric. That is to say, we are all being squeezed together by the atmospheric pressure pressing everywhere on our bodies. If someone raises his thumb away from the hand, the anatomical 'snuff box' makes its appearance between the two tendons at the base of the thumb, forming a hollow pocket. There are many other places in the body where skin hollows of this sort are maintained by the external pressure of the atmosphere rather than by the skin itself being tethered to underlying structures.

If we now come back to the minimum necessary arterial blood pressure we can see that it has to be at least 15 mmHg to allow fluid to leave the capillaries and to overcome the suction effect of colloid osmotic pressure. In an erect human the blood must be able to get up to the top of the body, i.e. the top of the scalp, at sufficient pressure to be able to maintain an equilibrium of pressure in the capillaries and thus nourish the top of the scalp. Therefore an absolute minimum pressure in the scalp must be 15 mmHg and because of the hydrostatic pressure difference between the level of the heart and the top of the head, an additional 15 inches or 20 mmHg equivalent pressure is required to raise the blood up to this point. In the case of a giraffe eating a tall tree it is quite obvious that the blood pressure needs to be far higher still. Indeed, enormously high blood pressures have been recorded in free ranging giraffes and the giraffe has the highest blood pressure of any known creature. In most situations it has been observed that an additional small pressure, known as the 'critical opening pressure' is necessary to prevent blood vessels which have some elastic in their walls from closing right down and, of course, an additional pressure is required to move blood through the network. So for an erect human being it would seem inescapable that the minimum blood pressure would be 15 + 20 + (5 to 10) = 40–45 mmHg (1/20th of an atmosphere). This is the very least a human being could possibly manage with for any significant amount of time.

If we think in terms of the survival of a species it beomes obvious that an excessively high pressure would be disadvantageous. If the body suffers a deep wound which severs an artery, blood would be lost more rapidly and catastrophically if the pressure was unduly high inside the system. Furthermore the work of the heart is principally in raising the pressure of blood from the filling side to the output side and an excessively high pressure would make the heart do an unnecessary amount of work. We already know that the average blood pressure of a fit healthy adult is of the order of 85 mmHg when measured at the level of the heart. This is some 40 mmHg above the calculated minimum value and indeed approximately twice this amount. Since the heart pumps in beats with around 70 strokes/minute the blood pressure is not steady but goes up and down with each heart pulsation, typically fluctuating between 110 and 75 mmHg from systolic (peak) pressure to diastolic (trough) pressure. In the newborn infant the pressure is rather lower than this and from early adult life in the population as a whole it tends to rise gradually. But it is reasonable to argue that the ideal blood pressure throughout life would be the same as that measurable in a teenager, i.e. 110/75 or about 85 mm mean pressure. It is well known that those who are fortunate enough to maintain this 'normal' blood pressure throughout life have considerably better expectancy of life and health than those whose blood pressure rises during their life.

If we look at the opposite end of the scale, we know from experiments on dogs that the highest pressure against which the heart can be made to pump is around 250 mmHg mean pressure, i.e. about 1/3rd of an atmosphere. This would correspond to a systolic/diastolic pressure of about 350/180. This level corresponds quite closely to the highest pressure ever recorded in a most severely hypertensive human individual. To summarise therefore, it would appear that the minimum pressure in the arteries is about 45 mmHg; the normal blood pressure is about 85 mmHg; and the absolute maximum pressure which the heart is capable of generating is about 250 mmHg. The great mystery which has exercised the minds of several generations of medical scientists during the last eighty years or so is 'What controls the blood pressure level both over short and long periods of time?'.

The last century has seen the discovery of an enormous number of stabilising systems controlling blood pressure. The best known of these is a system which depends on natural measuring devices, the baroreceptors, which are situated in the walls of arteries supplying the brain. These send nervous impulses which signal to the controlling centres of the brain second-by-second information about what the blood pressure is doing. This then allows the brain to take corrective action. For many years the kidneys have been known to play a very important role in blood pressure control and the association between kidney disease and high blood pressure was observed in the last century. If the blood supply to one kidney is impaired the kidney secretes a chemical material into the blood stream (renin) which has the power to raise blood pressure. It would not be possible in the space of a brief article to itemise all the other negative feedback stabilising systems. A very large number of experiments has been done on animals, and accident and disease have done a comparable series of experiments on human beings. These show that it is possible to strip away one control system after another, and yet the blood pressure remains approximately normal. For example, it is possible to have both kidneys removed from the body or destroyed by disease and, providing that life is maintained by an artificial kidney removing waste products and preventing overloading with fluid, the blood pressure will usually be normal. Similarly it has been shown in animals and human beings who have suffered complete transection of the spinal cord high in the neck, thus depriving the brain of any control over nerves to arteries and veins, that the blood pressure again remains reasonably normal. It is possible for people to suffer massive loss of limbs, e.g. both legs, with a consequent enormous reduction in the amount of vasculature and increase in vascular resistance — but the blood pressure remains normal. Yet during the course of a person's

life, in the absence of any disease process, the blood pressure is far from stable from moment to moment. During deep sleep, for example, the brain allows the blood pressure to go down to surprisingly low levels which may be 60 mmHg or even less — quite close to the calculated minimum — and on the other hand during peaks of physical exertion, extreme emotional excitement and sexual intercourse, the blood pressure may rise transiently to one and a half or almost twice the normal value. Despite these fluctuations the average value remains remarkably constant throughout life in the absence of recognisable disease and quite evidently the stabilising systems are exceedingly efficient.

Although, thanks to a tremendous amount of basic physiological research, we can itemise a very large number of mechanisms stabilising blood pressure, we do not know for sure what the ultimate 'reference standard' is. If you want to stabilise a direct current voltage, for example, it is normal practice to use some device such as a highly accurate reference cell or reference neon which maintains a constant voltage across it. The output of the stabilising unit is continuously compared with the reference voltage and adjustments made so as to stabilise the output. Despite an enormous amount of work there is no general agreement of what comprises the ultimate 'reference pressure' of the circulation though almost all investigators would agree that this resides either in the kidneys or in the brain since these are the two organs which seem to have most to do with blood pressure control.

The mystery of hypertension

One big problem is that all the mechanisms of blood pressure control that we know of in any detail are capable of becoming reset to any prevailing level of blood pressure, whether high or low. Historically this was first shown for the arterial baroreceptors mentioned above, but it seems to be true for mechanisms in the kidneys as well as for those connected with the nervous system. Thus if some abnormal stimulus succeeds in raising the blood pressure for a reasonably long length of time, e.g. several days, weeks or months, then the other stabilising mechanisms appear to accept the new conditions as the expected norm and thereafter stabilise the blood pressure at its new level. Since most emotional and strenuous physical activities during a person's life raise the blood pressure, it is tempting to attribute the tendency of the blood pressure to rise slowly during the course of life to subconscious emotional conflicts and other rather nebulous oft-repeated events. The problem is that some people have intense blood pressure-raising experiences but yet remain obstinately with a normal blood pressure (at rest) to the end of their life. This strongly suggests that there must be some reference standard, especially since virtually all the known blood pressure stabilising systems can be induced to shift their sensitivity range in almost all established forms of high blood pressure. This also applies to the very common 'essential' form of hypertension, which has at present no known or agreed cause. The high blood pressure is actively maintained by all the controlling mechanisms that we know. If someone with high blood pressure loses blood through an injury, for example, the blood pressure will transiently fall, but in due course the blood loss is made good by the body and the blood pressure will once again return to the high level.

It seems most likely that if we could only understand and find the ultimate reference standard by which blood pressure was set we could likewise understand the nature of the abnormality which underlies high blood pressure. In the last twenty years or so there has been steady progress in understanding and putting together as an integrated whole the very large number of mechanisms concerned with blood pressure stabilisation, but the key to the whole system still eludes us.

The riddle of heart failure

To the layman 'heart failure' means some inadequacy in the heart resulting in a failure to pump the blood round. To the doctor, however, although this may well be the underlying problem, the words 'heart failure' conjure up more the end result of something wrong with the heart. There is usually a rise of pressure in the capillaries either of the lungs (causing flooding of the substance of the lungs and sometimes even the air passages with fluid) or in capillaries in the rest of the body (leading to a leak of fluid out, thus causing swelling of the dependent parts). It is quite common for the first symptom of 'heart failure' to be swelling of the ankles. Often the failure is both apparently of the left side of the heart, apparently associated with damming back of the blood in the lungs, causing lung congestion and shortness of breath, combined with damming back of blood in the rest of the body, causing swelling of the ankles and other parts.

This however is far from being the whole story. If in an animal we artificially create some damage to the heart preventing its pumping properly, (for example by causing leakage of a valve or obstruction at some point of the circulation), the immediate effect is not, paradoxically, a rise in the capillary pressure at any point, but rather a fall, since the normal capillary pressure of 15 mmHg or so is considerably higher than the average static pressure in the circulation, i.e. that pressure which would be found if the circulation were to be instantaneously stopped and all pressures equalised. This indicates that the high pressure in the capillaries in 'heart failure' must be brought about either by an increase in the volume or by a reduction in the capacitance of the circulation. ('Capacitance' measures the amount of blood which can be contained at any particular static pressure.) In practice, heart failure is almost invariably due to an actual increase in the volume of the blood. Only in exceptional circumstances does capillary pressure rise to a severe degree without previous expansion of the blood volume.

The problem in heart failure is to understand the underlying mechanisms by which reduction of the ability of the heart to pump brings about retention of fluid in the bloodstream and expansion of the blood volume. All sorts of things contribute. People whose circulation is failing get thirsty and drink more and this will obviously tend to expand the volume of fluid in the body. However, this would clearly not suffice to produce continued expansion of the blood volume. It is (unfortunately) commonplace for people to drink twelve pints or more of beer daily. Such people in the end suffer damage to their livers, but do not normally develop heart failure. The immediate cause of blood volume expansion appears to be associated with the kidneys, which control the rate of excretion of water and salt. The kidneys are also, and perhaps not coincidentally, the organs which have led the field as the main culprits for causing high blood pressure. Somehow or other it appears that when the heart is not pumping enough blood round to meet the needs of the tissues, the kidneys receive some message instructing them to restrict the rate of excretion of fluid and salts until a new equilibrium is reached with an expanded blood volume. (This is teleologically advantageous because it helps to keep up the output from a damaged heart.)

Another big mystery in circulatory physiology is the nature of the organ or natural device which reports to some integrating centre, possibly the brain, that the heart is not pumping enough blood. We also do not know the precise paths by which the brain then passes its instructions to the kidneys, although the nerves supplying the kidneys

may well play some part. However even a kidney deprived of nerves will retain salt and water if something goes wrong with the heart, so this is far from being the whole story. It might be tempting to imagine that the problem is simply on the pressure detection side. If the heart is pumping inadequately then the pressure in the arteries will obviously tend to fall. It might then be argued that the fall of blood pressure was a trigger towards retention of fluid by the kidneys and thus expansion of blood volume. However in established heart failure the blood pressure is just the same as in normal people and when the lungs are engorged it is frequently higher than normal, so this simple view is not easy to sustain.

Conclusions

No conclusions are possible at the present time in the areas I have mentioned — i.e. automatic control of the resistance to the flow of blood through the tissues, the control of pressure in the arteries and the control of the volume of the blood in relation to the ability of the heart to pump. Nonetheless the answers appear tantalisingly close and my personal guess would be that within the next twenty years we shall have an agreed answer as to the reference standard for blood pressure regulation, know the principal cause of 'essential hypertension' and understand reasonably fully all the processes involved in blood pressure regulation and blood volume expansion consequent upon heart failure. I suspect that these problems will be closely interrelated. The foundations of our understanding have already been dug. We now need some inspired builders.

References

DICKINSON, C.J. (1981) Neurogenic Hypertension Revisited. *Clinical Science,* **60**, 471–477.

GUYTON, A.C. (1980) *Circulatory Physiology III: Arterial Pressure and Hypertension.* Saunders, Philadephia and London.

GUYTON, A.C., JONES, C.E., COLEMAN, T.G. (eds.) (1973) *Circulatory Physiology: Cardiac Output and its Regulation.* Saunders, Philadelphia and London.

THE RESPIRATORY SYSTEM

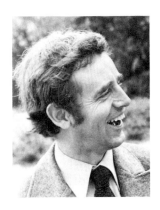

Malcolm Green

Consultant Physician in Chest and General Medicine, St. Bartholomew's and Brompton Hospitals, London. Honorary Senior Lecturer, Cardiothoracic Institute, London, and St. Bartholomew's Hospital Medical College.

The Respiratory System in Health

Our ignorance of the normal and diseased function of the respiratory system exceeds by many times our knowledge. Our study of this system, as with most of medicine, can be likened to exploring an iceberg: we may crawl around on the surface and even dig towards the interior, but the vast majority of the ice is hidden from us under the waters of our ignorance! Despite this, it is possible to fill a sizeable library with literature concerning our knowledge of respiratory function in health and disease. It is not my purpose to summarize this literature here: a few modern sources are listed at the end of this Chapter.

What is the respiratory system and what does it do? Even defining the respiratory system is difficult since it is an integral part of the body and nature does not make neat divisions between the various functioning parts. We can perhaps describe it as the lungs and associated structures, such as blood vessels, airways, nerves and covering membranes together with the chest wall, including muscles, bones and ligaments. The prime function of the respiratory system is to transfer oxygen from the air into the blood and carbon dioxide from the blood to the air. Associated with this, the lungs have other important functions, notably the conservation of heat and water and the removal of inhaled materials, be it dust, bacteria, viruses or other agents. In addition, the lung probably has other roles of which we know much less. It is increasingly apparent that it is a powerful biochemical organ with the ability to manufacture and degrade all manner of substances. The lung also appears to be an endocrine organ, secreting numerous active proteins. We are largely ignorant of the importance of these functions — whether they are under normal circumstances a minor by-product of the lung's activities or whether they are a major part of the body's biochemical and endocrinological system. Within this framework of the respiratory system a recent multi-author tome has attempted to outline the current state of knowledge of its 'scientific foundations'. The interested reader is referred to this for a relatively up-to-date statement of our current state of knowledge. Here I will merely highlight some of the areas of which we are most ignorant.

Structure

Anatomical studies of the body have been carried out for millennia. It might be thought, therefore, that this would be the most advanced area of knowledge. This is, however, untrue. For example, amazingly, there is argument as to how many airways there are in the periphery of the human lung. Only a handful of workers have studied the morphology of the human airways. It would seem simple to make casts of the airways, but fewer than half a dozen studies have done this. The very small airways cannot be casted but can be looked at down a microscope. However, both these techniques have led to problems. There are very few casts and the techniques of making them are varied. The methods of counting the airways (starting from the centre or from the periphery) have varied and most of the analyses have been made by only two authors (Horsfield and Wiebel) from one cast each. Assessing the size and number of peripheral airways down a microscope leads to horrendous problems of counting and sampling. The result of this is that estimates of the numbers of peripheral airways differ, according to different authors, by several orders of magnitude. This has important implications for our studies and understanding of the flow of air in and out of the tubes. It is generally, although not universally, believed that the resistance of the airways diminishes peripherally because of their increasing number. This means that the air has a lower linear velocity peripherally, and, indeed, at the extreme periphery movement of molecules is probably by diffusion rather than bulk flow.

With the advent of the electron microscope a new opportunity to study the cellular constituents of the lung has arisen. We have substantial knowledge by means of this and the conventional light microscope of the structure of the cells that make up the lung. However, the correlation of the function of the cells with their anatomy is much less clear. The function of many of the cells is only inferred, and for some of the cells (notably Clara cells and brush cells) no appropriate function has yet been assigned. Furthermore, the life cycle and natural history of these cells is still largely obscure. The problem is that anatomical studies do not allow us to tell whether a cell is getting bigger or smaller, whether it is migrating inwards or outwards, or generally how it is behaving in any confident detail.

An interesting anatomical feature of the lungs is the network of smooth muscle fibres which extends down the tracheobronchial tree. The larger airways are surrounded by a layer of circular muscle. As the airways become smaller peripherally, the muscle coat becomes relatively thicker and the fibres are arranged into a so-called geodesic network. At the very periphery the muscle fibres are not continuous but are still present, particularly at the entrances to the centilatory units themselves. These muscle fibres were described by Reisseisen in 1822 and have since been confirmed by many authors, who have all stressed their anatomical importance. Remarkably, however, no-one knows what their purpose is. It is postulated that they serve to stiffen the airways and prevent them from collapsing, or that they direct the inspired air preferentially into one part of the lungs or another. Neither of these, nor any other explanation, is very satisfying, although it is difficult to believe that this complicated arrangement of muscles is atavistic. At present our ignorance can perhaps be summarized by the suggestion that this musculature serves only to cause asthma.

Physiology

Most of our physiological knowledge of the lung is based on empirical observation of its behaviour in humans and animals under a variety of circumstances. From this, certain working hypotheses have been drawn up which currently appear more or less to fit the facts. However, our basic understanding of the arrangement of physiological mechanisms is minimal. An example can be taken from the forced vital capacity manoeuvre, commonly performed to study lung physiology and as a test of its function. The subject takes a maximal inspiration, blows out as hard and as long as possible and then takes a maximal inspiration. By suitable arrangement of measuring devices, the change in volume of the lungs (strictly the chest wall) and the rate of flow at the mouth can be plotted simultaneously: a typical example is shown in Fig. 1. It will be seen that the shapes of these relationships differ radically between inspiration and expiration. Further studies have shown that the inspiratory flow rates are effort-dependent: that is, the harder the subject drives his muscles, the greater the inspiratory flow rate he can achieve. However, expiration is quite different. From 80% of maximal lung volume down to full expiration the flow rate is limited at each given lung volume as shown in the diagram. Thus, for example, if a subject blows out, generating about half his possible muscle power, he can

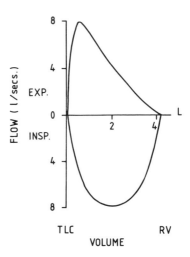

Fig. 1. Plot of gas flow rate measured at the mouth on inspiration (downwards) and expiration (upwards) against lung volume from maximum inspiration (total lung capacity – TLC) to maximal expiration (residual volume – RV). The subject takes a maximal inspiration and then blows out as hard and as long as he can to produce the expiratory flow volume curve and then immediately breathes in as hard and completely as he can to produce the inspiratory flow volume curve. Note the difference between the shape of the inspiratory and expiratory curves (see text).

achieve a flow rate at 50% vital capacity, which is the same as that achieved with more forceful expiration. In other words, he is unable to increase his flow above a certain level by further effort. Nobody has thought of any conceivable reason why this should have been predicted from a *de novo* analysis of the respiratory system. Indeed, it is extremely difficult to work out why it should occur. Knowing that it does occur, we can make certain analogies to waterfalls and other physical phenomena. These have allowed the generation of a large literature. Perhaps the most convincing concept that explains this phenomenon on a physical basis is the suggestion that a critical wave speed is reached in the airways which limits flow in much the same way that a critical wave speed in air causes a barrier to movement through air at the speed of sound. Even if this is the correct physical explanation, it is still obscure why this mechanism should be necessary in the lungs. It is, of course, possible that it is not necessary, but is just a chance consequence of the way the lung units have been put together.

The body exists in a gravitational field, and this includes the lungs. As might be predicted, therefore, there is a gravity gradient of pressure surrounding the lungs from the uppermost to the lowermost part. This pleural pressure gradient has important consequences for the function of the lung, since, for example, airways and blood vessels tend to close off earlier at the bottom of the lungs than at the top. The gradient can be most easily visualized by comparing it to the gradient of pressure inside a jar of the same height containing water. Clearly, the gradient in the jar is one centimetre of water pressure for each centimetre of distance below the surface of the water. In the human lung the pressure gradient is about 0.2 cm of water for each centimetre of vertical gradient, and thus the top-to-bottom gradient totals about 5 cm of water. It might be deduced that this is because the lungs have less weight than water, but this turns out to be an over-simplification because studies in animals have shown that the top-to-bottom pleural pressure gradient is about the same in rats and in elephants as it is in humans (4—6 cm water). Thus the gradient of pressure in the rat is nearly that of a comparable column of water, whereas in large animals it is much less even than in humans despite apparently similar lung tissue. This illustrates that we do not understand the nature of this pressure gradient, how it is produced, or why.

The driving force for respiration is the respiratory muscles and it would be hoped that we would have a clear understanding of their normal function. In fact, this field of respiratory physiology has been less studied than most. It appears clear that normal inspiration is achieved predominantly by contraction of the diaphragm, intercostal muscles and abdominal muscles. However, the interrelationships of these are hotly debated. For example, there is a widespread view that the diaphragm is the most important muscle of inspiration, being responsible for at least 80% of inspiration. Indeed, some workers have suggested that the only purpose of the intercostal muscle is to fix the rib cage and prevent it from collapsing inwards when the diaphragm contracts. Other workers have argued that the intercostal muscles have a much more important role, both in quiet breathing and in exercise, and may contribute as much, or even more, than the diaphragm. Until recently it was widely believed that the diaphragm was entirely a muscle of inspiration because of its position and measurements of its activity. However, there is increasing evidence that it is active during expiration and some have suggested that it may prevent the lungs from deflating too quickly, in the same way as the triceps prevents excessively fast flexion of the forearm by the biceps. These questions remain unresolved.

Gas Transport

The prime function of the lung is to transport oxygen into and carbon dioxide out of the body. These functions have been studied in detail by a number of workers for many years. Despite this, we are still remarkably ignorant of the mechanisms by which these processes take place. Oxygen is inspired at the mouth in the form of air, which has an oxygen concentration of 21%. A lesser concentration reaches the alveoli at the periphery of the lung. Observations of the effect of inspiring various pure gases or mixtures and analysing the expirate at the mouth allow us to speculate as to the mechanisms within the lung. These are complex and poorly understood. It is agreed by all that there is inhomogeneity, that is, that the concentration of the gases is not uniform throughout the lung. How this lack of homogeneity arises is not clear. The two main alternatives are either that parts of the lung are more fully flushed with air than other parts (regional inhomogeneity) or that the gas already in the lung is pushed out to the periphery of the lung and followed by the new gas, which mixes only slowly with the old gas in the lungs (stratified inhomogeneity). The controversy between these two mechanisms, which probably both apply to a greater or lesser extent, has swung in favour of one or the other each decade during this century. The debate is not settled and a recent article concluded, in the jargon of the field, 'it is likely that some important parameters have not been properly considered in the model analysis'.

Perhaps we are more certain as to how oxygen passes into the blood from the alveoli? Early this century it was thought that the tissue separating the air and the blood was critical and limited the rate at which the gases diffused and that in disease this was increased to cause an 'alveolar capillary block'. This concept was rejected in the 1960s in favour of the belief that diffusion occurred extremely quickly through the membranes even in disease and that the transfer of oxygen depended merely on the relative levels of ventilation and perfusion of a given unit. More recently, it has been argued that diffusion can, at least in disease and possibly even in health, be a rate-limiting factor. This concept may yet prove to be at least partially correct.

The control of ventilation

The control of ventilation is an example of complex but well-adjusted autoregulation. Curiously, the respiratory centre is most sensitive to carbon dioxide and adjusts ventilation to keep carbon dioxide levels in the body constant. It is relatively less sensitive to oxygen under normal circumstances for reasons that are not clear. Possibly a rise of carbon dioxide is more toxic than a low oxygen level, or this arrangement may have occurred by chance. Everyone knows that ventilation increases on exercise. Surprisingly,

however, the reasons for this are poorly understood. It might be thought that the increased need for oxygen or production of carbon dioxide would stimulate ventilation, but measurements show that the changes in ventilation precede and prevent such changes in blood gases. Perhaps there are neurological messages from the muscles, or it may be that chemicals or hormones are liberated. Possibly it is not the steady level of gases in the blood which is relevant, but their tiny oscillations during the breathing cycle. All in all, we do not know.

The Respiratory System in Disease

Ideally, the practice of respiratory medicine should be based on rational principles derived from a comprehensive knowledge of the anatomy, physiology, biochemistry and other functional mechanisms of the system. Unfortunately, as we have seen, our understanding of the latter disciplines is patchy to say the least, and our ability to project that knowledge to the diseased state is in most cases almost non-existent. Instead, over many years disease patterns and progress have been observed and pathological, biochemical and other studies made. Thereafter a more or less satisfying theoretical framework is built up to accommodate these facts, where possible. Despite this, however, a large part of diagnosis is simply pattern recognition and treatment rests on empirical observations of the effect of certain interventions on the apparent natural history of the disease. These problems can be illustrated by considering some of the more important respiratory diseases.

Asthma

About 20% of the population shows evidence of allergy, that is, increased sensitivity to external allergens such as dust, pollen, animals and the like. The most common manifestation is a positive skin test to a tiny dose of the allergen. Skin reactivity is clinically unimportant, but a large number of such 'atopic' people have clinical manifestations, particularly hay fever and asthma. Hay fever probably affects 10–15% of the population at some time, and asthma some 5–10%. Thus these conditions are exceedingly common and very tiresome for the sufferer. In addition, asthma can be dangerous: it causes some 1000 deaths each year in the UK. We have no idea why some people should be allergic, and furthermore, no idea why some allergic people develop hay fever and others asthma. Presumably the allergic state is due to an exceptional sensitivity of part of the body's immunological mechanisms, that is, the defences against external agents and chemicals. However, the nature of the tie-up between the allergic state and the body's immunological defences is obscure. It is difficult to see why 20% of the population should have this hypersensitivity: on genetic grounds it might be thought that there should be some advantage to the species from such a widespread tendency. None has been identified, and indeed it is difficult to think of any conceivable biological advantage. Alternatively, it could be that allergy is an important part of the immunological mechanism, but that the system is relatively poorly adjusted to need, so that say 20% of the population has 'too much' allergy, 20% 'too little' and 60% about right! It may be that this rather 'design-pessimistic' explanation is correct, since it now appears that many, perhaps all, non-allergic people can be induced to become allergic to certain substances if they are exposed to sufficient quantities over a period of time. This is particularly relevant in industry, where heavy exposures to inhaled substances such as toluene diisocyanate (a component of plastics, paints, etc.), solder flux fumes, salts of platinum and other substances can cause severe and persistent asthma in otherwise non-allergic subjects.

Hay fever and asthma appear to have many similarities of mechanism, although the details of the interaction between the inhaled antigen and the susceptible subject to cause either are poorly understood. As mentioned above, one of the important features of asthma is the contraction of the smooth muscle of the airways causing constriction of the tracheobronchial tree. Inflammation and swelling of the lining of the airways is probably also important, but the sequence of events between the inhalation of an allergen and the constriction and inflammation of the airways is mysterious. Interesting cells called mast cells appear to play an important part, perhaps by liberating toxic chemicals such as histamine and the leukotrienes. It is believed that nerves also play a part and that some of the airway constriction may be due to nervous reflexes.

For reasons which are not clear, asthma tends to be worst at night, and many sufferers wake at night or in the early morning wheezing and coughing. Their symptoms not infrequently improve during the day, and paradoxically there may be no signs of the condition when they visit a doctor in the afternoon. Many patients with asthma are allergic to housedust, and in particular a tiny mite which lives in bedding, pillows and carpets. It has been suggested that sufferers inhale this allergen from their bed and thus their symptoms are worse at night. Although this is possible, it is not the whole story. Figure 2 shows the peak expiratory flow rate (a measure of airways function) of an otherwise fit non-allergic 47-year-old farmer. He had developed a specific allergy and asthma due to grain dust. After a spell away from grain dust he was entirely fit, with a normal peak flow of 500 l/min. On day 2 at 10.00 a.m. he poured grain dust in and out of a dish in a carefully controlled environment for 60 minutes. He had no further exposure to this dust and his lung function was carefully monitored in hospital thereafter. As can be seen from Fig. 2, he developed an immediate reduction in his lung function, indicating constriction of the airways. This improved

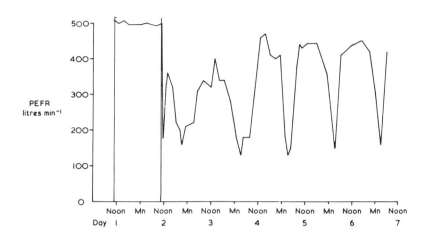

Fig. 2. Peak expiratory flow rate (PEFR) measured 4-hourly day and night for a period of 7 days in a 47-year-old farmer with a specific allergy to grain dust. At 10.00 a.m. on day 2 he is exposed to grain dust for 60 minutes but has no further exposure thereafter (see text). Mn = midnight.

but became worse again in the night. On the four subsequent days his lung function was essentially normal, but each night, without any further exposure to grain dust, he had a substantial fall in his lung function and all the symptoms of asthma. It seems, therefore, that a single exposure to an allergen can cause severe symptoms of asthma at night for at least a week subsequently: in some unknown way a persisting mechanism is triggered which is regulated by a circadian rhythm within the body. The causes of this phenomenon are obscure, but it is clinically important in that asthma may persist for many days and even weeks after the exposure. This makes the detection of possible causes doubly difficult.

Our understanding of asthma is complicated by a group of asthmatics (called intrinsic) who develop asthma later in life and who appear to have no manifestations of the allergic tendency. Their asthma tends to be more severe and more difficult to control. Most studies of the mechanisms of asthma ignore this group as being too difficult to understand for the present.

Fortunately, there are several highly effective treatments for asthma. A group of compounds called beta stimulants has a rational basis in that it dilates respiratory smooth muscle. Other treatments, however, are more empirical: disodium chromoglycate appears to inhibit some of the functions of mast cells, although how and why is unknown. The most powerful treatment for asthma is corticosteroid therapy. These substances are naturally secreted by the adrenal gland and large doses are highly effective at suppressing asthma. The reasons for this are obscure.

Chronic bronchitis and emphysema

Whereas asthma causes constriction of the airways which is generally intermittent and reversible, chronic bronchitis and emphysema are characterized by the fixed irreversible obstruction of the airways which results in limitations of the airflow into, and more particularly out of, the lungs. These two conditions are probably at opposite ends of a spectrum of so-called 'chronic obstructive lung disease' (COLD). Cigarette smoking has been identified as a most important contributing factor to COLD; which is seen only very rarely in non-smokers. On the other hand, the susceptibility of smokers to COLD is very variable and it has been suggested that other factors are also important. These may be genetic but it is also possible that virus infections are a potent additional causative agent. Similarly, it is not clear why some cigarette smokers tend to develop chronic bronchitis with associated cough and sputum production, whereas others tend towards emphysema with more conspicuous breathlessness and destruction of lung tissue. Some have argued that this depends on the postulated differences between the biochemical make-up of different persons' lungs, which may metabolise the products of cigarette smoking and other agents differently, but evidence for this is lacking.

A currently fashionable hypothesis suggests that cigarette smoking predominantly attacks the small airways in the periphery of the lung — those of less than about 2 mm internal diameter. As mentioned above, it is generally believed that overall these small airways have a very low resistance to airflow due to their very large number. Thus cigarette smoking could gradually constrict and obliterate the small airways over many years before clinical symptoms appear. Indeed, it is calculated that perhaps 90% of the small airways could be destroyed before breathlessness became clinically important in a relatively sedentary middle-aged man. On this basis it might be possible to identify at an early stage those smokers whose small airways were becoming damaged by performing sophisticated tests which are believed to reflect the function of these small airways. Unfortunately, even if such individuals could reliably be detected, the only useful treatment or advice at present available is to urge them to stop smoking. Furthermore, even if all the technical problems associated with this approach could be

overcome it is unlikely to be epidemiologically fruitful. Although cigarette smoking is by far the most important identified cause of COLD, Table 1, taken from a study of British doctors, shows that it accounts for only about

Table 1. Excess deaths in male smokers by cause (total 485 deaths per 100,000 smokers per year, age-standardised). From Doll and Peto (1976).

Heart disease	31%
Diseases of blood vessels (strokes, etc.)	21%
Lung cancer	19%
Chronic bronchitis and emphysema	10%
Others	19%

10% of the excess deaths attributable to cigarette smoking. Thus 90% of the deaths attributable to cigarette smoking would continue and, indeed, persons who showed no evidence of damage to small airways might even be encouraged to believe that cigarette smoking was not harmful for them!

Lung cancer

A discussion of cigarette smoking leads inevitably to the question of lung cancer. The chances of dying from lung cancer are twenty-five times greater in a man smoking thirty cigarettes per day compared to a non-smoker. Table 1 shows that lung cancer accounts for 19% of the excess deaths due to cigarette smoking. Whilst these facts now appear incontrovertable, we are ignorant as to how cigarettes predispose people towards lung cancer, why some subjects are more susceptible than others and how to treat lung cancer once diagnosed. There does appear to be some genetic susceptibility towards the development of lung cancer in cigarette smokers, as it has a tendency to run in families. However, it is known that cigarette smoke contains several substances which will cause cancers in animals, particularly on the skin of mice, notably polycyclic aromatic hydrocarbons and *N*-nitrosamines. The latter are regarded as hazardous in food at one part per billion, but occur in very much larger concentrations in tobacco.

By far the best treatment for lung cancer is preventative: to stop people smoking. Once lung cancer has been diagnosed, our ability to treat it is extremely poor. It appears that on average lung cancers tend to grow slowly, having probably been present for 5—15 years before diagnosis. It is conventional to remove lung cancer at operation if this is technically feasible, as it is in about 20% of patients. It has, however, been questioned whether this leads to overall better survival, since only about five patients out of every 100 presenting with lung cancer are alive after five years. It has been calculated that about the same number would be alive at five years if no treatment of any sort were given! On the other hand, it is, for obvious reasons, very difficult to test this hypothesis.

Although millions of pounds have been poured into research on treatment for lung cancer and thousands of scientific papers have been written, there is no solid evidence that any treatment 'cures' this type of cancer. For a time it was believed that radiotherapy could prolong life, but this is now widely questioned and most doctors believe it is mainly useful in reducing symptoms. Convincing data one way or the other are lacking. More recently, powerful and relatively toxic drugs have been developed which can certainly suppress or even cure some cancers. Un-

fortunately, they do not appear to be at all effective on lung cancers, with the exception of a particular type called small cell carcinoma. In this type of lung cancer it appears probable that the drugs can prolong life in some patients by a matter of months or even occasionally years, and most doctors now seem to believe that it is worth offering their patients this possibility, although again our ability to predict which patients will respond well and which patients will develop severe or even sometimes fatal reactions to the drugs is virtually non-existent. All in all, our ignorance of lung cancer and its treatment is depressing.

Tuberculosis

It is perhaps encouraging to end with a disease where out ignorance is slightly less, namely tuberculosis. Tuberculosis is one of the oldest and epidemiologically most important respiratory diseases. It has been identified in Egyptian mummies 5000 years old and has caused the death of countless people down the ages. With improving control of malaria, tuberculosis has become one of the world's most important communicable diseases. In the more developed countries the incidence of tuberculosis has fallen steadily this century, but it is still an appreciable problem, particularly among lower socioeconomic groups and people of Asian origin. We have much more knowledge about tuberculosis than most other respiratory diseases. We know that it is caused by an infecting organism, *Mycobacterium tuberculosis*, which is transmitted from person to person. There are, however, many mysteries. For example, it has been shown in Great Britain that it is possible to confer a considerable, although not complete, degree of immunity to tuberculosis by injection of a non-virulent organism, Bacillus Calmette-Guerin (BCG), in a manner similar to smallpox vaccination. However, a large scale programme for BCG vaccination carried out recently in India has been surprisingly ineffective. There appear to be other national differences. Thus immigrants to the UK of Indian origin have a much higher tendency to develop glandular tuberculosis than do the indigenous population, who more frequently develop respiratory tuberculosis. Furthermore, glandular tuberculosis can be much harder to treat and the glands can increase in size even on apparently effective treatment. The cause of these differences is obscure. There is some evidence that there may be minor differences between the types of infecting organisms and possibly there are differences in the body's immune reactions to tuberculosis in different races. It has also been suggested that vitamin D may be important in preventing glandular tuberculosis and that this may be relatively more plentiful in the indigenous population. However, this would not explain why immigrants of African origin do not appear to be particularly predisposed to glandular tuberculosis.

The modern drug treatment of tuberculosis is highly effective but it is based on empirical observations. Drugs have gradually been discovered which, when tested in patients with tuberculosis, appear to kill the organism but not the patient. In an elegant series of studies carried out over 25 years, the British Medical Research Council and collaborators tried various combinations of antituberculous drugs and went a very long way to showing which are the most effective combinations with the fewest side effects. Again, these results are the product of careful observation in controlled trials and could not be predicted from our knowledge of tuberculosis or the chemical nature of the drugs themselves.

Conclusions

Doctors are able to help patients in many ways. They can frequently make a diagnosis, usually by a process of pattern recognition, using information from history, clinical examination and investigations. Once a diagnosis has been made it is sometimes possible to initiate effective treatment which may cure the disease, or perhaps more frequently alleviate the symptoms. If the disease is progressive the doctor can provide comfort and support. To perform these the doctor is able to call upon a substantial body of useful and relevant knowledge. On the other hand, his areas of ignorance are vast. It is exceedingly uncommon to find a disease whose pathophysiology can be understood comprehensively in terms of the fundamental disciplines of anatomy, physiology and biochemistry. Indeed, as we have seen, our comprehension of these in relation even to the normal respiratory system is in many respects woefully lacking. Our ability to project the knowledge we have to the diseased state is exceedingly tenuous. However, by accumulating empirical knowledge, conducting carefully structured studies and observing and quantifying the natural history of diseases and the results of our interventions, progress is continually being made. It is reasonable to believe that by this process we will steadily uncover more of the iceberg, reducing thereby our ignorance of the respiratory system in health and disease.

Further Reading

BATES, D.V., MACKLEM, P.T. and CHRISTIE, R.V. (1971) *Respiratory Function in Disease.* 2nd edition, W.B. Saunders, Philadelphia, London and Toronto.
CROFTON, J. and DOUGLAS, A. (1981) *Respiratory Diseases.* 3rd edition, Blackwell, Oxford.

DOLL, R. and PETO, R. (1976) Mortality in relation to smoking: 20 years' observations of British doctors. *British Medical Journal*, **4**, 1525.

EMERSON, P. (1981) *Thoracic Medicine*. Butterworths, London.

FLENLEY, D.C. (1980) *Recent Advances in Respiratory Medicine*. Churchill Livingstone, Edinburgh and London.

Royal College of Physicians of London (1977) *Smoking* or *Health*. Pitman Medical, Tonbridge Wells.

SCADDING, J.G. and CUMMING, G. (1981) *Scientific Foundations of Respiratory Medicine*. William Heinemann, London.

THURLBECK, W.M. (1978) *The Lung Structure, Function and Disease*. Williams and Wilkins, Baltimore.

THE NEED FOR IGNORANCE IN CANCER RESEARCH

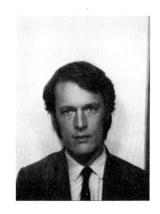

Richard Peto

Reader in Cancer Studies, University of Oxford.

He has worked chiefly as a clinical trial statistician and as a chronic disease epidemiologist for the past 15 years. His long-term hope is to continue moving towards an overview of the important causes of human disease that is not too far removed from the fine detail of the observed correlates of human disease, to encourage the search for further such correlates (including particularly the biochemical correlates of future disease onset rates, as these may help elucidate the role of infective, nutritional and hormonal factors), and finally to engender proper randomised intervention studies, perhaps of certain nutritional factors, that are relevant to this overview.

The most extraordinary thing about cancer is that multicellular organisms such as bristlecone pines, whales and humans can exist at all without developing multiple cancers within a few weeks of conception. Any cell in a tissue such as the liver has a genetically determined program which, together with the signals it receives from the rest of the body, tells it when to divide, when not to divide, when to differentiate and when to die. In a healthy body, cells should, and do, die all the time in unimaginable numbers; for example, of the 1,000,000,000,000 or so platelets in your blood, 100,000,000,000 will die tomorrow, and of course a similar number of new ones will be born. Accidental changes can be made in the genetic program of one individual cell in a tissue which will be inherited by both daughters when that cell divides, and if such a 'somatically heritable' change was made which conferred even the slightest selective advantage onto the altered family of cells then one might imagine that that change would be selected for very vigorously within one person's body, with disastrous neoplastic consequences. Of course we know that any individuals who could not keep Darwinian evolution in check among the cells of their own body would die of cancer long before they had children, so the real question is by what conceivable mechanisms can we keep Darwinian evolution among the cells of our bodies in check for our three score years and ten? Animal cells grown in glass dishes are subject to overgrowth by transformed clones, so why aren't animal cells grown in animals equally susceptible? One partial answer is that perhaps very, very few of the apparently viable cells in our bodies are really viable in the long term (the stem cells) and that all the rest have very firm instructions indeed that no matter what advantageous change they invent they must all die after, perhaps, a fixed time or a fixed number of further cell divisions, so their 'advantage' will die with them. If, as a safety precaution, there are several independent self-destruct mechanisms in each cell that should be moribund, then the risk of such a cell altering its genetic information in time to bypass all of them at once may be so remote that we need worry about cancer developing only from the 'stem' cells. However, even the stem cells seem to be rather better protected against cancer than one might imagine. When mammalian cells are grown *in vitro* it seems that a single heritable change, produced either spontaneously or by chemicals, etc. often suffices to transform them and to allow one cell to overgrow its unaltered neighbours. This may, however, be an artefact of the currently available cell culture conditions, in which perhaps only cells which are already halfway towards being cancerous can thrive. In contrast, *in vivo* it seems as though rather more distinct heritable changes are needed to change an epithelial stem cell into the seed of a growing cancer. (Our non-epithelial cells are even more amazingly cancer-proof than our epithelial cells are, so 90% of the human cancers that do eventually arise affect the epithelia that line our air ways, milk ducts, guts, glands, etc.) We have as yet no reliable idea of what these various cellular changes may be, but they are clearly under reasonably rapid evolutionary control (over a period of a few million years), otherwise longevity and large body size could not have been attained. Indeed, there is quite a real sense in which human epithelial cells can be said to be a

billion times more cancer-proof than mouse epithelial cells. For epithelial cells in both mice and men, the cumulative probability of cancer increases about tenfold with every doubling of age. Since our lifespan is about $2 \times 2 \times 2 \times 2 \times 2$ (= 32) that of laboratory animals, while the number of cells of which we are composed is perhaps 1000 times the number of which a mouse is composed, our individual cells must have to have evolved ways of being about $10 \times 10 \times 10 \times 10 \times 10 \times 1000$ times more cancer-proof than individual mouse cells are for our lifelong risk of cancer to be about the same as the lifelong risk for a mouse (which, to the degree of approximation presently relevant, it probably is).

By what conceivable mechanisms can our epithelial cells continue to be a million or a billion times more cancer-proof than are the epithelial cells of rodents? The protective processes probably do lie in the cells rather than in the whole organism, because human cells grown individually or in cultured tissues are extremely difficult to transform from a semi-normal to a semi-cancerous condition, while such 'transformation' can be achieved relatively easily with cultured rodent tissues. We know that DNA-damaging chemicals are often carcinogenic, but DNA is chemically rather similar in mice and men and even though the marvellous repair mechanisms which constantly seek out and correct local damage in DNA are more rapid and accurate in humans than in rodents, it is difficult to believe that these differences alone could account for this million- or billion-fold difference.

There are other lines of evidence that suggest that alteration of a normal into a malignant cell requires not just the 'early' changes that can be brought about by the action of a DNA-damaging chemical (or, perhaps more commonly, by some oxidative accident), but also certain other 'late' changes, some but not necessarily all of which can be brought about by classical 'promoters'.

Perhaps it is these 'later' stages on which evolution has chiefly worked so effectively to give us our longevity (John Cairns, a molecular biologist whose discoveries chiefly relate to the early stages of carcinogenesis, once commented in frustration that 'The key to understanding carcinogenesis is to understand the later stages of carcinogenesis; the early stages are just trivial molecular biology'). If evolution, in just a few dozen million years, can manipulate these late processes so profoundly, reducing the risk per cell by a few orders of magnitude, will an understanding of them be of any practical value to us? After all, just half an order of magnitude reduction in the rates at which these 'late' processes occur in partially altered cells would knock 70% off the cancer problem, which would be a useful start!

Alternatively, and possibly to more immediate effect, perhaps we can merely bear in mind the general conclusion that such biological knowledge as we have suggests that minor changes can probably produce major changes in cancer onset rates and then see whether, without understanding exactly how human carcinogenesis generally takes place, we can discover some dietary, hormonal, infective, occupational or other environmental factors determined by out lifestyle that importantly affect the risks of cancer.

For example, smoking currently causes about one-third of all cancer deaths and the research that led to this did not depend on any cellular biology at all (beyond the ability of doctors to distinguish moderately reliably between cancers arising from different parts of the body). It was merely noted from routine monitoring of certified causes of death that lung cancer death certification rates were rising rapidly, the rise being more rapid in men than in women and so presumably not wholly artefactual. Because of this, a study was initiated in which lung cancer patients and other patients were asked a mass of questions about their work, place of residence, eating, drinking and smoking habits

and the only big difference to emerge was that whereas only about half the other patients smoked cigarettes, nearly all the lung cancer patients did so. In other words, lung cancer patients seemed to be drawn overwhelmingly from among the cigarette-smoking half of the population. Because of this, prospective studies began which concentrated more directly on the exact smoking habits of tens or hundreds of thousands of apparently healthy people, any deaths among whom over the next decade or more were then monitored. This revealed that smoking was associated with a far wider range of causes of death than just lung cancer, the strongest associations being with death from cancers of the mouth, throat, larynx or lung and with death from chronic obstructive lung disease. Another important association was with death from vascular disease. Subsequent epidemiological research has confirmed that much, though not all, of the excess mortality associated with smoking is actually caused by smoking, so that smoking causes not only one-third of all U.S. and U.K. cancer deaths, but also an even greater number of deaths from causes other than cancer. These discoveries have already been of some practical importance and will eventually be of even greater public health importance. Historians in future centuries, in which smoking is no longer normal, may have some difficulty understanding the slowness with which societies in the 20th and 21st centuries responded to the discovery of the health effects of tobacco!

The present importance of the story of this discovery, however, is that it did not depend on any serious understanding of the mechanism(s) of carcinogenesis, nor on reliable identification of the importantly causative component(s) of tobacco smoke: indeed, neither has yet been achieved. This indicates that there are two alternative or rather complementary approaches to the prevention of cancer, the mechanistic strategy and the black box strategy. The former is the classical method that a pure scientist might recommend: understand the mechanisms of carcinogenesis and the preventive measures will follow. The latter, which has yielded by far the most important results so far in the prevention of chronic disease, merely seeks many correlates, or inverse correlates, of the risk of onset of various types of cancer among people of a given age, in the hope that among these many correlates or inverse correlates a few real causes or real preventive measures will be discovered. Preventive measures that affect the later stages of carcinogenesis may, moreover, have effects sufficiently rapid to be assessed reliably in a randomised intervention study of practicable size, complexity and duration. Again, however, this is part of the approach that treats the human body as a 'black box'.

Thus far, not only has almost all of the important knowledge about how to prevent cancer come from 'black box' epidemiology, but so too has the most direct evidence that most human cancer is avoidable. For, it has been observed that the onset rates of most types of cancer among people of a given age in different populations can differ quite widely. This may be true if the populations are defined by race, by religion, by occupation, by social class, by area of residence within one country, by sexual, dietary, drinking or smoking habits, or by reproductive history and it is certainly true if the populations are defined by country of residence. Moreover, when people migrate from one country to another they generally change their pattern of internal cancer onset rates, so the large international differences in internal cancer onset rates are not chiefly genetic. For example, after cancer of the lung, cancer of the large intestine is the commonest type of fatal cancer in North America, and it is equally common among U.S. whites and U.S. blacks, but is only one-tenth as common (by a given age) among blacks in West Africa, from where most of the U.S. blacks originated. This suggests that at least 90% of the U.S.

mortality from cancer of the large intestine might be avoidable by means sufficiently practicable for some populations already to have adopted them and the same is true for many other types of cancer.

'Black box' epidemiology has also suggested a rather surprising constraint on where one ought to start looking for avoidable causes of the commonest types of cancer (apart from lung cancer) in developed countries. For, over the past half century there has been, apart from the massive effects of smoking, surprisingly little change in U.S. or U.K. age-specific rates for most types of cancer. So, the long-established aspects of the American lifestyle must include some important determinant(s) of why U.S. mortality rates from cancers of the breast, large intestine, etc. differ so greatly from those in Japan, Africa and various other countries. For a recent review of current knowledge bearing on such matters, see Doll, R. and Peto, R. (1981).

Thus, a black box approach by scientists ignorant of the cellular mechanisms of carcinogenesis has thus far yielded:

(i) an avoidable cause (smoking) for about one-third of all US and UK cancer deaths;
(ii) the large majority of the several dozen other known causes of human cancer (all of which are, however, far less important in the US and UK than tobacco, and which collectively account for barely ten per cent of all cancer deaths in developed countries, although betel quid chewing, hepatitis B infection and probably, aflatoxin are major causes of cancer in certain underdeveloped countries);
(iii) evidence, based on large, non-genetic international contrasts, that most of the non-tobacco induced cancers in virtually every country (developed or not) are also potentially avoidable, though not peculiarly modern, diseases.

In these circumstances, it is difficult to agree with the editor of Nature who wrote, in a recent leading article (*Nature* 1981, 289, 431) that 'it will be time enough to talk about causes when the mechanisms have been worked out'!

Unfortunately, the low scientific repute of a 'black box' approach, as compared with a 'mechanistic' approach, to cancer research that this sort of quotation reflects has meant that many really obvious lines of epidemiological study, especially of dietary, hormonal or infective factors, remain unexplored. (For example, there has not even been any remotely systematic search among the hundreds of measurable aspects of human blood biochemistry and immunology for the important correlates and inverse correlates in the blood of healthy people of future cancer risks!). There is a danger that too great a commitment to the search for mechanisms will divert attention from the search for causes, and an *Encyclopaedia of Ignorance* might be a good place to complain about this.

Further Reading

DOLL, R. & PETO, R. (1981), The causes of cancer: Quantitative estimates of avoidable risks of cancer in the United States today. *Journal of the National Cancer Institute USA*, 66, 1191–1309. (Also available as an Oxford University Press paperback.)
A review for educated non-specialists of how we know cancer to be avoidable, what we currently know about how to avoid it, and what we are likely to discover over the next few years about how to avoid it. (The aim is to present a *quantitative* perspective.)

PETO, R. (1977), Epidemiology, multistage models and short-term mutagenicity tests. In: *Origins of Human Cancer*, (Hiatt, H., Watson, J.D. and Winsten, J., eds.), 1403–1428, Cold Spring Harbor publications, New York.
A review of some current knowledge and uncertainties about the mechanisms of carcinogenesis, together with reasons for distrusting some of what we think we know.

CAIRNS, J. (1975), Mutation, selection and the natural history of cancer. *Nature*, 255, 197–200.
An excellent example of imaginative, thoughtful, testable speculation.

CAIRNS, J. (1981), The origin of human cancers. *Nature*, 289, 353–357.
More imaginative, thoughtful, testable speculation.

CANCER

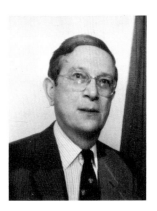

N.M. Bleehen

Professor of Clinical Oncology and Radiotherapeutics, University of Cambridge.

Formerly Professor of Radiotherapy, Middlesex Hospital Medical School. He has written various publications on medicine, biochemistry and radiotherapy.

There can be few diseases which evoke more emotion from the public than cancer. Ignorance, both about the nature of the disease and the possibility of the very real successes of some therapy, results in almost universal fear. It is a group of diseases where the doctors also largely remain ignorant about its etiology, prevention and treatment. Cancer is the second commonest cause of death in the United Kingdom, although about a quarter of all patients who develop cancer are cured of their disease. In addition, it should not be forgotten that as a result of treatment, many achieve very long term symptomatic relief.

Cancer is a disordered proliferation of cells which will invade normal tissues, destroying them as they go. It may arise in most of the normal tissues of the body and its behaviour will depend on the site of origin. Some cancers are only very locally invasive and can easily be controlled by local measures. Others are rapidly invasive and spread, by so-called metastases, to other parts of the body distant from the primary tumour. This may occur through blood or lymphatic channels, or sometimes across body cavities. Once this spread has occurred, cure of the patient becomes much more difficult and local methods of treatment, such as surgery or radiotherapy, are less successful. The word cancer is a synonym for 'malignant neoplasm or tumour'.

Some tumours are not malignant and are said to be 'benign'. They are not invasive nor do they metastasize to other parts of the body. They may sometimes be removed surgically with a successful outcome.

The management of any cancer must therefore take into careful account the site of origin of the disease, its size and the extent, presence or absence of distant metastases. These assessments are made on the basis of conventional clinical examination — special investigations such as X-rays and biochemical tests. These are then interpreted in the light of previous experience. Unfortunately, none of these tests are absolutely certain and our ignorance in this field largely results in the failure of therapy. Additionally, where there is a choice of possible treatments, the actual criteria for choosing a particular form of treatment may be uncertain. Some of these uncertainties and extents of our ignorance are discussed in this chapter.

Cancer has been recognized for at least 3000–4000 years. Thus the Ebers Papyrus from Egypt which dates from around 1500 B.C. mentions ulcerated tumours. A few cancers, particularly of the bone, have been identified in mummies dating from even earlier. In the 3rd–5th Egyptian dynasties (c. 5000 years ago). Treatments described in the papyri of this time include surgery with a knife or red hot iron, and possible palliative treatments with mixtures of boiled barley and dates.

Hippocrates, known as the founder of medicine, who lived in the island of Cos around 460–370 B.C., knew and described cancer of the breast, uterus, stomach, skin and mouth. He classified the tumours into the hard cancer and the ulcerated cancer and thought that these were associated with an excess of 'black bile', one of the four humours manufactured by the spleen and the stomach. This black bile, or melanchole, remained the principal theoretical cause of cancer for a further two millenia. Hippocrates did not advocate any specific treatments, but associated with it one of his cardinal contributions to clinical practice, that of 'primum non nocere' — that is, if you can do no good, at least do no harm by unwise intervention.

Even following the era of experimental medicine, dating from the 17th century work of William Harvey on the circulation of the blood, no real improvements in therapy appeared, other than technical advances in surgery, until the turn of this century.

We thus enter the twentieth century without any real knowledge as to the cause, or causes, of cancer and any effective treatment other than surgery, which was frequently mutilating and rarely successful. Advances in technology and biological research have now provided us with further treatments. These include radiation therapy, resulting from the discovery of X-rays by Roentgen in 1895 and the isolation of radium by the Curies at around a similar time. Exploitation of the biological effects of ionizing radiation on normal and malignant tissues very rapidly produced a new modality of treatment which was able to cure some cancers not easily managed by surgery and to palliate many others.

There has long been a dream to have a medicine which will cure all cancers. Unfortunately, chemotherapy still lags far behind this aim. However, since the Second World War, numerous drugs have been developed and tested, a few of which are therapeutically successful in the management of a variety of cancers. Thus some of the diseases where management has been changed by the introduction of new chemotherapeutic agents include many of the lymphomas, testicular tumours, chorionic carcinoma and some tumours in children. We are now in a situation where some of the rarer diseases may be controlled by such chemotherapy, whilst useful palliation can be obtained in others. This particular field of clinical cancer therapeutic research is a rapidly expanding one and is promising much for the future.

Thus, the three principal modalities of treatment we now use for our patients are surgery, radiotherapy and chemotherapy. There are others that are also employed which are much less well authenticated and are the subject of active clinical research. These include immunotherapy, the use of agents to improve the host's resistance to their tumour, and hyperthermia which employs methods to increase the temperature of tumours to several degrees above normal body temperature in an attempt to destroy them. In addition to these authenticated and 'respectable' but experimental techniques, there are many others still being used. There is perhaps no disease which has provoked so many quack therapies as cancer, largely because of the fear and desperation of the patients and their relatives.

Cancer research is an extremely active field of biomedical work. This research will range from fundamental investigations into the molecular basis of the malignant deviation of the cancer cell, through to biochemical, pathological, epidemiological and prevention research. Each of these is important as it attacks the problem at different levels. Clearly, identification of the basic defect in the cell, if such exists, will be important because this should provide a basis for a rational reversion back to a normal state. However, we continue to treat patients in the absence of such information and patients continue to be cured in the absence of this information. Those of us who are directly involved in the therapy of patients believe that we have to continue to improve the results of our semi-empirical treatments by equally empirical advances until such time as the basic science allows us to be scientifically precise. As a clinical oncologist, I will concentrate most on our ignorance concerning methods of curing cancer.

Surgery

Surgical techniques in themselves are not likely to produce further major advances in the treatment of cancer. Indeed in a disease such as cancer of the breast, little advance has been made in the past eighty years. As a physician, I am not competent to judge where the future technical advances may take place. However, at present the main area of ignorance in the surgical management of cancer relates to the treatment of the occult metastases. There are many local treatments which fail because of the presence of these metastases at the time of apparently successful local resection of the tumour. Much work is now being carried out to decide on the place of chemotherapy and other adjuvant treatments to control this sub-clinical spread at the time of primary surgery. These concepts will be discussed later in this chapter when chemotherapy is considered.

Radiation Therapy

Radiation therapy relies on the ability of certain forms of ionizing and particulate radiation to damage biological tissues. We are still uncertain as to the exact mechanism of this damage and why tumour control may occur in spite of normal tissue damage which is also produced by these treatments. Radiation therapy is normally given over a period of days or weeks with the total radiation dose being fractionated into individual treatments. The treatments are usually given five times a week or sometimes three times a week or less. It is now believed that this fractionation enables normal tissues to recover from damage more rapidly than the tumour. This results in a therapeutic threshold in which the final damage to the tumour is more than that to the normal tissue.

Laboratory methods for determining the proliferation characteristics of both tumour and normal tissues exist, however these are very difficult to translate meaningfully to the clinical situation in man. Techniques to enable us to do this might be of considerable value in planning more rational radiation fractionation treatments. Currently, we base the fractionation more on the 24 hour day and 5 day working week than on any biological rhythm likely to be present in the patient. Times of treatment relate to times of convenience, and may be altered because of such biologically trivial events as weekends, bank holidays and religious festivals. The problems of translating appropriate laboratory techniques to the clinic remain to be solved. Most are invasive and may perturb the situation in such a way that the information obtained is worthless. Considerable efforts in clinically orientated research are going on to develop new techniques. These may include some of the advances in biophysical techniques currently in progress, as well as conceptual leaps which have yet to be made.

One of the major contributions from radiation biology towards radiotherapy has been the identification of the concept of the 'oxygen effect'. As far back as 1907, Schwartz demonstrated that pressure on skin, with consequent reduction of its blood supply, might protect that skin from X-ray damage. Subsequently, in the 1950s the work of Gray and his colleagues, showed that many tumours almost certainly contained cells deprived of oxygen and nutrients, because of their remoteness from the capilliaries and small blood vessels. It was thought that these hypoxic cells were the cells that might survive radiation treatments and therefore result in failure of treatment. Considerable effort has been made since that time in an attempt to improve radiation therapy by increasing the oxygenation of tumours. One technique that has been used is to treat patients breathing oxygen under pressure in hyperbaric oxygen tanks. These studies, in a variety of diseases, have now been carrying on for nearly thirty years and it is only recently that some evidence has suggested that an improvement in results, for example in carcinoma of the larynx and cervix, may be obtained. We remain, however, ignorant of the role of this treatment in many other diseases. These treatments using hyperbaric oxygen are very cumbersome, time consuming for patients and staff, and are unlikely to be generally acceptable. Other methods are therefore being investigated.

Radiation with neutrons is one such technique. These particles are not thought to be as dependent on oxygen for their biological effect. Early tests at Berkeley, California in the late 1930s, resulted in major tissue damage, largely because of ignorance of the biological background for the fractionation of the treatments. Subsequent research has led to a more rational basis for therapy and new clinical trials are in progress. The machines required to produce these particles are cyclotrons and are considerably more expensive than most normal therapy machines. Preliminary results of this work have shown promise but have yet to confirm their place as established therapy.

One problem concerned with this type of treatment is our ignorance as to the optimum way to design the clinical research studies concerned. Formal clinical trials requires a comparison of at least two different forms of treatment. In this case, the treatment being compared with neutron therapy is conventional ionizing radiation therapy from the machines producing X-rays. In the absence of the methods already mentioned for measuring the kinetic parameters of these tissues and also the detailed *in situ* biological response, it becomes very difficult to choose what might be the optimum therapy regime for one modality. Much of the choice will remain the clinical dogma of the therapists concerned and may be less convincing to the others who stand in the side lines waiting for the results!

Both the techniques of hyperbaric oxygen

and neutron therapy are either cumbersome or expensive and alternative methods for overcoming the problem of the hypoxic cell are being actively pursued. One such method employs drugs which diffuse into the neurotic parts of a tumour and mimic the radio-sensitizing action of oxygen. Such hypoxic cell radiosensitizers have been identified and are undergoing clinical trials. In experimental systems, improved control of tumours can be obtained without a comparable increase in normal tissue damage. Unfortunately, such treatments have yet to show comparable value in clinical practice.

Our ignorance in this situation is exemplified by the fact that several promising drugs have been identified which will act as useful hypoxic cell sensitizers in experimental animals. The toxicity of these drugs has been well identified as far as these model systems are concerned. However when at least two of these drugs, which have now been taken into the clinic, have been investigated their usefulness has been severely hampered by a side effect that had not been identified in the experimental model. Neurotoxicity is a major dose limiting factor in man, and this was not at all apparent in the preliminary animal testing of these drugs. As yet, we still have no satisfactory model which will pick up this sort of toxicity in the hundreds of new radiosensitizers that now have been synthesized to follow on from the first generation drugs.

Chemotherapy

The toxicity testing of drugs is an extremely important aspect of modern drug development. It is no less important where the treatment of cancer is involved, although of course a smaller therapeutic threshold may be accepted in this situation than in the treatment of a simple infection by an intibiotic or a headache with an analgesic. Adequate toxicity testing by current techniques is very time consuming and expensive. Most drug regulatory authorities will insist, quite correctly, on as much detailed testing as is possible. However, as the above example shows, this may not necessarily give the full answer. We also know that toxicities with other drugs may appear which were not originally detected by the screening methods currently employed, as for example with thalidomide. Much work is required to provide more certain methods of evaluating the toxicity of different classes of drugs. This is essential if we are to improve the results of treating cancer by chemotherapy.

Modern anti-cancer chemotherapy commenced during the Second World War and was a by-product of poison gas warfare. A military transport vessel containing mustard gas sank and the effect of the released agent on the blood cells of servicemen exposed to it was noticed. A possible anti-cancer value was postulated and the first nitrogen mustard drugs were developed in 1945. Since that time, probably in excess of 600,000 compounds have been developed and screened on experimental models. Of these, probably around 1% had some anti-cancer activity and 75 have been submitted to prolonged therapeutic trial in man. Only 30–40 are in general use in the clinic.

The biochemical specificity of many of these drugs still remains to be understood. However, a major problem in their design has been the absence of any clearly formulated and documented biochemical differences between tumour and normal cells which might then be exploited. Those that have been described have either failed to stand the test of time or have been disappointing in their lack of specificity. This has resulted in a toxic effect on normal as well as cancer cells. However, as with radiation therapy, recovery of normal cells enables a small therapeutic threshold to be obtained.

Various techniques are employed to try and improve the therapeutic threshold. One may use combinations of drugs with individual toxicities for different tissues. Many of the drugs act at different stages of the cell proliferation cycle. If we were able to assess these stages in patients' tumours during therapy, then true kinetic scheduling of the drugs might be possible. Various empirical attempts have been made to effect this, using sequences of drugs. However the evidence for their being any more effective than other less 'scientifically' designed regimes remains unconvincing. Should suitable techniques for improving drug scheduling be available, then improvements in therapeutic gain must ensue.

A major area of ignorance is the reason for differences in response to treatment between different patients with a similar tumour and also between different types of tumours. Thus, patients presenting with the same pathological type of lung cancer and apparently the same extent of disease may give very different responses when treated with radiation and drugs. This may result in cure of one and rapid death of the other. Obviously an extremely practical and useful advance in drug therapy would be the ability to predict the individual sensitivity of tumours to a range of likely drugs. This approach has been the subject of much research over many years and several techniques are now being claimed to assist such prediction. Attempts are being made to grow individual tumour cells from pieces removed from the patient and then expose them to different drugs. Their response is assessed by a variety of endpoints. The major problem with these techniques is that not all tumours are accessible to such removal and even when they are, many cells so removed will not grow under the artificial laboratory conditions. These current techniques, therefore, are only applicable in a relatively small proportion of patients. Having obtained growth under laboratory conditions, there is as yet no convincing evidence to show that in the majority of tumours the responses obtained are predictive of the results that would be obtained in man. Nor is it certain that better results are obtained by using the

drugs that have been predicted by the test rather than those that have been used empirically. With the current uncertainties about chemotherapy, major advances in these predictive techniques which could be easily applied to the majority of patients would be invaluable.

A further problem about chemotherapy is that, in the main, most drugs will act systemically throughout the body. If it were possible to target the drug selectively to tumours, this would have profound therapeutic implications. Once again, little advance has been made in this field, although numerous techniques have been applied. Perhaps most hope in this situation rests on the belief that it may be possible to identify specific antigenic components in tumour cells. Various candidates for such antigenic substances have been identified, although as yet none appear to be specific enough. If they do exist, then it may be possible to link cytotoxic drugs to antibodies which could then home in on to the tumour cells. Of particular relevance in this situation has been the production of uniquely specific antibodies using the hybridization techniques for monoclonal antibody production developed by Milstein. Considerable work is going on in this field but at this time we are still ignorant as to whether or not specific tumour antigens truly exist, or whether they just represent variations of expression of the normal differentiation antigens present in other cells.

It has already been mentioned that many of the failures of cancer therapy are because early metastatic spread of disease has already occurred by the time the patient first presents himself for treatment. This spread may be undetected clinically by conventional methods and the patient undergoes apparently radical treatment only to die subsequently because of the further growth of the metastases. Clearly, any technique which would identify these microscopic metastases earlier than currently possible would be of considerable advantage. In a very few tumours this is now possible. Thus in chorionic carcinoma, a malignant change in the placenta of women, secretion of the hormone human chorionic gonadatrophin can be monitored and levels measured in patients in whom no tumour is actually clinically detectable. By following these levels, it is possible to monitor the results of therapy. For most of the common tumours such substances are not produced. Should there be specific tumour products of the sort discussed above, then the use of antibodies to detect these products circulating in the blood, might then be used to monitor the results of therapy.

As mentioned earlier, much effort is currently being made in an attempt to treat these occult metastases in patients who have undergone radical surgery or radiotherapy. Chemotherapy is then given post-operatively for a period of months or years. These adjuvant treatments are not without their immediate toxicity. There is also the possibility of long term side effects because of the potentially carcinogenic nature of some of the drugs used. It would therefore be very desirable to be able to identify those patients who have a residual microscopic tumour burden by measuring any tumour products that are available. Equally important, it would be desirable to know when to stop these adjuvant treatments. At present, the duration of such courses is largely based as much on the tolerance of patient and physician as the viability of the residual tumour.

Numerous clinical studies investigating adjuvant treatment, particularly in such a common disease as carcinoma of the breast, are now in progress. These studies illustrate our ignorance of the situation extremely well. We know that perhaps a third of the patients with carcinoma of the breast will be cured of their cancer. However, it is difficult to talk with certainty about a cure, because some patients show a tumour recurrence more than twenty years after treatment of their breast cancer without any apparent tumour development in the intervening years. Clinical trial design will permit the assessment of suitable methods of treatment. However, it must be appreciated that in this particular situation it may be necessary to treat many hundreds, indeed thousands of patients in such a formal study and observe them for a very long period of time before adequate answers can be obtained. The value of tumour markers that could be used to anticipate clinical recurrence therefore cannot be overestimated.

The chemotherapeutic agents discussed above are largely destructive in their action; that is they are used to kill tumour cells more than normal cells. However, hope exists that it might be possible to identify agents which would reverse the malignant change and cause differentiation back to the normal state. As yet we are unable to do this although various classes of agents have been looked at. Obviously the most useful approach would be if a specific molecular defect were identified which could then be approached by molecular engineering techniques. We are perhaps not as far away from this as we were ten years ago due to the advent of remarkably specific methodologies developed by molecular biologists. Nonetheless, the problems involved with such approaches remain enormous.

Immunotherapy

The concept of immunological resistance to tumour growth was proposed by Ehrlich at the turn of the century. This was made fashionable by Bernard Shaw's description of Sir Colenso Ridgeon, in his play *The Doctor's Dilemma*, who advocated stimulation of the phagocytes. Many attempts have been made since that time to improve the host's resistance to tumours, but in the main these have all lacked any convincing success.

These have either related to an attempt to boost the host's natural resistance by a variety of non-specific agents or attempts to interact with putative specific antigens in tumours. As we have already discussed, the evidence for these remains uncertain. It is therefore not surprising perhaps that very little in the way of convincing data has emerged from a vast amount of effort in this field. The subject, however, continuously revives itself as new circulating immune cells are identified by immunologists and agents which modify them are described. Thus the recent flurry of interest in the use of interferon in cancer treatment, with successes still largely unsubstantiated, possibly relates to the stimulation of one recently identified blood cell, known as the natural killer cell. Its activity in patients is thought to be increased by interferon. At present the results of immunotherapy range from the frankly incredible reports of uncritical enthusiasts to the sombre and realistic assessments of their more scientific colleagues. It is largely ignorance of specific immunological differences between tumour and normal cells which is perhaps the greatest barrier at this time to the realistic implementation of such techniques.

Hyperthermia

The final modality of treatment which perhaps should be considered is that of hyperthermia. The ability of tumours to withstand temperatures of a few degrees above that of normal body temperature appears to be less than that of the normal tissues. This probably relates more to the metabolic environment of these tumours than any specific differences between the tumour cells and the normal cells. Thus the increase in acidity known to occur in tumours, and their poor oxygenation, may well relate to some of this thermal sensitivity. Additionally, an impaired blood supply permits greater accumulation of heat from external sources in the tumour than

in the normal tissue. One reason for excitement about such a technique is that it may well be complementary to the conventional methods of radiation and chemotherapy. Hyperthermia does appear to enhance the effects of radiation treatment and also some drugs. Unfortunately, this may occur both in normal tissues and tumours. More information is therefore required before one can hope for any major therapeutic advances in this field.

Perhaps the most important region of ignorance here is our inability to deliver and measure the defined amounts of heat required in the tumour. It is relatively easy to heat the whole patient's body up to a specific temperature, although the physiological response of the patient may then be more difficult to control. What is much more difficult is to raise the temperature of a tumour volume in a patient to say 42–44°C whilst maintaining a lower temperature in the normal tissues immediately surrounding it. The difference in the blood supplies of tumour and normal tissue may help in this situation but the physical methodology for so delivering the heat are as yet very imprecise. Even more difficult is the accurate measurement of the temperature in these tissues. Virtually all present techniques are invasive and interact with the radiofrequency and microwaves used in the heating methods. Advances in this field to combat our ignorance undoubtedly will occur over the next few years. They are largely a matter of technology and the finance required to solve the difficulties. Whether or not these will then have a major impact on therapy and result in the cure of tumours otherwise not cured in man, will remain to be seen.

Conclusions

The above discussion has largely concentrated on methods of treatment and monitoring the results of treatment. We are clearly ignorant about many of the factors that might be associated with the response of the tumour and its removal when it has been damaged by the treatment. Methods to enhance this clearance of damaged tumour would possibly improve treatment results, particularly if the damaged tissues still maintained a potential for re-growth. Methods for reducing the effects of treatments on normal tissues also would be advantageous in improving the therapeutic ratio. Research is now in progress using certain protective agents which were originally designed as radiation protectors for military use. These also seem to have a protective effect on some chemotherapeutic agents. Development of new classes of these agents is required.

The emphasis on therapy implies a certain pessimism about the prevention of cancer; this is not intended. Certainly many of the risk factors involved in the development of cancer have now been identified. Numerous carcinogenic agents are known, such as certain dyes which will cause bladder cancer. It is relatively easy to remove these from industrial processes. However, major morbidity and mortality ensues from other identifiable components of our environment, which as yet we have not been able to eliminate. Cigarette smoking is an extreme example where we have very good information to link the large numbers of patients developing lung cancer with the long term smoking of cigarettes. In a study on British male doctors, the relative risks of developing lung cancer were assessed for smokers versus non-smokers. Those who smoked up to 14 cigarettes per day showed an 8-fold increased risk of developing lung cancer, whilst for those smoking 25 cigarettes or more per day, it was 25-fold. Since that study there has been a considerable reduction in the cigarette smoking habits of doctors, but unfortunately educating people about the harmful effects of smoking has so far made very little impact on the problem. We appear to be totally ignorant about successful ways of coping with this social problem.

The risks associated with other environmental pollutants which might be carcinogenic are also difficult to assess. Epidemiological studies have helped us to understand the importance of some of these, for example, the association of asbestosis with a particular form of lung cancer, mesothelioma. Similarly it has recently been proposed that there is a relationship between drinking coffee and cancer of the pancreas, but this hypothesis has not yet been substantiated. It has been postulated that perhaps three quarters of all cancers are preventable if only the external carcinogenic influences could be identified with certainty and then removed. This perhaps is an over-enthusiastic and somewhat unrealistic estimate of the situation. Even if they were identifiable, it seems very doubtful that we would be able to prevent them or their spread.

An encylopaedia of ignorance may inevitably read like a catalogue of pessimism. This is certainly not intended in this account of cancer treatment. Rather, it is intended to be a declaration of optimism for further therapeutic success. Time and much effort will surely justify this belief.

Further Reading

CAIRNS, J. (1978) *Science and Society*, W.H. Freeman, San Francisco.
DEELEY, T.J. (1979) *Attitudes to Cancer*, SPCK.
ISRAEL, L. (1981) *Conquering Cancer*, Penguin, London.

IMMUNITY TO VIRUSES

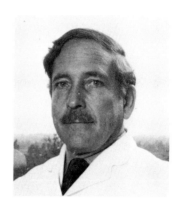

Anthony Clifford Allison

Director of the Institute of Biological Sciences, Syntex Research, Palo Alto, California, USA.

He has spent most of his career as a member of the Scientific Staff of the Medical Research Council at the National Institute for Medical Research, Mill Hill, and the Clinical Research Centre, Harrow, where he was Head of the Cell Pathology Division. From 1978 to 1980 he was Director of the International Laboratory for Research on Animal Diseases, Nairobi, Kenya. His major research interest has been the immunology of infectious diseases.

Chemotherapy has so far been less efficacious against viruses than against any other micro-organisms. However, the recent development of acycloguanosine, a non-toxic drug that is highly effective against herpesvirus infections, shows that this may not always be the case in the future. Nevertheless, for the present the principal method of controlling virus infections is active immunization which may be achieved by the introduction of a suitable vaccine into the body. The vaccine contains a form of the organism, or its toxins, which retains the antigens of the original but lacks its harmful effects.

Studies of immunity to viruses have been of historic importance. The first vaccine was that used by Edward Jenner against smallpox in 1798. He showed that virus isolated from cows could protect humans against smallpox, hence the term 'vaccine' which is derived from 'vacca', the Latin word for cow. In 1967 the World Health Organization initiated a global vaccination campaign against smallpox, systematically immunizing contacts of cases. The disease was eradicated ten years later, one of the great achievements of applied medical science.

A second major success was vaccination against yellow fever virus, which is transmitted by mosquitoes and caused widespread serious disease in West Africa and Central America. The occurrence of yellow fever and

TABLE 1. Some human virus invections

Type of virus	Virus	Site of infection	Host protection
Poxvirus	Smallpox	Generalized	Vaccination with live virus
Herpesvirus	Herpes Simplex 1	Primary in oropharynx	Acycloguanosine
	Herpes Simplex 2	Genital	Acycloguanosine
	Varicella-zoster (chicken pox, shingles)	Primary generalized, later along the path of a nerve	Immune globulin
	Epstein-Barr virus (infectious mononucleosis)	Primary of oropharynx and B lymphocytes. Associated with lymphoma and nasopharyngeal cancer	None
Enterovirus	Poliovirus (3 strains)	Primary of the intestine and oropharynx. Sometimes spreads to neurons of the central nervous sytem	Vaccination with live or killed virus
Myxovirus	Influenza virus (many antigenic types)	Respiratory	Vaccination with killed virus
Paramyxovirus	Measles	Generalized	Vaccination with live virus
	Rubella	Generalized	Vaccination with live virus
Flavivirus	Yellow fever virus	Generalized (liver)	Vaccination with live virus
	Hepatitis B virus	Hepatitis	Vaccination with killed virus antigen

malaria were amongst the major factors that foiled the French attempt to construct the Panama Canal; also naval and military personnel serving in the Caribbean area often died of yellow fever. Mosquito control and then vaccination against this disease, the latter introduced during the second World War, have dramatically reduced casualties from yellow fever.

The improvements in hygiene and living conditions this century have also helped to reduce the mortality from several infectious diseases, including measles which is a virus infection. However, they have actually aggravated the effects of poliomyelitis, by delaying the age at which persons became infected and thus increasing the likelihood of the development of the paralytic form of the disease following the gastrointestinal infection with this virus. The development and use of killed and live poliovirus vaccines has been the critical factor in the sharp reduction of cases of paralytic poliomyelitis in industrialized countries during the past two decades. Several virus diseases of domestic animals have also been effectively controlled by vaccination, for example Marek's disease, a common malignant proliferative disease of lymphoid tissue which is caused by a herpesvirus and can be prevented by vaccination. This is the first case of effective vaccination against a type of cancer. Some human cancers are associated with viruses, and the possibility of preventing them by vaccination will be explored in this article.

The Immune System

There are two major mechanisms of immunity against viruses: one which is specific, the other, non-specific. Specific immunity is produced by the conventional immune responses mediated by the B- and T-lymphocytes of the immune system. This type of immunity is effective only against the same virus or antigenically related viruses. Lymphocytes have specific immunoglobulin receptors on their surfaces allowing them to recognize antigenic determinants. There is a great diversity in the specificity of these receptors in different B-lymphocytes. When B-lymphocytes with receptors for virus antigens bind to these antigens, the cells are stimulated to divide, and the expanded clones of cells eventually differentiate into antibody-secreting cells. There are five major classes of antibody, IgG, IgM, IgA, IgE and IgD. B cell differentiation is facilitated by a product of T-lymphocytes. Hence one of the roles of T-lymphocytes in virus infections is to help in the formation of antibodies against virus antigens, especially antibodies of the IgG and IgA classes.

Another role of T-lymphocytes is to kill virus-infected cells. A subpopulation of T-lymphocytes, which has receptors for the virus antigens expressed on the infected cell surfaces, multiplies in response to the infection and differentiates into cytotoxic cells. These can efficiently kill virus-infected cells provided that the latter have the same major histocompatibility antigens as the T-lymphocytes (HLA antigens in the case of human cells and H-2 in the case of mouse cells). Thus the lymphocytes apparently recognize viral antigens associated with major histocompatibility antigens.

Non-specific immune mechanisms rely on T-lymphocytes and are mediated by interferon. Cloned cytotoxic T-lymphocytes meeting virus antigens (associated with the right major histocompatibility antigens) will liberate a special type of interferon termed γ-interferon. The interferons are a family of glycoproteins which exert antiviral activity through cellular metabolic processes involving synthesis of both RNA and protein. Three types of interferon are now recognized: α- and β-interferons are produced by most cell types; they are acid stable, antigenically distinct and have molecular weights of 18,000 and 38,000 daltons respectively; γ-interferon is released by lymphocytes stimulated by antigens or mitogens, and has a molecular weight about 25,000 daltons. Interferons bind to receptors on most cell types (see Fig. 1) and activate an enzyme synthesizing short chains of adenosine residues linked by 2'-5'-phosphodiester bonds (instead of the 3'-5'-phosphodiester bonds characteristic of nucleic acids), with terminal adenosine triphosphate.

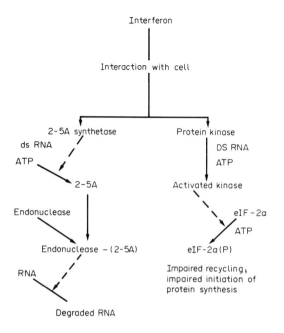

Fig. 1. Effects of interferon on virus replication.

These trimers and tetramers, known collectively as 2-5A, in the presence of double-stranded RNA activate a ribonuclease which can degrade viral genetic and messenger RNA, inhibiting the replication of both DNA and RNA viruses. Interferon also induces the synthesis of a protein kinase which can catalyse the phosphorylation, and consequent inactivation, of a factor required for elongation of polypeptide chains during their synthesis.

Mechanisms for exploring immunity against viruses can be analyzed in cell cultures, in experimental animals and in humans with selective deficiencies in their immune system. The results of such studies are discussed below with reference to the steps in virus replication. If replication is prevented the infection may be arrested.

Virus Replication

The first step in virus replication is the attachment of virus coat proteins to receptors on the surface of the host cell (see Fig. 2) and the fusion of the virus coat with the host cell plasma membrane. Fusion is mediated by specific virus coat proteins, termed fusogenic proteins — such as haemagglutinins or haemolysins, and the process is favoured by the acidic microenvironment within the endocytic vacuoles. The fusion liberates the virus genome (RNA or DNA), which can then replicate in the host cell cytoplasm or nucleus. Some mechanisms of resistance may operate at this stage, for example the absence of receptors for virus coat proteins on some cells will restrict the host range of viruses. Thus, several human viruses can infect primates but not laboratory or domestic animals. For example, poliovirus can bind to primate cells and initiate infection, whereas this does not occur with bovine or chicken cells. However, poliovirus RNA can be introduced into bovine or chicken cells and multiply in them with the formation of typical virus, showing that the block is at the virus binding and uncoating stage and not the later stages of replication.

The attachment of antibodies to proteins of the virus coat can prevent their binding to host cells and fusion with the plasma membrane. With many viruses such neutralization is the principal mechanism of acquired immunity. It is often due to circulating antibodies, mostly of the IgG class but also of the IgM class shortly after primary infection. The neutralizing effects of antibodies are increased by the fixation of complement (a group of serum proteins involved in the immune response), which adds early complement components to the virus coat protein-antibody complex and further hinders the attachment to host cells and uncoating. Antibodies of the IgA class, secreted at mucous membranes into bronchial, intestinal, genito-urinary and mammary secretions, can also prevent attachment of viruses to host cells, thus protecting sero-mucous surfaces against virus infections. An additional function of IgG antibodies is to facilitate the attachment of viruses to phagocytic cells

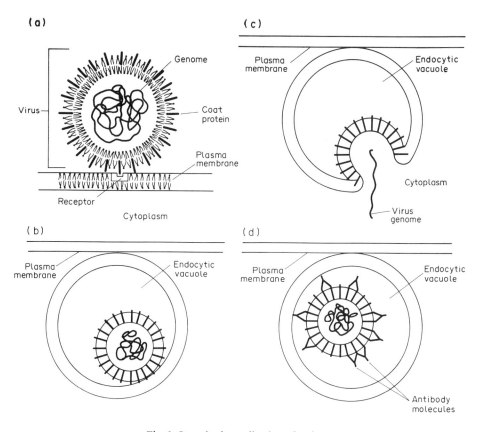

(a)

Virus

Genome

Coat protein

Plasma membrane

Receptor

Cytoplasm

(b)

Plasma membrane

Endocytic vacuole

(c)

Plasma membrane

Endocytic vacuole

Cytoplasm

Virus genome

(d)

Plasma membrane

Endocytic vacuole

Antibody molecules

Fig. 2. Steps in the replication of a virus.

(for example macrophages), in which they are often unable to replicate. This occurs through the receptors on phagocytic cells for the Fc part of the IgG antibody molecule (see Fig. 3).

During the replication of most viruses, viral antigens are inserted into the host cell plasma membrane where they can combine with antibodies. Provided that the antibodies are of the right subclass and that their density on the surface of the infected cells is sufficient, the infected cells can be lysed by complement. The cells can also be lysed by 'natural killer' cells which bind to the Fc parts of the antibody molecules on the surface of the virus-infected cells. Natural killer cells are present in the circulating population of leukocytes (white blood cells).

Mechanisms of Immunity

Serum antibodies

Experiments on laboratory animals have provided further information about the role of different mechanisms of immunity in each of the major groups of viruses. To elucidate the role of circulating antibodies against viruses, active immune responses are suppressed by X-radiation or drugs and attempts are then made to protect the animal passively by transfer of antibodies of different classes, either before infection or after it is established. If early or late passive protection can be achieved, it can be concluded that serum antibodies can prevent infection or facilitate recovery from an established infection. Such antibodies may have neutralized the virus,

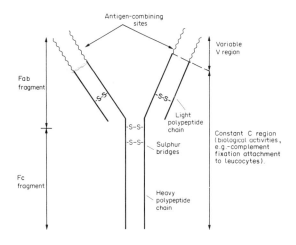

Fig. 3. Basic structure of the antibody molecule (IgG).

allowed antibody-dependent cytotoxicity of virus-infected cells, or facilitated the uptake of virus by phagocytic cells. The importance of the latter mechanism is demonstrable in newborn mice, which have macrophages able to support the replication of several viruses, in contrast to those of adult animals. Protection of newborn animals against viruses is much more efficiently effected by transfer of antibody and syngeneic adult peritoneal cells than by antibody alone.

Experiments of this type show that serum antibodies, particularly of the IgG class, play a major role in recovery from most virus infections and protection against reinfection. This is true of enteroviruses, adenoviruses, myxoviruses, paramyxoviruses and arthropod-borne viruses. For example, antibodies against the tip of the influenza haemagglutinin molecule, which vary in different strains of the virus, can protect people against this infection. Antibodies of the IgG class prevent the spread of Coxsackie viruses from the primary sites of infection to the heart and pancreas, where the infection can produce serious damage.

Comparable conclusions can be drawn from observations on the type of infections observed in children born with inherited defects in their capacity to synthesize immunoglobulins. While poliomyelitis infections have been common in England in the past, agammaglobulinaemic children (unable to synthesize antibodies) were much more likely to develop paralytic poliomyelitis than normal children. Poliovirus passes from the primary site of multiplication in the intenstine to the brain through the blood stream, and small amounts of serum antibodies can prevent this passage, as experiments in monkeys have shown. Agammaglobulinaemic children are also prone to other chronic enterovirus infections of the central nervous system, such as those produced by echoviruses.

Although pre-existing serum antibodies can prevent infection they are much less effective against established infections, for example those produced by herpesviruses. Herpes simplex virus (Type I) can persist in nerve ganglion cells for years in individuals with serum antibodies and produce recurrent infections of the face. A second type of herpes simplex virus (Type II) produces common, persistent genital infections, which can be transmitted during childbirth to babies, producing fatal infections. Other herpesviruses include cytomegalovirus, which can produce serious defects in foetuses and newborn children, and the Epstein-Barr virus which infects lymphocytes, causing them to proliferate in a disease known as infectious mononucleosis (glandular fever). This virus also appears to be associated with some types of cancer. It can be shown that once a herpesvirus infection is established in an animal, serum antibody cannot prevent the spread of the infection, which occurs by direct transfer of the virus from one cell to another without the virus being accessible to antibody. However, transfer of immune T-lymphocytes to syngeneic infected animals can bring about recovery. Whether this is mediated by cytotoxicity of virus-infected cells, liberation of γ-interferon or some other mechanism is at present unknown.

Interferon

Potent and specific antibodies against interferon (α and β) aggravate herpesvirus infections in laboratory animals, so it is reasonable to conclude that these types of interferon reduce the severity of the infection. Some children do not produce γ-interferon, and they are unable to recover from infectious mononucleosis, suggesting that this type of interferon plays an important part in bringing about recovery from this disease. Other children prone to recurrent respiratory virus infections have been found to have defective production of α- and β-interferons. Potent interferons are now being produced by recombinant DNA technology and these can be used to reduce the severity of some virus infections.

Recombinant DNA technology

Recent advances in biotechnology have helped in the study of immunity against viruses. By fusion it is possible to obtain cells which produce antibodies recognizing a single antigenic determinant. Such monoclonal antibodies have been produced to several virus antigens. They are useful reagents for defining the determinants of the virus antigens required to initiate infection, as well as for defining serological variants. Virus genes and complementary DNA sequences of RNA viruses have been cloned in *Escherichia coli* with the production of virus antigens in the bacterium. Antigens produced in this way have been used successfully to immunize animals against virus infections. This may become the method of choice for the production of some virus antigens, such as those of hepatitis B virus.

Hepatitis B virus can be carried in the blood for years and transmitted by blood transfusion, by contaminated syringes or other instruments, or by sexual contact especially amongst homosexuals. The introduction of a serological test and the use of disposable syringes has greatly reduced the prevalence of the disease in industrially advanced countries. This is another example of applied virus immunology. It is now possible to purify the virus antigen from infected plasma, ensure that it is not contaminated with infectious virus and immunize susceptible persons. The antigen is scarce and expensive, so only persons at risk, such as the medical staff working in kidney dialysis units, can be vaccinated with it. Thus the production of this antigen by recombinant DNA technology would be a useful advance in knowledge.

An alternative approach is to use the known sequence of bases in the hepatitis virus DNA to deduce the sequence of amino acids in the virus antigens. From the amino acid sequences of proteins it is possible, using computer programmes, to predict their probable configuration and which groups, exposed on the surface, are likely to be the major antigenic determinants. This is one area in which we are still ignorant, and one which will be explored during the coming decade.

Virus Vaccines

The vaccines of the future are likely to be virus coat protein subunits prepared conventionally, by recombinant DNA technology or by synthesis, and the use of live viruses for vaccination will probably decline due to their having certain disadvantages. The vaccine viruses may occasionally produce undesirable infections, especially in persons whose immune systems are not functioning normally. Nevertheless we are still ignorant of the best way to use the vaccines so as to elicit the desired immune responses, whether they are humoral or cell mediated.

This problem has been investigated with the use of adjuvants. If a substance is poorly antigenic it is frequently possible to improve the specific response to it by mixing or combining it with an adjuvant. In experimental work Freund's complete adjuvant has been used. It is a water in mineral oil emulsion containing heat killed tubercle bacilli. It produces strong inflammatory reactions at the site of injection.

The component of tubercle bacilli that has adjuvant activity, increasing cell-mediated and humoral immune responses, has been chemically characterized as muramyl dipeptide. A synthetic programme has produced analogues which are more potent adjuvants and do not induce fever or other undesirable side effects. The mineral oil component of Freund's adjuvant can be replaced by vesicles of natural lipids termed liposomes, which are biodegradable. Virus coat antigens can be inserted into the liposomes to construct virus-like particles which are highly immunogenic. Synthetic peptides corresponding to key antigenic determinants on the surface of the virus can be coupled to protein carriers to increase their capacity to elicit immune responses.

Conclusions

All of these technical developments have already been made, and it is likely that they will come to be widely used to increase the range of immunity against viruses in the next decade. We are still ignorant of which viruses will be controlled in this way. One candidate is the hepatitis B virus; the hope would be to first break the cycle of transmission in Western countries and eventually in Third World countries. Since hepatitis B virus is thought to play a role in the causation of primary cancer of the liver, immunization against the virus should reduce the incidence of the cancer. Likewise, if the Epstein-Barr virus does participate in the causation of cancer of the nasopharynx and immunization proves practical, the incidence of this type of cancer should be reduced. China would be a good place for such studies, because it has a large, well controlled population and carries out public health programmes, such as the People's War against the snail transmitting bilharzia, with determination and precision. If it were possible to control these virus diseases by immunization and show that the incidence of the two types of cancer were greatly reduced, this would be another substantial scientific and public health achievement.

Further Reading

ALLISON, A.C. (1979) Infectious diseases. In: *Medical Immunology* (Irvine, J., ed.), 77–102. Teviot Scientific Publications, Edinburgh.

BORDEN, E.C. and BALL, L.A. (1981) Interferons: biochemical, cell growth inhibitory and immunological effects. *Progress in Hematology*, 12, 299–339.

BURNS, W.H. and ALLISON, A.C. (1975) Virus infections and the immune responses which they elicit. In: *The Antigens* (Sela, M., ed.) volume III, p. 480. Academic Press: New York, San Francisco, London.

MERZ, D.C., SCHEID, A. and CHOPPIN, P.W. (1980) Importance of antibodies to the fusion glycoprotein of paramyxoviruses in the prevention of spread of infection. *Journal of Experimental Medicine*, 15, 275–281.

ZINKERNAGEL, R.M. and DOHERTY, P.C. (1979) MHC-restricted cytotoxic T-cells: studies on the biological role of polymorphic transplantation antigens determining T-cell restriction, specificity, function and responsiveness. *Advances in Immunology*, 27, 51–177.

HEALTH CARE

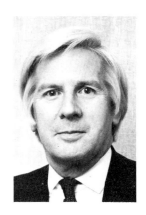

George Teeling-Smith

Director of the Office of Health Economics, London.

Professor Associate in Health Economics at Brunel University and Honorary Fellow of the Pharmaceutical Society of Great Britain. He has been a temporary adviser to OECD, WHO and CIOMS.

We are extraordinarily ignorant about many aspects of the organisation of health care and medical services. The first and fundamental unknown is how many people should be employed in health care and how much should be spent on a nation's health. All that we do know is that however much medical care is provided, it will all be enthusiastically used by patients and there will still always continue to be a reservoir of unmet medical demands. In other words, the potential demand for health care is unlimited, at least when it is made available free or at nominal charge to the user, as it is under the National Health Service in Britain and under Medicare and Medicaid in the United States. How much a nation spends on health, therefore, seems to be arbitrary. Although Britain has almost doubled the number of its medical and nursing staff over the past 30 years, it still spends only about 5 per cent of its National Income on its National Health Service. Countries like Sweden and the United States, on the other hand, spend between 8 and 10 per cent on corresponding services. No one can state whether either of these two levels of expenditure is appropriate. Both the low spenders in Britain and the high spenders in America and Sweden think that more money is needed to improve the quality of their medical services.

The reasons for this basic ignorance over how much should be spent on health will become apparent in the course of this essay. The first point which starts to explain the unlimited pool of medical demand is that it is normal to feel unwell. When the public are asked how they have felt over the previous four weeks, for example, at least four out of five will say they have had some symptoms of illness. In Britain, over a two-week period in the late 1960s, a random sample of the general public reported an average of four symptoms each (Wadsworth *et al.*, 1971 and Dunnell & Cartwright, 1972). At present most of these symptoms are successfully treated by the individuals themselves or else are ignored without any harm being done. However, they could instead all be taken to the doctor and if that were the case the doctor would, of course, be expected to provide treatment. Hence the unlimited potential demand from patients and the first reason for the uncertainty as to how much medical treatment is really necessary.

The next problem is faced by the family doctor, who seems to be surprisingly uncertain about how much of the sickness that he sees he should be able to treat himself and how much he should refer on for a specialist opinion in hospital. In a survey in the 1960s, two similar general practices in Edinburgh reached startlingly different conclusions on this point (Scott & Gilmore, 1966). One referred only one patient in 200 for a specialist opinion. The other referred one patient in four. This 50-fold variation in the number of referrals has never been investigated or explained. It is disagreeable and inconvenient for a patient to be referred to a consultant when it is not strictly necessary in medical terms. Yet it seems clear that some general practitioners are doing just that. Perhaps more seriously, it is a gross misuse of scarce medical resources for a patient to be investigated unnecessarily in hospital. This seems to be an area where medical ignorance is making life uncomfortable for the patient and adding needlessly to the cost of medical care. A more rational policy of hospital referral could help

to keep down medical care expenditure. The present irrational practices help to explain the bottomless reservoir of 'demand' for medical care at the hospital level.

Once the patient has been referred to the specialist, it then becomes a subjective judgment on his part as to whether or not the patient needs to be admitted as an in-patient. Obviously, if the person is seriously ill there is no question about the need for admission. But if the patients are reasonably fit, there seems to be a great deal of uncertainty about whether they should be admitted to hospital for treatment, observation or investigation. Sometimes they are admitted simply because it is easier to carry out diagnostic investigations or treatment on someone who is in hospital. What is often forgotten in such cases is that hospital stay is exceedingly expensive. It costs as much to stay in most hospitals as it does to stay in a first class hotel. Thus unnecessary admission to hospital adds substantially to health care expenditure — whether paid for by the individual himself, by a health insurance scheme, or by the taxpayer at large.

There is, in this context, suspicious evidence from a study in Exeter in the South-West of England that in areas where patients are more often referred to a hospital specialist they are also more likely to end up as in-patients (Ashford & Pearson, 1970). The mere fact that a person is seen by a hospital doctor, rather than in the actual state of his health, seems to be an important factor in determining whether or not he will end up in a hospital bed. Once again, there is no obvious explanation for this variation which clearly has important economic implications. The same sort of uncertainty applies once a person has been admitted to hospital. There are enormous variations between countries, between the regions within countries and between individual hospitals and doctors as to how long a patient is kept in hospital for a particular condition. For example with a simple hernia or varicose vein operation some doctors discharge their patients after one or two days (Doran *et al.*, 1972). Others keep them in hospital for two weeks. The same sorts of huge variation apply for most diagnostic investigations and for most medical and surgical treatments. Taking an overall national picture, the average length of stay in hospital in Sweden and the United States is only half that in Great Britain.

Ironically, there is a good deal of evidence about how long patients need to stay in hospital. A number of very carefully controlled investigations in Britain have all shown that shorter lengths of stay seem to be just as effective medically as more prolonged periods. In the case of hernia, for example, it has been shown that the patients who were sent home after one day did just as well as those kept in hospital for a week or longer. Serious conditions such as heart disease have also been shown to need much shorter spells in hospital than the present average (Harput *et al.*, 1971; Hayes *et al.*, 1974). With diseases such as tuberculosis, when effective medicines are available, there seems to be no medical or epidemiological justification for hospital treatment at all (Dawson *et al.*, 1966). What is unknown however, is how patients and doctors can be persuaded that they are occupying hospital beds unnecessarily for so many conditions.

Sometimes, of course, patients are kept in hospital unnecessarily for 'social' reasons. For example, they may live in over-crowded conditions at home where recovery from an operation would be difficult. This is, however, no excuse for using very expensive hospital facilities in place of home nursing or hostel accommodation. In other cases, patients are kept in hospital merely for the convenience of doctors, who find it easier to see them there — or who may simply not be available to authorise their discharge to go home. A study as long ago as 1966 hinted at these sorts of explanation for the unnecessary use of hospital beds (Ministry of Health). In yet other cases, and even more alarmingly,

doctors have admitted that patients have been kept in hospital simply in order to keep otherwise empty beds filled. This is a splendid example of Parkinson's Law in operation. It probably explains, for example why so many more beds are occupied in the Liverpool area of Britain — where beds are abundant — than in Sheffield — where they are scarce. But, all in all, it is obvious that we are extraordinarily ignorant about exactly why hospital beds are occupied unnecessarily and exactly how many could be eliminated if their wasteful use were to be cut out.

Apart from the general problem of the misuse of hospital beds, there is another much more specific problem which contributes to our uncertainty about the value of medical care and to the unlimited potential demand for medical services. This is the subject of pathological and radiological investigations. In pathology, these are the diagnostic examinations which involve taking various specimens from the patient and either examining them under the microscope or, more commonly, performing a range of chemical tests on them. In radiology, it involves taking pictures of parts of the inside of the body, employing increasingly sophisticated techniques including the use of computers to 'construct' a clearer and more accurate X-ray picture, for example of the brain.

The number of such tests has multiplied drastically in the decade between 1969 and 1979. About ten or twenty times as many tests are performed now as ten years ago and they have in general become more detailed. Thus the scope for finding an 'abnormal' result has enormously increased. However, these abnormalities are statistical rather than necessarily medical. That is, when the person varies in his specific test result from the average reading for the community as a whole it may have no more medical significance than the fact that he is significantly above or below the average height for the population. In other words, in many cases the medical profession is ignorant about whether or not the 'abnormal' result is related to the person's symptoms or disease. Doctors do not know whether the abnormality could or should be corrected by some medical or surgical intervention.

Despite this, it is obvious that doctors are increasingly enthusiastic about having these sorts of tests carried out. Among sceptics of the health service organisation, there are nasty suspicions that some of these tests may do no more than provide job satisfaction for the doctors who order them and technicians who carry them out. At best, they may be no more than an indication of the doctors' uncertainty about the correct diagnosis. Either way there is unfortunately little or no evidence that the tremendous proliferation of pathological and radiological tests has produced a corresponding improvement in the prognosis of those subjected to them. What is certain is that they have contributed substantially to the scope of medical activity and hence to the potential expenditure on medical care. Next there is the even more delicate question of how much surgery actually improves the health of the patient. Undoubtedly there are many types of operation which do, even if they are not invariably successful. For example kidney transplants and brain surgery can save lives. The replacement of diseased arthritic hips with artificial joints can transform the life style of the previously crippled victim. Stomach surgery, for example, to relieve an obstruction caused by cancer or to remove a bleeding ulcer or an inflamed appendix, is often essential. Many routine repairs, such as for hernias and haemorrhoids, are necessary and generally successful.

On the other hand, there is doubt about whether all of the surgery performed to 'cure' cancer actually improves the prognosis. At least one carefully controlled trial on cancer of the bronchus showed that those who had the surgery fared no better than those given more conservative treatment (Scadding, 1966). Heart surgery, particularly in the United States, is the subject of much controversy. There is evidence from Germany that many healthy appendices are removed by over-enthusiastic surgeons (Lichtner & Pflantz, 1971). There is even the story of the surgeon who made a great reputation for himself by having patients with a smaller cut and scar than those of anyone else carrying out appendicitis operations. It was a long time before he was caught out, when it was discovered that all he did was to nick the skin and sew it up again. He never went near the supposedly 'diseased' appendix, which nevertheless gave no more trouble once its owner believed that it has been removed. Finally, there is even greater doubt whether most tonsillectomies and hysterectomies are really necessary. They are both fashionable operations, but there is little or no hard and fast evidence of their necessity or value. Clearly surgery is an area where there are many unknowns. In some cases it looks as if the surgeon is doing no more than providing an elaborate and costly form of psychotherapy.

Another matter for concern in this field is the question of whether the prestigous teaching hospitals give patients a better chance of success and survival in surgery than do the peripheral district hospitals. Studies have been carried out which certainly suggest this (Morris, 1975). Of course, the underlying problem is to decide whether teaching hospital patients do better because they are selected to be 'better risks' or whether — as many people believe — their outcome is better because the hospitals are better equipped and because the surgeons are more experienced and skilful. It is certainly possible that the teaching hospitals, so far from getting the 'easy' patients, actually deal with more difficult cases than the peripheral hospitals and hence are doing doubly well in getting better results. The same questions, of course, apply in a less dramatic way to medical treatment in hospital as well as to surgery.

On the question of the outcome of medical care, there is the whole subject of doctors' apparent lack of success in controlling mortality in middle age. Death rates among infants and children continue to fall as the result of medical progress. The rates among those in their 'teens and twenties are kept relatively constant despite medical progress but this is readily explained by the increasing death rate from accidents — mainly motor-cycle accidents. In contrast, for those in their forties and fifties death rates still seem to be constant simply because medicine is being relatively unsuccessful against the main causes of middle-aged death — heart disease, circulatory diseases and cancers.

It appears that for this age group 'unhealthy' living is counteracting the progress made by medical science. For example women are smoking more cigarettes and men continue to eat and drink too much, while at the same time taking too little exercise. No one knows how to change people's pattern of behaviour in order to persuade them to live more healthily. A great deal of money and effort has been put into 'health education' with surprisingly unsuccessful results so far. No one seems to know how doctors or others can change people's way of life so that they get the full benefits of medical progress and technology. It is, of course, likely that in due course medical science will itself be able to counteract the effects of unhealthy living. Thus, perhaps instead of persuading people to smoke, eat and drink less we will simply have to wait until we can prevent or cure the ill-effects of such excesses.

Finally, looking at the whole enigma of health, one comes to the subject of absence from work attributed to illness. This has increased in the past 20 years in almost all Western countries, despite the technological progress in medicine and the increasing amounts of manpower and money devoted to the medical services. Indeed by this measure, the population seems to consider itself more and more unhealthy as it spends more and more on increasingly sophisticated medical care. This brings us back full cycle to the starting point of this essay. Why is demand for medical care unlimited, and why does it seem to increase as medical progress should be making us all 'healthier'? This situation is the opposite of the one which the politicians Beveridge and Bevan expected when they introduced the National Health Service in Britain in 1948. They expected demand for medical care to dwindle away once treatment had been made freely available to cure the reservoir of illhealth. In fact the reverse has happened. The reservoir of illhealth seems to have got steadily larger as it has been more and more expensively drained. In Britain health care expenditures have increased more than 20-fold since the late 1940s.

We are only now beginning to recognise clearly that this has actually happened and to understand the problem which it poses. It must be clear from the various examples selected in this essay that we now know we are profoundly ignorant about much of the underlying nature of illhealth and about the proper way to tackle it. Indeed we do not know what a truly 'healthy' society would be like. It is obvious that anyone who thought that the problems in the organisation of medical care might be simple ones needs urgently to think again. It seems that we must accept, as many people do today, that the World Health Organisation's definition of good health — 'a state of complete physical, social and mental wellbeing' — is an unattainable chimera. No amount of medical progress can lead to a healthy utopia, but no one in the present state of knowledge can exactly explain why.

References

ASHFORD, J. and PEARSON, N.G. (1970) Who uses health services and why? *Journal of the Royal Statistical Society,* **133/3** Series A.

DAWSON, J.J.Y., DEVADATTA, S., FOX, W., RADHARKRISHNA, S., RAMAKRISHNAN, C.V., SOMUSUN-DARAH, P.R., STOTT, H., TRIPATHY, S.P. and VELU, S. (1966) A five year study of patients with pulmonary tuberculoses — a current comparison of home and sanatorium treatment for 1 year with isoniazid plus P.A.S., *Bulletin of the World Health Organisation,* **34**, 533.

DORAN, F.S.A., WHITE, M. and DRURY, H. (1972) The scope and safety of short-stay surgery in the treatment of groin herniae and varicose veins; a report on 705 cases, *British Journal of Surgery,* **59**, 333.

DUNNELL, K. and CARTWRIGHT, A. (1972) *Medicine Takers, Prescribers and Hoarders,* Routledge and Kegan Paul, London.

HARPUT, J.E., CONNOR, W.T., HAMILTON, M., KELLETT, R.J., GALBRAITH, H.–J.B., MURRAY, J.J. and SWALLOW, J.H. (1971) Controlled trial of early mobilisation and discharge from hospital in uncomplicated myocardial infarction, *Lancet,* **II**, 1331.

HAYES, M.J., MORRIS, G.K. and HAMPTON, J.R. (1974) Comparison of mobilisation after two and nine days in uncomplicated myocardial infarction. *British Medical Journal,* **3**, 10.

LICHTNER, S. and PFLANZ, M. (1971) Appendectomy in the Federal Republic of Germany epidemiology and medical care. *Patterns Medical Care,* **9**, 311.

MINISTRY OF HEALTH (1966) *On the state of the Public Health.* Her Majesty's Stationery Office.

MORRIS, J.N. (1975) *Uses of Epidemiology,* 3rd Edition. Churchill Livingstone (see Table 3.7).

SCADDING, J.G. (1966) Comparative trial of surgery and radiotherapy for the primary treatment of small-celled or oat-celled carcinoma of the bronchus. *Lancet,* **11**: 979.

SCOTT, R. and GILMORE, M. (1966) *The Edinburgh Hospitals in Problems and Progress in Medical Case* (McLachlan, G., ed.) Oxford University Press.

WADSWORTH, M.E.J., BUTTERFIELD, W.J.H. and BLANEY, R. (1971) *Health and Sickness: The Choice of Treatment,* Tavistock Publications, London.

ENIGMAS OF HEARING AND DEAFNESS

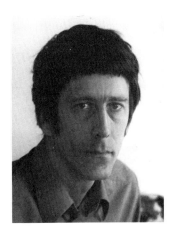

M.P. Haggard

Special Professor of Audiological Sciences, University of Nottingham and Director of the Medical Research Council's Institute of Hearing Research.

His publications and professional affiliations include the areas of acoustics, phonetics and audiology as well as experimental psychology. He describes himself as both practically and philosophically oriented and as having learned, just in time, how to suppress one or the other streak in the appropriate company.

Normal and abnormal hearing may be studied in a number of different domains. In the anatomical domain we can describe normal anatomy and its pathological variations whether gross or microscopic. In the physiological domain we can describe the physical and chemical mechanisms subserving normal functioning and the particular ways in which these are impaired in disease. In the psychological domain we can describe in information-processing terms the repertoire of general and basic auditory abilities which people have and the disabilities consequent upon impaired sensory function (i.e. generally the gaps in this repertoire but occasionally also hypersensitivities of a troublesome nature). Finally, we may appreciate the way in which educational, economic, social or cultural variables depend on these abilities and hence the handicaps to which the disabilities lead. The chief causal links are shown in Fig. 1. Each domain and level of description of this scheme is scientifically valid and autonomous. Greatest application value results from considering more than one domain at a time; medical education sometimes overlooks this. I shall concentrate here on the physiological and psychological domains.

The beneficial application of knowledge depends upon its orderly (and generally maximal) diffusion within society. Health depends upon knowledge (physiological,

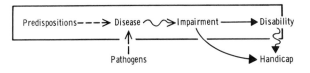

Fig. 1. The terminology of disability as approved by the World Health Organisation (1980). While the WHO rubrics define impairment as possible without an identifiable pathological underpinning, it is clear that where it exists a separate level of description is required; i.e. where anatomical correlates are available 'impairment' should be reserved for externalized physiological manifestations. The frame indicates the confines of the individual organism and the wavy arrow indicates a rather variable relationship.

microbiological, behavioural, etc.) circulating at three levels: (1) in the popular culture, (2) among planners and administrators who determine the content of food, water and other public facilities and (3) among practitioners whom the public recognize and have access to, most generally and notably medical doctors. Any strategy for enhancing this knowledge and widening its circulation must balance the probable accessibility of answers to questions with the probability of the answers actually being deployed within society or within the relevant professions. Those obtaining the knowledge have inevitably become to an ever greater extent separated from those applying it, so gaps in the application of multidisciplinary professional knowledge do not always correspond precisely with gaps in the scientific disciplines. In this essay I shall therefore attempt to clarify some perspectives upon hearing and deafness that are required to make good use of what is already known or may become known and shall not restrict myself to teasing fellow scientists about the shaky empirical or philosophical foundations of hearing science. As audiology is a relatively new and specialized field a summary of what is known is necessary to illuminate the challenge of what is not.

Fundamentals: What do the Hair Cells do?

To understand what is entailed in deafness one must first understand what is entailed in hearing. Hearing plays an important role in receiving signals about the mechanical events in and the composition of objects in the environment because size, density, stiffness and to some extent shape, affect the transmission and reflecting of sound waves. This in turn enables hearing to play a dominant role in communication and hence in social behaviour. The linguistic information in social communication is coded by a dynamically organized skilled performance, speech production, into a spectro-temporal form. This is possible because the articulatory organs can create a range of sound sources and of resonant cavity configurations to modify them. To a first approximation the dimensions of these sources and resonator structures are inversely proportional to the frequencies of major components of the output; consequently, the most essential ability for normal reception of spoken language is the ability to distinguish the frequency components of complex sounds and their changes with time. This is by no means the only important problem in the theory of hearing but it is the central one and the one which most revealingly links anatomical, physiological and psychological domains.

Sound enters the inner ear (cochlea) by a relatively straightforward process of impedance matching by the eardrum and the tiny bones of the middle ear. Alternate compressions and rarefactions of the air are converted to movements of the fluid (perilymph) in the scala vestibuli and scala tympani of the inner ear. These in turn cause a pattern of deflection to travel along the basilar membrane towards its inner end (i.e. from base to apex of the coiled-up cochlea). In the cross section representation in Fig. 2 this travelling wave would cause the entire structure to bend upwards and downwards. The sensory end-organs (hair cells) are mounted on this

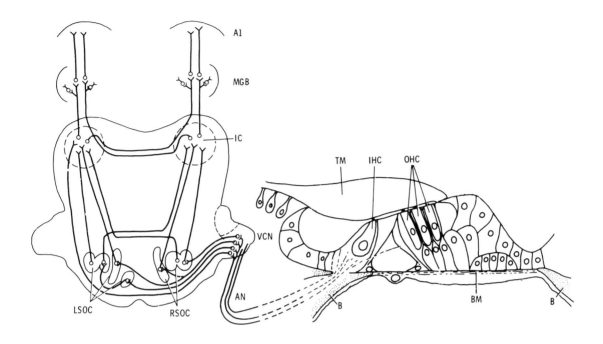

Fig. 2. General anatomical layout of the peripheral and central auditory systems. A cross section of the organ of Corti in the cochlea (bottom right: redrawn after Manley and Kronester-Frei, 1980) has been connected to a schematic of the auditory central nervous system (redrawn from Harrison and Howe, 1974; not to scale). In the cochlea are labelled TM – tectorial membrane, BM – Basilar membrane, IHC – inner hair cells, OHC – outer hair cells and B – the bony spiral supporting structures. The basilar membrane is held straight by pressure equalization of the different fluids above and below the organ of Corti. Travelling waves propagate along the membrane (in the direction out of the page in the case of the right ear), displacing the entire structure alternately upwards and downwards. The majority of afferent fibres originate in IHC and access the central nervous system via the auditory nerve (AN) and ventral cochlear nucleus (VCN). The remaining connections illustrate the high degree of cross connection between the two sides of the brain (by comparison, for example, with the visual or somatosensory systems). The lateral superior olive in the superior olivary complex (SOC) is the first stage of interaction of binaural inputs. Above this stage, nuclei receive afferent inputs both ipsilaterally and from contralateral nuclei that have received inputs from both sides. The functions of this complicated arrangement are not yet well understood but appear to play some role in spatial perception, selection and orientation, for which in the case of the auditory system no simple spatially structured coding (such as position of stimulation or movement of the structure containing the sense organ) exists. The inferior colliculus (IC) and medical geniculate body (MGB) have been investigated with single unit recording techniques and the preservation of various binaural and monaural aspects of stimulation established, without any clear overall picture of their function emerging. Al, the primary auditory cortex, appears to mediate the analysis of complicated patterns of time frequency and space. The efferent fibres from the crossed olivo-cochlear bundle to (chiefly) the OHC are not shown.

membrane in the fashion shown in Fig. 2. Deflection of the hairs due to shearing motion between basilar and tectorial membranes (and possibly due to fluid motions directly) causes the hair cells to depolarize and release trans-

mitter at the synapse with the auditory neurone. Thanks to the investigations of Georg von Bekesy, by 1950 the basic principle of mechanical functioning of the inner ear was generally accepted: the gradations of mass and elasticity properties of the basilar membrane lead to the travelling wave having a low-pass filter action with a band-pass component. This distributes the place of maximum excitation for frequency components of a stimulating signal along an axis from the basal (outer; high frequency) end of the spirally structured cochlea to the apical (inner; low frequency) end. To explain most phenomena in hearing we require a more detailed scrutiny of the anatomy, physiology and biochemistry of the inner ear. Von Bekesy realized the first problem; that the mechanical principle alone was insufficient to account for fine frequency discrimination. He thought this was handled by inhibition in the central nervous system; this view is now known to be incorrect because auditory nerve fibres display finer selectivity than is observed in cochlear mechanics, sufficiently fine to explain most psychoacoustical data on frequency resolution. Rapid advances were made in the late 1960s and 1970s, when computer scheduling of stimulation sequences and computer analysis of nerve fibre response statistics made it possible to plot rapidly functional relationships between stimulation patterns and the discharge patterns of auditory nerve fibres. The discrepancy between their selective tuning and the mechanical filtering of the basilar membrane has led to the postulate of a 'second filter' mechanism. It has now become possible to record from inner hair cells. Directly on presentation of the stimulus they already show similarly fine selectivity characteristic of auditory nerve fibres. This renders any mechanism of purely neural interaction unnecessary as the basis of selectivity and places the second filter logically between the pattern of basilar membrane motion and the electrical events which release transmitter substance at the synapse between hair cell and afferent fibre. A wide range of mechanisms is still possible. On the principle of parsimony, any hypothesis to fill the gap will be favoured insofar as it ascribes a coherent set of plausible roles

to aspects of the anatomy whose precise roles are as yet uncertain.

The known but unexplained aspects of the structure of the inner ear are chiefly (1) the shape, mass and composition of the tectorial membrane, (2) the configuration of the outer cell hairs with probable attachment by some of the curved formation of hairs to the tectorial membrane (see Fig. 2); the inner hair cells possibly do not touch the tectorial membrane but nestle in an indentation, (3) the surprising and so far unexplained fact that about 90% of auditory nerves fibres innervate inner hair cells, leaving the more numerous outer hair cells with little afferent contact with the central nervous system.

Current hypotheses to embrace these facts range from the purely hydromechanical through some more plausible mixed hypotheses to a purely molecular biophysical explanation. At the mechanical extreme it has been suggested that the complicated spatial structures of the basilar and tectorial membranes provide a mechanical input to the hair cells involving higher order derivatives of the basilar membrane displacement pattern and that this input is highly frequency-specific. Among the mixed hypotheses it has been suggested that the different hair cell types respond to different variables (e.g. velocity and displacement) and that some form of interaction occurs.

One hypothesis ascribes to the outer hair cells (which contain actin-like proteins) a motor role in a mechanical feedback system; in other words the more numerous inner hair cells would amplify the pattern of movement at low sound levels to a level sufficient to stimulate inner hair cells. Although still highly speculative, this is not totally implausible; a sizeable minority of people's eardrums emit low levels of acoustical energy when not engaged in receiving it, consistent with spontaneous oscillation of an active feedback loop. This is not related in most cases to the clinical symptom of subjective tinnitus (noises in the head or ears) which often accompanies hearing loss and can in some instances be more distressing. Other types of data from which the role of the outer hair cells might reasonably be inferred are conspicuously lacking. Experiments on the role of the efferent fibres, which innervate predominantly outer hair cells, have not been successful in defining their role; cutting the main efferent nerve bundle does not appear to reduce frequency selectivity markedly. Thus the outer hair cells and the mechanical feedback loop may be concerned with sensitivity to low sound levels rather than with frequency analysis as such. A purely biophysical explanation of frequency selectivity would ascribe to each hair cell the ability to configure a molecular tuned circuit to enhance its selectivity to individual frequencies close to but not uniquely constrained to the frequency which is mechanically represented maximally in its vicinity. Thus for each of the probable stages within the transduction process remaining unspecified, a hypothesis claiming an important role in fine frequency selectivity has been proposed. Findings in recent years have tended to favour the micromechanical feedback loop.

The immense technical problems of acquiring direct evidence from the small and vulnerable cochlear structures imply that at present we can only give preference to hypotheses that incorporate most of the known micro-anatomical facts and which are consistent with other biologically relevant aspects of the auditory system's performance. Notable among these is the remarkable ability to reconcile good frequency resolution with adequate temporal resolution and to maintain both over a power range of about 10 log units. Whatever they do, the outer hair cells are quite likely to be involved in this dynamic stability and the poverty of afferent innervation makes it likely that some form of interaction with the inner hair cells takes place.

The foregoing story does scant historical justice to five decade of progress since vacuum tube instruments inaugurated auditory physiology. I have omitted to mention parts of the auditory system other than the organ of Corti and the detailed comprehensive accounts of input-output relationships for the auditory system that have been established by psychological (behavioural) methods in man and animals for speech and non-speech sounds. This account does, however, show that the 'solution' apparently offered by von Bekesy in the late 1940s to the core problem of hearing must be seen as a step that spares new students the need to read most of the previous literature. The true solution still eludes us. What is clear is that the second filter mechanism, whatever it is, is physiologically vulnerable to a wide range of agents — drugs, noise, anoxia.

Hearing Pathology

Classifying deafnesses according to the disease processes causing them has been successful only in a few cases. This is partly because diagnoses are often presumptive (i.e. depending largely on ruling out the positively identifiable conditions) and partly because in only a few instances do clear treatment indications follow. Functional classification is therefore a necessary first step whether we are concerned with advising patients, with treatments or with gaining further knowledge. This classification has remained somewhat primitive, being preoccupied until recently with distinguishing conductive deafnesses (i.e. those involving mechanical obstruction or disconnection in the external or middle ear) from all other forms, for which the contrasting term 'perceptive' was used. The latter term gave way to the preferable but still rather catch-all term 'sensorineural' in the 1960s. This classification is achieved largely in the impairment domain. The inability to hear faint pure tones is usually expressed as a greater or lesser positive value on the scale of decibels Hearing Level. This refers to the extra intensity required relative to the norm for young adults with no identifiable ear pathology for a faint sound to reach threshold. It is the most generally accepted and probably still the most generally useful measure of severity of deafness; when taken together with other information it also has some differential diagnostic value. The hearing threshold *per se* is not of great adaptive importance, but provides a rather direct measure of basic functioning of the middle and/or inner ear (in all but a few difficult-to-test cases); it should hence be taken as an impairment measure. As such it affords some suggestions of the extent of pathology on the one hand and of disability on the other but a precise quantification of neither. (Nowadays for difficult-to-test patients, it is also possible to extract from averaged evoked electrical responses various objective indices of impairment that have been mapped onto behavioural thresholds in testable patients).

It is profitable in clinical assessment to distinguish seven categories of deafness based on the most impairing 'site' of dysfunction; this is not necessarily the exclusive or original site of pathology. The assessment is arrived at from combinations of results of audiological tests in which people respond to sounds with systematically varied properties. The seven main types are: (1) External or middle ear conductive, (2) Inner ear hydromechanical, (3) Inner ear sensory, (4) Auditory nerve, (5) Brainstem auditory pathways, (6) Auditory cortex, (7) Non-organic. This last category (sometimes called 'functional' hearing loss) is used when no peripheral or central pathology can reasonably be attributed. Once misunderstanding of test instructions is ruled out, the exaggeration of a genuine hearing loss is the most common form of 7; straightforward malingering is rare, but other forms also exist. Type 4 is not uncommon, but may present first with non-auditory symptoms, e.g. a disseminated sclerosis; another example of type 4, the acoustic neuroma (or more

precisely schwannoma of the VIII nerve) can have primarily auditory symptoms but is often asymptomatic and is rare as a lifethreatening condition. Types 5 and 6 are relatively rare: patients of type 6 usually present with other obscure problems of auditory pattern perception but with little loss of hearing for faint sounds.

The distinction between 2 and 3 can be helped by considering again Fig. 1, the crosssectional diagram of the inner ear. From the base to apex of the inner ear and along the dimension orthogonal to the page there propagates a travelling wave of amplitude approximately proportional to the amplitude of the stimulating pressure changes; this reaches its maximum at a point characteristic of the stimulating frequency. If the mechanical properties of the basilar membrane or tectorial membrane are abnormal, and particularly if a static fluid pressure difference between scala media and the other two channels (scala vestibuli and scala tympani) causes distension of the membrane, the above proportionality will be changed and an example of type 2 will arise. This is thought to be the critical aspect of the pathology in Meniere's syndrome, which involves vertigo, tinnitus, a feeling of pressure and hearing loss (often initially at low frequencies and fluctuating). As the site is in the inner ear in both types 2 and 3, relatively sophisticated behavioural or electrophysiological tests may be necessary to separate them. Type 3 can be caused by intense noise exposure; it is also by far the most common and the main, but not the exclusive, basis of loss of hearing in old age. The commonness of types 1 and 3 tends to preempt the attention of the non-specialist practitioners through whom cases are referred, with the risk that other forms may go unidentified and unreferred or be given inappropriate treatment.

Determining the functionally effective site of lesion can be an important step to establishing aetiology; it can be established largely by behavioural ('subjective') tests at relatively low expense. Types 1, 4 and 5 are often subjected to radiographic and/or electrophysiological confirmation because surgery may be called for; for most types a truly aetiological decision usually requires other types of information also, e.g. the history of symptoms. By 1975 clinical audiology had progressed in a few specialized centres in Europe and North America to a stage where classification among five or six of these seven sites of lesion could be made with reasonable certainty in the majority of clinical cases; but the diffusion of the knowledge on which such good practice must be based has been, and remains, slow.

Application of Knowledge about Hearing and Deafness

We may distinguish five reasons for the historical inertia in pursuing and applying the study of auditory function. Conductive conditions have similar incidence in the clinical caseload of a general hospital ear, nose and throat department to all other ear conditions combined. However, population studies show that conductive conditions are outnumbered by sensorineural conditions in the population. This discrepancy is probably due to conductive conditions being pathologically more visible and psychologically more symptomatic; they are more frequently asymmetric, leading to noticeable head-turning behaviour and are often accompanied by organic symptoms (e.g. fluid discharge, discomfort or pain), to which it is more socially acceptable to admit than to a communication disorder.

A second reason for the historical inertia is that the professional structure for health services to the deaf is in most countries based institutionally upon otolaryngology — a regional speciality that is oriented chiefly to surgery because of the surgical training required for large parts of it. Surgery can in

some cases prevent the most serious consequences of middle ear conditions, but for the foreseeable future it has very restricted applicability to types 2 (cochlear conductive) and 4 (neural) and virtually no application at present conceivable to type 3 (sensory). Here the hair cell dysfunction leads to a marked disability in the understanding of speech sounds, particularly in unfavourable environments such as noise and reverberation, even where the speech is loud enough to be audible. This is due to disturbed frequency selectivity, as explained above. Middle ear conditions are better understood than the others by general physicians and otolaryngologists alike. Indeed, the emphasis upon frequency resolution and the contemporary auditory physiology summarized above has not yet entered the basic medical curriculum and is unfamiliar to many otolaryngologists.

As a third reason for slow development of well-articulated concepts of deafness we cannot overlook society's attitude to disability. Protagonists sometimes exaggerate the stigma and handicap associated with deafness, an understandable reaction to the taking for granted of the chief communication channel by an unimaginative public. The disability can be partly offset by the right rehabilitative support, by accepting the ultimate limiations imposed by the impairment and yet striving to minimize, to an extent that the individual's personality can sustain, the consequent disability and handicap. However, the false association of deafness with senility and stupidity and the genuine problems which deafness creates for social communication are more likely to affect an individual's personality as seen by others than are disorders of physical mobility. This makes individuals more likely to deny and to hide deafness than other disabilities. The improvement of general attitudes to disabilities which began in the 1970s is now helping to rectify the balance.

The fourth reason for inertia in adopting a full functional classification involves the overlap of categories, in many cases leading to uncertainty in diagnostic assessment. For example, pathology in the middle ear can, if not checked, lead to pathology in the inner ear, making 'mixed' deafness (type 1 plus type 3) quite common. Likewise, an acoustic neuroma as well as compressing the auditory nerve in the internal auditory meatus may exert pressure on the vulnerable blood supply to the inner ear, leading to mixed symptoms including those of cochlear disorder, but the original site of lesion here is the auditory or vestibular nerve and the pathology is entirely different. Overlaps and ambiguities about sites of lesions are common in other areas of medicine and do not constitute a rational argument against the refinement and adoption of the scheme of functional classification for patient populations as a whole, even if other methods may eventually lead more directly to hypotheses about pathology or to aetiological diagnoses. The effect of such uncertainties and of the possible inability, given central pathology, to perform behavioural tests is to encourage many diagnosticians to abandon the attempt to classify initially between sites 4, 5 and 6 on the basis of behavioural evidence. It further becomes tempting when considering the individual to skip electrophysiological measures of impairment and leap from a global assessment to a surgery-relevant hypothesis based upon radiological evidence alone. The balance of medical benefit with ethical and financial cost for this tactic has not been established.

The fifth contribution to the vicious circle of ignorance is the limited range of treatment options currently available for the various disease states that lead to the most prevalent handicapping dysfunction — type 3 inner ear sensory deafness involving loss of frequency resolution. For example there is controversy over the general effectiveness of vasodilators or of mild electrical stimulation to improve circulation as possible therapies for hair cell dysfunction which may be due to a reduction of blood supply. the therapeutic hypotheses themselves are reasonable. The uncertainty probably arises from inadequate definition and restriction of the pathology in the treatment groups, generally inadequate investigative precision and from the limited reversibility of the auditory pathology by the time it comes to treatment. The otolaryngologist or audiological physician is therefore at present left with the recommendation of a hearing aid as the main and in most cases, the only line of management. Scientific principles are emerging for individual fitting of aids (including the electronic processing of the amplitude envelope and frequency spectrum), but the development of rigorously specified clinical strategies for aid prescription requires extensive and long-term validations which have generally not been done. The recent developments in the science and technology of hearing aids are founded in physics and ultimately in applied mathematics, not in applied biology: hence they are beyond the range of interest and competence of most medically and surgically trained personnel unless specifically trained. No professional structure exists* to prescribe aids rationally in a different fashion for the different forms and severities of deafness. Findings available today suggest this should be possible on a rigorous basis for subvarieties of types 1, 2 and 3. Until that structure emerges there will be little incentive for spreading systematic assessment on the basis of the seven-category scheme or for developing it further for the differential prescription of aids.

Thus we see that a fairly comprehensive scheme of functional and structural classification of hearing disorders has developed in spite of rather than because of the institutional arrangements for deploying such

---

* I.e. in the UK. In North America audiologists trained to Masters or Doctorate level exist. In certain university and government establishments they have avoided the pressures of commercialized medicine sufficiently to develop rigorously founded schemes of assessment and rehabilitation.

knowledge and despite a certain social reluctance to accept deafness as a medically referable condition.

The Problem of Multiple Causation

Is our ignorance of causes and effective treatments an inevitable result of the essentially statistical and inaccessible nature of the phenomena under examination, or have the appropriate questions simply not yet been posed and answered? If I did not believe that a set of questions with usable answers awaits formulation and gradual answering, I would not be a hearing researcher and would not be writing this chapter. Yet there are difficulties in some areas that approach the character of insurmountable barriers. The microscopic scale of the cochlea makes it difficult to extract samples of tissues for biochemical analysis; it also entails that pathologies originating in bone, the fluid system, the blood supply or the soft tissues of the cochlea spread to the other systems and obscure their own origins. This restricts both the general scientific demonstration of pathogens and the attempt to establish a major aetiology in the individual patient. The administrative and ethical difficulties in acquiring post mortem pathological material paired with good audiological descriptions of function are extreme.

A limit in using a functional site classification as a step to pathological inference is that a single pathological process may act at more than one site. The processes of hair cell receptor function described above require a considerable energy supply. This is brought via the blood stream and the stria vascularis which pumps ions into the scala media to maintain a bias voltage of +80 to +100 millivolts with respect to the scala tympani. Hair cell deflection is assumed to modulate a direct current flow through the hair cells. This energy supply is clearly a vulnerable link in the chain of hearing and in principle it should be possible to delimit functionally a

deafness arising at the stria vascularis; sensitivity should be affected, but selectivity less so if the hair cells are unaffected. However, the evidence for such a dissociation in humans is as yet negligible; for example, drugs that build up in the stria tend also to damage the hair cells. Likewise, failure of the blood supply in the cochlear region is likely to affect not only the stria vascularis but also the auditory nerve.

The multiple contributors of damage to the hair cells are not simply cumulative but interact synergistically, rather as two discrete disease states may interact in causing mortality. The effects of ototoxic aminoglycoside antibiotics (e.g. kanamycin, gentamycin) are potentiated by diuretics (e.g. frusemide, ethacrynic acid) and potentiate the effects of noise. It is likely that deficiencies of the blood supply and diet likewise potentiate the major effects of noise and age. When pathogens are neither few and absolute nor direct and rapid in their mode of action, to identify them in principle is hard enough. To then use this knowledge via health education to build up rational behaviour patterns as a basis of prevention becomes a formidable challenge. We all know of some smokers who died of lung cancer; this makes the evidence for that association personally acceptable even if it may be logically ambiguous. However, with the exception of the clear effects of noise, the social environment is unlikely similarly to support health education related to probable factors in hearing losses. The social environment does not define for us the extent of the hearing loss in another person, only his partially related disabilities. Far less does it define the subtle combinations of multiple continuously graded pathogens and predispositions preceding them. In these circumstances to proscribe every suspected or even likely pathogen would appear to the public as a restriction of life to mediaeval proportions with mystical taboos.

In the clinical appraisal of the individual the in-depth biochemical and immunological investigation to establish the prime cause of a type 2 or 3 hearing loss can sometimes be rewarding, but not always. In a few cases it is possible to establish highly probable causes such as allergic reaction, metabolic abnormality or ototoxic drug intake at a stage where control of intake leads to reversal of the condition. A more typical therapeutic predicament is met in Meniere's syndrome, which involves a hearing loss of type 2 (inner ear hydromechanical) steadily augmenting to involve type 3 (inner ear sensory). Here it is often possible to slow and control the progression of the condition, but not to reverse it. It is not possible in most cases to establish categorically that an individual has no relevant degree of risk on main causal factors. For this reason and because of synergism, most cases of deafness in the elderly must be presumed to originate from some additive and interactive combination of three factors: excessive noise exposure (type 3; preventable, not reversible), general cardiovascular disorder with poor blood supply to the organ of Corti and the stria vascularis (type 3; probably partially preventable), and the accumulated operation of minor changes due to ageing (types 1; external or middle ear conductive; 2; 4; auditory nerve and 6; auditory cortex) the extent of each probably being separately genetically determined. In the part it has been customary to use the term 'presbycusis' to describe variants of this complex. This is a useful term only if it is recognized as shorthand and not taken at the one extreme as a catch-all excuse for suspending further investigation on everyone of age greater than 60, nor at the other extreme taken as an explanatory specified pathology. I believe this attitude to the basis of hearing loss in old age is scientifically, medically and socially more acceptable than other views at present, but I cannot dignify it with any more pretentious a label than 'attitude', for as a theory it is largely an admission of ignorance.

The Compounding of Disability and Secondary Prevention

To think clearly about the relationship between the four domains of study we have to accept a terminology that allows causality to operate chiefly in the direction of the ordering of the four domains given earlier: organic pathology → physiological impairment → psychological disability → social handicap. However, one process that is challenging and crucial for health provision involves influences apparently acting in the reverse direction. It is now known that near-total deprivation of sound input by simulated conductive deafness in young mice leads to abnormal and deficient cellular development in the first nucleus of the ascending auditory system; impairment now apparently leads to pathology and we enter the realm of psychosomatic medicine! More precisely, deprivation of experience through a remediable or partly remediable pathology in the ear may lead not only to a disability but to a secondary yet irremediable pathology in the brain. Prevention of this deprivation effect is called secondary prevention.

The importance of early learning can hardly be doubted. For example in a Japanese childhood, the distinctive contrast of the 'r' and 'l' sounds of English is not usually encountered: this leads to the inability to perceive the acoustic-phonetic differences between such sounds even among expert Japanese speakers of English who have been taught to produce the sounds acceptably. Thus cultural experience enhances and limits human perceptual abilities in a way that appears to become 'hard-wired' with time.

A wealth of such illustrations of the importance of early experience has created an intellectual climate in which early identification, ascertainment and provision of aids is widely accepted as a necessary prelude to compensatory education of prelingually deaf children. Evidence on the effects of formal instruction of very young deaf children is controversial; appraisals by educators have been ideological rather than empirical. The benefits of early identification may be parsimoniously ascribed to the provision of compensatory amplification in conjunction with an ensured amount of communication with another person, particularly with one who checks in a spontaneous and relatively natural fashion that the communication is being successful. Wholly rigorous demonstrations of beneficial effects of early compensatory amplification are still lacking, so the general acceptance of the value of early detection and provision is based chiefly upon the intellectual climate created by evidence from animal experiments of developmental sensory deprivation. However, there is some circumstantial clinical evidence: before the mid-1960s early identification was not emphasized and hearing aids were not fitted to children of less than 1–2 years. It was only rarely then that severely prelingually hearing-impaired children achieved near-normal skills of speech production, of speech reception (with an aid) or of general language use, only for example when a resourceful parent encountered a specialist holding the then unpopular view favouring early remediation. Nowadays these achievements are not uncommon.

Occasionally the salutary scepticism about the cost-effectiveness of screening programmes in some fields spills over into prelingual deafness screening and the absence of rigorous supporting evidence for its benefits is noted. Clearly, it is only fair to evaluate ultimate benefits where the screening itself is effective and where some rational differential educational management is based upon differential assessment. For example, it seems acceptable that amplification and training in oral skills (i.e. speech production, speech reception with amplification and lip reading) should be emphasized for those known to have usable residual hearing, while manual skills (sign language) should be emphasized in those who do not. The value of early versus late identification in these two instances is really two separate questions, dogged by the complication that the more profoundly deaf child is more likely to be detected early. The questions have not been properly answered because they have not been separately posed for the appropriate provision. They have not been posed separately because educational discussion has for long been dominated by an absurd controversy between those who regard oral education as universally and unambiguously better than manual communication and those holding the opposite view. Also, a reasonably precise assessment of hearing function in the infant has only become available in the 1970s with electrophysiological methods. Rigid thinking about deaf children as a single category has prolonged our ignorance of these inter-related questions of the best style of compensatory provision and the importance of beginning it early. In this instance enlightened opinion would already regard a controlled trial involving delay of compensatory provision as unethical, because in children both the circumstantial evidence and the theoretical support favouring early intervention are good enough to justify action by community health services. Thus rigorous evidence must now accumulate at the slower rate offered by failures of screening, with some variables inevitably uncontrolled.

Impairment apparently leads to pathology and hence compounds the total disability; can this also occur later in human development? Does the sensory deprivation from a mild or moderate hearing loss in mature people or animals lead to a decreased ability to use information if it is later made (partially) available again? This question applied to the elderly is not purely academic. Although the severity of the typical deafness in the elderly is less dramatic than in the prelingually deaf child, the prevalance rate for deafness of clinical significance in the elderly, (over 20%) is some two orders of magnitude higher than that for prelingual deafness in children, which is about 0.1–0.2%. Informal evidence suggests that people fitted in middle age with hearing aids while their loss is still mild succeed in making better use of them than do those who defer the moment of accepting an aid. The delayers hypothetically lose some of the speech-perceiving skills that make an aid worth having. Their delaying may be due jointly to the presumed social unacceptability of deafness and the insidiousness of its onset. Certain behavioural tactics such as learning to lipread would offset the disability in a non-industrialized society where aids are not available, but they may compound the eventual disability by delaying the provision of aids available in an industrialized society. In some cases the disability leads to a communication barrier and to a descent into depression and isolation. Re-enter synergism. The disabling effects of a longstanding impairment due, for example, to noise will be compounded by the central and peripheral effects of ageing. In many cases, paradoxically, it is the compounding factor of ageing which leads to referral for a hearing aid just as the suitable period for learning how to use one is passing; i.e. those who seek help are often not those who would benefit most! This paradox justifies an epidemiological approach of secondary disability prevention.

Wholly rigorous evidence that beneficial effects of preventive fitting of hearing aids were due to sensory deprivation *per se* as opposed to the tertiary isolation and depression effects in the later aid-seeker would be difficult to achieve. From the practical point of view even the well-controlled trial assessing the combined effects of secondary disability and tertiary handicap would be enough. If successful, this would justify appropriation of resources to change the present purely responsive approach to fitting hearing aids into an aggressive approach based upon secondary prevention. Yet the problems in making even such a gross demonstration

valid are considerable. Early aid-seekers (or those who might fully accept an aid before they would actively seek one) may differ from others in some subtle genetically or environmentally determined variable of hearing or of personality. Non-seekers of aids could not be induced to use aids experimentally for more than perhaps a few hours, ruling out an experimental approach, so the demonstration would require elaborate psychological assessments on the seekers and the use of statistical control methods. Resources have not yet been put into this research of the required scale and finesse. The strength of the circumstantial evidence does not yet appear to justify action. The hypothesis is probably correct, but the cost of confirming it is currently high in relation to other health priorities. Also, the limited success of preventive medicine among the sectors of society apparently needing it most has been noted in enquiries into inequalities in health.

In this essay I have tried to show how some scientific issues fit into the professional fabric of services for deaf people. There is a balance between an understandable inertia in unleashing demand for costly services until their effectiveness is proven and an equally understandable frustration at not being able to provide new evidence because the services are insufficiently monitored or scientifically oriented to furnish it automatically. There are certain fundamental enigmas that will take considerable time and resources to solve, some of which could lead eventually to quantum leaps in the nature of service offered. Considering the reasons for gaps in our knowledge of hearing and deafness shows up the slender scientific foundation of some aspects of present services for the hearing-impaired, but this should not be allowed to detract from efforts to improve the circulation and application of knowledge already available.

Further Reading

BALLANTYNE, J. (1977) *Deafness*. Churchill Livingstone, Edinburgh.

BERLIN, C.I. (ed.) (1980) Studies in the use of amplification for the hearing impaired. *Excerpta Medica.*

VAN DER BRINK, G. and BILSEN, F. (ed.) (1980) *Psychophysical, Physiological and Behavioural Studies in Hearing.* Delft University Press, Delft.

CONRAD, R. (1979) *The Deaf Schoolchild.* Harper and Row, London.

DEPARTMENT OF HEALTH AND SOCIAL SECURITY (1980) *Inequalities in Health.*

HARRISON, J.M. and HOWE, M.E. (1974) Anatomy of the afferent auditory nervous system of manuals. In: *Handbook of Sensory Physiology* Vol. V(i) (Keidel, W.D. and Neff, W.D. (eds.), Springer, New York.

JERGER, J. (ed.) *Modern Developments in Audiology.* Edition II.

MANLEY, G. and KRONESTER-FREI, A. (1980) The electrophysiological profile of the organ of Corti. In: *Psychophysical, Physiological and Behavioural Studies in Hearing* (Bilsen, F. and Van den Brink, F. (eds.), Delft University Press, Delft.

MUTATION

J.H. Edwards, F.R.S.

Professor of Genetics, University of Oxford.

Formerly Professor of Clinical Genetics, University of Birmingham.

His main interests are the classification of rare syndromes, fetal disease, chromosome mapping, the interpretation of data from linked records, and the integration of human genetics and genetic counselling within the established specialities.

Mutation could claim to be the subject on which there is more ignorance, both open and concealed, than almost any other subject in biology. Furthermore due to the anxieties engendered by what cannot be seen, and the exploitation of nuclear reactions for profit in peace and cheap weaponry in war, the matter is exposed to the full glare of public and private misunderstanding, both by intent and by default.

First, we must clarify the words we need to use. The genetic message consists of a string of four symbols. This string is usually segmented into some twenty or so substrings, the chromosomes, and is conveyed from parent to child in the germ cells, each child receiving two similar sets, one from each parent. Within each individual, these paired strings pair, break, and rejoin, so that each individual passes on in his or her gametes a selection of the two strings: this selection is made by chance. That is, given two input strings from the mother and father, divided by commas with sub-strings

ABCDE, FGHIJ, KLMNO, ...

a b c d e, f g h i j, k l m n o, ...

their children would receive such strings as

ABcde, fghIJ, KLMNO, ...

and this is a normal rearrangement, in part due to the independence of the sub-strings, or chromosomes, and in part due to the actual cut-and-rejoin processes between matching chromosomes. This provides the mechanism of normal variation, so that children differ from each other and from both parents. In fact, the cut-and-join is slightly more complicated than the two-strand model indicates but the consequences are effectively the same.

The method is complicated: the unit characters are the bases which are fairly small containing a dozen or so atoms. As well as rearranging they have to multiply; this they do by each string having a paired structure, one being the replica of the other. Of the four bases, Thymine (T), Cytosine (C), Guanine (G) and Adenine (A) each has their obverse (A with T; C with G). They multiply by separating when their obverse bases are assembled to form a pair of identical paired strings. For various reasons T is sometimes coded as U (Uridine), but in this context these may be regarded as synonyms.

For example the paired string:

    AGCTGTCTAATA
    TCGACAGATTAT

will separate to give the two strings

    AGCTGTCTAATA
    TCGACAGATTAT

which then form new obverse strings

    AGCTCTCTAATA
    t c g a g a g a t t a t

    TCGACAGATTAT
    a g c t g t c t a a t a

where the small letters denote the 'new' strings. In practice these form a cable, the 'Double Helix', however, this complication does not affect our model.

Both the division and the cut-and-join process, which is largely restricted to a single cell division in the germ cells, are very complicated, and provide adequate scope for errors. For example an error may occur in replication:

AGAT . . . — AGAT . . . — AGAT —
  t c t a   . . . .   c c t a

instead of   t c t a
and later

    c c t a   will replicate to
    GGAT —   mutation (A to G)

Alternately, cut-and-splice errors could be more complicated, with bits missed out, or bits duplicated. As the coding parts of the genetic message are in the form of three letter words unpunctuated by any gaps, any duplication or deficiency not involving a multiple of three bases would degrade the message beyond recognition. All these events are mutations. The thread of life, the string of bases, started in a small way about 3,000,000,000 years ago. Now, due to constant duplications, deficiencies and changes, we, who claim to be the highest organism, share with other mammals a heritage of about 3,000,000,000 bases from each parent. This is a large number.

If we reproduced by dictating our genetic message at a base a second, each act of fertilization would take 70 years. On average, since the primaeval slime we have added about a base a year, with little change in the number in the last hundred million years. It is the accumulation of these differences or mutations, which is the source of evolution. This can be regarded as a process for the elaboration of new texts, whose consequences, the members of the next generation, may or may not survive. If they survive they may or may not succeed in conception and in rearing offspring themselves.

Death is the only proof reader: the proofs cannot be corrected. There are, of course, various correcting mechanisms built into the system, but these can only work at a very limited level; a printer ignorant of English could be advised to put u after q, and, the automatic correction of uq to qu would usually improve the text but not always. However, such correcting procedures are necessarily limited, and of no relevance to the increase in mutation rate from radiation or chemicals, since the relevant data are on misprints after such treatment. Since evolution can only act by selection, and selection can only act on differences, we have a basic text-producing mechanism in which variations must have their source in mutation. Each new variation may well live or die with its host, and since the genetic message is duplicated it will have a 50% chance of being passed on to each child.

As a species we have evolved because we varied in the past, and this variation is the consequence of mutation. Variation is the basis for the differences between children, for the large differences between cousins, and for the far larger differences between men and mice. If there were no mutation in the past we would not be here: nor would we be here if the amount of mutation had exceeded our capacity to 'clear' mutants by their selection.

Mutants, like any textual change, may or may not disturb the meaning: most will be of small effect in degrading the message, but a sufficient number will degrade any message. But even in the simple problem of misprints a separation between 'good' misprints which improve the text, 'neutral' misprints which only degrade the text slightly, and 'detrimentals', which lead to either ineffective or misleading instructions, cannot be defined easily. Even 'neutral' mutations would be difficult to define, since often a word or phrase might tolerate either of two misprints with little loss of sense on their own, but jointly be confusing and potentially detrimental.

Even in an established language considerable experience is needed to proof read, or to adjudicate on the 'neutrality' of an error. The genetic language is but poorly known. Something is understood of the 'genes', the units which produce defined products for export from the cell nucleus. They are the 'nouns' of the genetic language. They represent less than a tenth of the text in higher organisms, and are not only embedded in extensive prefixes and suffixes, but usually contain extensive infixes, or non-exporting segments of DNA of unknown function. These have only recently been discovered (for a clear introduction see Chambon in the Scientific American May 1981). Most of the variation in our genetic material is probably in the poorly understood text between the 'nouns' for we have no reason to assume any preference of mutations for the fraction of the text occupied by 'nouns'.

It is not even clear whether the differences which distinguish, for example, man from the chimpanzee, are to be found in the 'nouns' at all: certainly the gene products, or proteins, are extremely similar in both species, and if in some way the 'nouns' in the fertile ovum of a chimpanzee could be exchanged for their equivalent human forms, it is possible there would be little obvious effect.

The 'nouns' show a mean difference between individuals of around 1 in 1000 bases, or a mean difference on average of about 3,000,000 bases. In each pair of different bases one was usually parent to the other but misprints may take place, for example:

$$
\begin{array}{cccc}
A & A & & A \quad G \\
 & & to & \\
T & C^* & & T \quad C
\end{array}
$$

Where C* is a new mutation or misprint, which is derived from T, the normal pair with A. TC*TC then produces the obverse AGAG, in place of AAAG, so that there are now two forms in the population, the ancestral (AAAG) and the mutant (AGAG). This must have happened sometime, and, if we knew when, we could define the distribution of ages of these events. Most would have preceded the division between species, but some, especially those which are seriously disabling, would be of fairly recent origin. For example Sickle cell anemia, the second commonest lethal recessive in the world (another haemoglobin disorder, Thalassaemia, is commoner), could well have arisen from a single mutant event in the early Christian era. The recessive disorders peculiar to the Ashkanazi Jews and the Finns must have arisen as unique events after their separation from the Sephardic Jews and the Hungarians.

As the system of reproduction involves loss there is a chance of minority terms being lost. For example if 50 individuals, with 100 genes, 90 of one form and 10 of another, each produce two effective gametes which lead to viable offspring, there is a chance of approximately $(1/2)^{10}$ or 1 in 1000 that all the minority forms would be lost. In any population exposed to a bottle-neck — and colonization often involves very thin bottle-necks -- there is a major loss of variability from chance. This variability is constantly being replaced by mutation.

We have little idea of the mutation rates in mammals, since the 'mutants' on which most work has been done do not have a known relationship to a gene which can be studied directly at the biochemical level. The constancy of some proteins, such as albumin and, in most racial groups, haemoglobin, suggests that the mutation rate must be very low, of the order of about one base pair per gamete per generation.

Given that we have evolved to where we are, what effect will varying the mutation rate have on our health? Would a doubling produce any serious effect? On what basis are the recommended maximum doses of radiation made? Should we not perhaps encourage evolution by introducing a little variability?

A human adult consists of about 10^{15} cells, of which only a small fraction, of the order of a millionth in the male and far less in the female, have the potential of posterity through forming gametes: in practice, in a stable population, only two will, on average, make the grade to the extent of producing an adult who will reproduce.

The remainder of these cells are either end cells, for example nerve cells, and will not reproduce, or stem cells such as those involved in replacing the blood, hair, skin and gut lining, which are constantly reproducing, or cells which divide occasionally or in response to need. The red cells alone are being produced at more than a million a second. Each cell with the capacity to divide, and most cells probably have this capacity (since most tissues have some capacity to regenerate after injury) and the capacity to divide uncontrollably. This condition is known as cancer.

Many agents are known which will increase this basic risk of living; it is a risk which is inseparable from having a body with the capacity to adapt and to repair injuries. Radiation is one of many such agents, as was first discovered by the pioneers of radiography, and since quantified in mice and man. The best data available are from following the radiation of an inflammatory disease of the spinal joints, a disorder of young males which rarely shortens life.

Unfortunately the excellent data on this unfortunate consequences of radiation therapy, supported by similar data on those exposed at Hiroshima and Nagasaki, have lead to cancer being regarded as the major problem of radiation. This has been asserted in a leading place in the Flowers' report and forms the basis of many projections of the consequences of various types of nuclear accident involving power stations, and of nuclear weapons. Further publicity has been given to this undoubted risk by the prolonged controversy over the exposure of workers in an American shipyard working on nuclear submarines, a controversy largely conducted in the weekly and Sunday press. Since about 20% of adults may expect to die from cancer, and since there have already been substantial damages awarded to workers exposed within the recommended safety limits, this relatively minor problem of cancer-risk, as opposed to genetic risk, continues to receive a steady press.

The facts are that while cancers are a slight risk, even for the most exposed workers with the current safety limits, it is a risk which is many-fold less than the excess risks run by the average smoker. The mutation leading to a cancer will at least develop within a lifetime of the exposed, and will not be passed on to future generations. Even if, as is possible, the risks are underestimated, the nuclear industry is clearly one of the safest industries. Cancers are well documented in advanced countries usually with the preservation of microscope slides of the tumour. All industries have their hazards, and this hazard, in spite of its emotive name, hardly competes with the hazards peculiar to most other industries, especially those related to fossil fuels.

However, while the consequences of a mutation to a non-germinal cell will occur within the lifetime of the worker, and manifest themselves as a well studied type of disease, the germinal mutations are of quite another variety. We would expect the majority to show up for a few centuries if they relate to a specific metabolic defect, or, if they merely reduce the level of developmental potential in a general way, never to show up as a specific disorder. Some mutations will disrupt whole chromosomes, and be manifest in the next generation, and others, through more subtle rearrangements, may show up in the second generation. The dominant disorders are very badly understood at the level of the gene and there is no evidence that these are likely to be the major problem.

The natural dose of radiation from both outer space and from the disintegration of various naturally occurring isotopes is easily measured, and shows considerable variation. Roofing, as expected, reduces exposure while some building materials, such as the granite used for housing in Aberdeen and elsewhere, produces far more radioactivity than it absorbs thus imposing an additional radiational burden on most Aberdonians greatly exceeding what they have received, or are likely to receive, from any source short of War.

Given the impracticality of conducting many scientific and medical activities without some increase in radiation, and the commercial attractions of nuclear power, there has necessarily been a demand for advice on permissible levels and for an administrative framework for the supervision of those exposed.

This advice is largely based on measurements of the natural background radiation. The common sense view is that since we are surviving this degree of nuclear bombardment, and the various areas and populations exposed to slightly higher levels seem none the worse, then workers exposed to radiation should merely be protected from exceeding some arbitrary upper limit based on this being n-fold the population exposure from natural causes. We merely agree on some number n which is a compromise between the impossible and the intolerable.

Fortunately there seems to be expert agreement among physicists that the damage is proportional to the total energy absorbed and is unlikely to be related to critical wavelengths, as for example is sunburn. This view accords well with the considerable experience of the use of radiation to destroy cancerous tissues. The evidence on the degree of intentional damage is entirely consistent with proportionality of dose to a first approximation. The rarity of adverse effects on the children of those who have been exposed, although based largely on absence of reports on large populations at risk rather than systematic studies, is certainly consistent with the view that artificial radiation has no specifically harmful effects beyond those of natural radiation.

The units of radiation, the roentgen, the rad and the rem, which for practical purposes for most types of radiation may be regarded as identical, provide the usual measure. Natural radiation occurs at a rate of about 100 millerems (or a tenth of a rem) a year. To double the mutation rate of those few systems adequately studied in mice requires about 100 rem, or a thousand years of natural exposure concentrated into one generation. In man the limited data are consistent with this.

So at worst the crippled survivors of nuclear war would have accumulated the same consequences as their ancestors accumulated in the last mellenium or so.

Attempts have therefore been made to find a framework of guidance for accepted levels of radiation by learning from the consequences of therapy, of accidents, or war, and of analogy from other species. These attempts have hardly succeeded in providing estimates within an order of magnitude of their aim.

But what are the immediate consequences of a mutation? If the mutant unit is big enough, such as the whole chromosome whose excess presence is responsible for Down's syndrome, sometimes called Mongolism, the consequences can be severe. A predisposition to this disorder is known to be achieved by low levels of radiation. It affects over 1 child in 1000 and is of one of the most catastrophic immediate consequences: a duplication of almost 100,000,000 bases takes place. At the other extreme, the change of a single base may lead to a subtle change in a highly ordered protein, such as haemoglobin, so that its physical properties

cause the deformed red cells found in Sickle-cell disease: a disorder which is fatal if the defect is conveyed through both parents. On the other hand, as with a text or musical score, there are positions in which a single letter, or note, may be of little consequence.

The simplest question we can therefore ask is, assuming that we are dealing with a shrapnel type injury from single fragments, what increase in the radiation doses can be tolerated? A community could probably tolerate a doubling of the 'natural' dose if this proved to be essential for commerce or defence. However, the consequences of doubling in relation to genetic damage will probably be largely due to recessive damage, and this will not show up for a few centuries, when children are born who are descendants of an ancestor who had the mutation.

This is about the state of the present recommendations. Their acceptance during this twilight period of ignorance can hardly lead to catastrophic consequences in a few generations, during which, provided the depth of this ignorance is realised, sufficient should be known to modify these primitive, but sound, guidelines.

Further Reading

BERG, Kare (ed.) (1979) Genetic Damage in Man Caused by Environmental Agents.

COGGLE, J.E. (1971) The Biological Effects of Radiation. The Wykeham Science Series 14.

FLOWERS Report (1976) Royal Commission on Environmental Pollution. 6th Report. Cmnd. Paper 6618, HMSO.

NEWCOMBE, H.B. (1875) Mutation and the Amount of Human Ill Health. Radiation Research. Academic Press, New York.

NOVITSKI, E. Human Genetics.

SOBLES, F.H. (1969) Radiation as a Tool in Fundamental and Applied Genetics. In: *Fifty Years of Genetics* (John Jinks, ed.) Chapter 17.

DESTINY AND THE GENES: GENETIC PATHOLOGY AND THE INDIVIDUAL

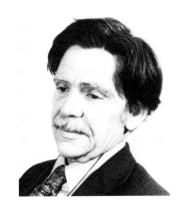

Philip G.H. Gell, F.R.S.

Professor Emeritus, University of Birmingham.

He has worked for the Medical Research Council and as Reader and Professor of Experimental Pathology, University of Birmingham. He is now officially retired but working in the Department of Pathology, University of Cambridge (Virus group).

The most profitable areas of ignorance to discuss are those in which we feel we have sure knowledge but in fact do not, concepts accepted as scientific by everyone except scientists; such problems for example as those of allergy, analytical psychology and the genes. It is this last area which I wish to examine, since it is a fruitful source of beliefs unsupported by evidence, both in the public mind and elsewhere. Ultimately I attempt to bridge with a few ideas and speculations the hiatus in knowledge between the functioning of the genes in man and the personality of the individual. Can we extract any useful pointers on this question from the minute amount of information we do have about genes in man and by analogy from the still very small amount of information we have about genes in animals of less thorough comparable complexity?

To what extent are we the prisoners of our genes? The fact that we can make so few useful generalizations about the area between a genotype, defined in terms of a particular gene product, and overt behaviour and personality has been a rich source of rubbish, as any area half explored by science usually is. My main aim therefore is to examine my own ignorance, which I believe to be shared by the rest of us on this subject, by way of indicating what little we do know of how or whether our nemesis is right there in the nucleus.

179

Other sorts of constraints on freedom, including blind chance and the pressures of the environment, function partially at least by interacting with what is there in the first place, the genotype. It is only this interaction which is interesting. The interplay of the genes with one another, with the environment and if you like with derived extrapolations such as original sin, the Freudian instinctual drives and the will generate an interacting system which must be understood if one is to go any way towards answering the question with which I started this paragraph.

How do the genes actually work? How does a run of DNA exert an influence on such a piece of work as man? First of all we can stress that the only things which genes can or will ever give rise directly to are runs of amino-acids, forming proteins. These proteins may be actual enzymes which function in the economy of the body or they may be substances which control the level of activation of other genes in the nucleus: a large part of the genotype seems to be devoted to this controller function. The link between these proteins of precise function and such faculties as intelligence, aggressiveness, altruism and so forth is bound to be difficult to analyse, if not in principle unanalysable.

Owing to the impracticability of controlled breeding programmes in man, we have to rely upon chance genetic defects for most of our information, since only rarely and in the simplest situations is there any demonstrable dependence of a behavioural trait on any biochemically defined product of an allelic gene. Defects arising from the genetic apparatus are of several kinds, of which the first and most obvious kind is that due to a single aberrant mutant gene, as occurs for instance in haemophilia. Such incompetent genes, though easy to identify, are unimportant in evolution and do not show much interaction with other genes, hence such cases, the exception rather than the rule, do not give us much insight into the normal function of the genotype. More information can be gained from cases where whole chromosomes or chromosome pairs are affected: in particular we have information about some defects which affect the sex chromosomes. A little while ago a great deal of interest was aroused in the so called hypermale syndrome, where there is an extra Y, i.e. male chromosome in the genotype, so that the formula is XYY. Patients with this defect were supposed to have a predisposition to criminal delinquency involving violence: in fact people began to talk about 'the criminal chromosome'. This was however a characteristic aberration of simplistic genetics. In the words of Becker (1974) 'More and more information now demonstrates the complexity of the interaction betwixt genetic and environmental factors in the development of human behaviour'. Nevertheless, it was not so long ago even in scientific circles that serious consideration was given to the hypothesis that progressive antisocial behaviour might be directly and exclusively genetically determined. The question arose after a high incidence of XYY chromosome configurations was detected in aggressive male criminals (Jacobs et al., 1965). In 1969 in the USA a symposium was devoted to the XYY configuration and its implications in personality development. The Report on the XYY Chromosome Abnormality (1970) gives an account of the conclusions arrived at by this symposium, among which are 'while a greater prevalence rate of XYY males amongst several groups of institutionalized criminals of mentally disordered dependents is not to be disputed the widely publicized belief concerning aggressivity and natisocial behaviour as typical characteristics of such individuals are premature and subject to error. The fact that criminal behaviour is a complex and multi-determined phenomenon makes it extremely unlikely that the extra Y chromosome is the only or even the major cause of this'. In fact, it appears as if people with XYY were different only in being rather more apt to lose their tempers under stress, more apt to let this result in physical action, and being in most cases unusually large and strong, more apt to do damage in consequence. The 18th century, which didn't know much about chromosomes, would have called them 'choleric', suffering from an excess of black bile: no more.

In Turner's syndrome there is a chromosome actually missing, the formula is XO, and the subjects are essentially females, with some genital defects. In addition a proportion (about 70%) have an apparently lowered I.Q., the rest being normal. Psychological examination shows that this low I.Q. results from a bizarre group of defects, including (Becker, 1974) . . .'poor orientation in space and time, inaccurate writing of words and numbers, dyslexia and dyscalculia, difficulties in word mobilisation and vague or imprecise word usage, symptoms which depend upon a poorly developed body image, poor left—right discrimination, difficulty in space—form perception, and poor concentration'. Such defects, definable fairly precisely in terms of behaviour, — 'body image' is a much more exact concept than 'intelligence' — evidently arise from unbalancing effects of minor inadequacies in many genes which should have been represented as alleles on the missing chromosome, all of which make some contribution to 'body image', that in its turn has a profound influence on the development of intelligence.

These two examples illustrate the complications we have to deal with if we try to talk about the heritability of imprecise concepts like intelligence. A similar complexity is evident if we consider the field now developing as genetic pathology, which is concerned with the influence of the genotype on disease susceptibility. It is clear that certain diseases run in families, but most of these do not show an obvious pattern of inheritance like say haemophilia, but seem to crop up in some families quite sporadically. It is only of recent years that we have been able to make sense of this situation. This is because such diseases have multiple causes, and the presence of a

particular gene is only one of these causes. This gene may however conspire with factors in the environment both internal and external to favour the development of a disease such as juvenile diabetes or arthritis. In the former for example, if a child with the gene happens to contract a not uncommon virus infection, and if he is on a certain type of diet, he may develop an antibody which reacts deleteriously with certain cells in the pancreas; if this antibody is produced in quantity or repeatedly so that a considerable number of cells are destroyed he will then develop diabetes. So even in the presence of the gene there is a further chain of necessary events, some gene dependent, some aleatory, which must occur before the disease is developed: the presence of the gene is not sufficient. A large number of diseases nowadays, some common such as rheumatoid arthritis, some less common but devastating such as disseminated sclerosis or lupus, some quite rare, such as Sjogren's syndrome or myasthemia gravis fall into this group, but it is evident that they all involve some component of the immune system, hyperactivity or under-activity or perverse activity. How does this happen?

To understand this we have to discover how the genome influences immune responses. For the successful development of an immune response, antigen, e.g. from a micro-organism, has to be presented in a physical complex with a genetic marker on the host's own cells. These markers, which vary from person to person but are under genetic control, are more, or less, able to complex with particular antigens, and so to present them efficiently — such is the current hypothesis at least. Now, in many diseases a positive immune response may paradoxically be associated with the production of disease. In the case quoted (juvenile diabetes) this occurs possibly because there is a purely fortuitous similarity of one particular antigen of the virus, (and a virus will carry dozens of different antigens), to that of an antigen of the human pancreatic cell which produces insulin, so that the antibody 'cross-reacts' to damage that cell. In other diseases a failure to respond to an antigen in one way, e.g. by antibody production, may leave the body only able to respond with tuberculin type hypersensitivity which can be actively damaging. In yet a third way, presentation of antigen in a certain way may lead to the generation of cells (suppressor cells) which damp down the immune response instead of promoting it which is the normal way of tailing off the immune response, but can get out of balance. The immune system is complex and there are many other possible situations, but the upshot is that a whole group of diseases may be associated with immune responses, positive or negative, whose deleterious nature is under genetic control. These genetic factors with other non-genetic ones may, as I have said, conspire to facilitate the development of the disease.

It must be stressed that many people without the gene may develop the disease but rather fewer in proportion to incidence of the gene in the population at risk. Supposing for example that 10% of the population have gene A, whilst 20% of the population have gene B but of those that have the disease, perhaps 0.01% of the population, equal numbers have gene A as have gene B, then we can say that there is a statistically significant association of the disease with gene A.

Thirty or forty different diseases in man have been investigated from this point of view, varying from tuberculosis and rheumatoid arthritis to some of the very rare conditions mentioned above, and with all of these we can put down a percentage varying from 99% to 0% for an association with a particular identifiable gene of man. All these genes are in the region of the genome associated with immune function, since there happen to be easily identifiable markers on the cells of normal people coded from this region. There are four loci in this region in man which are polymorphic systems, that is to say at each locus there may be thirty or forty different

possible genetic variants. The HLA—B region is the one most commonly associated with these diseases, although the importance of the HLA—DR/DW region, which is probably analogous to the immune response region in the mouse, is beginning to be recognised too. Particular numbered alleles of the HLA—B region may be associated with particular diseases, that is to say that there is a statistically significant increased incidence of that particular allele in patients with that disease, although many patients lacking that allele may also have the disease. The presence of some of these alleles is not all loss. For instance the B8 allele although it is associated with a number of diseases due to perverse antibody response is also associated with an improved ability to recover from infections. In a quite different gene system, the Fy antigens of red blood cells, one genotype common in Africa confers resistance to *Plasmodium vivax* (tertian) malaria, probably because the cells lack a receptor for the parasite.

It is clearly a rather paradoxical situation that we have this relatively weak association of individual genes with what should be simple biochemical lesions causing diseases. There are various possible reasons for this. It may be that we are looking at the wrong gene, not the gene actually responsible for the disease incidence but merely at one which is linked to it, being rather close to it on the chromosome in a state known as linkage disequilibrium. There still might be a gene, most likely in the HLA—DR region, which is both necessary and sufficient to the development of the disease but on the evidence this is rather unlikely. Another possibility is that the association with the disease is really quantitative; if it is all a matter of complexing antigen with gene product for presentation to the immune system, gene products may just differ among themselves, some being markedly better or worse at complexing with antigen but all being capable of doing so. We can contrast the situation with B8 where all immune processes are intensified, with the effect of certain other alleles which are much more specific for particular diseases. Moreover since we have never been able to show the inevitable association of any genes in this group with disease (as is the case with haemophilia, etc.) the great majority of people with a suspect gene do not have any sign of the disease. There are almost certainly multiple extra-genetic causes and there may also be other genes in a genome which favour or inhibit the action of the suspect gene. It is clear that this is still an area of pretty considerable ignorance, but a dispensable ignorance which should be cleared up in a few years time, since we know what to look for and how to look for it. Nevertheless even in a situation of disease susceptibility, which is basically a matter of biochemistry, the influence of the genome will be partial and complex.

I should like to turn now to the more general question of behaviour in man, to attempt to trace how close is the link between genes, which we can consider biochemically, and the phenotype — the product of all the genes and a whole lot of other factors as well. So complex a matter as behaviour is obviously determined by a number of different genes working together. To what extent can it be analysed in genetic terms? Even in insects it is rare to find behavioural differences which are simply gene-determined, apart from those which are due to gross defects on a par with haemophilia in man. Behaviour determined polygenically is all the more readily modifiable by the activity of other genes in the genome and by environmental experience working in the nervous system. A nice example of this modifiability is provided by the work of Lagerspetz and Lagerspetz (1974). They bred strains of highly aggressive mice, showing clearly enough that a function like aggressiveness is broadly under genetic control, which surprises nobody. However these authors say 'As described earlier non-aggressive mice could be produced

in four different ways, by selective breeding for non-aggressiveness, by having aggressive animals defeated, by grouping aggressive animals for long time-periods, and by giving live animals, even descendants of the aggressive TA line, sexual experiences. The latter three methods imply that even in small laboratory animals like mice social experiences may cause complex and psychologically interesting effects and interactions. They also show that genetic disposition for aggressiveness can be modified by different social factors. In man the development of behaviour rests to a larger extent on learning than in other animals. It seems probable that in humans environmental influences account to a high degree for the variations in aggressiveness'.

Thus both interactions between genes and environmental effects have to be taken into account when we are considering the area between genotype and phenotype, what Waddington, who has done so much to map this field, called the 'epigenetic space'. In this connection Franck (1974) writes: 'the appearance of genetic changes which impair to a catastrophic degree the probability of survival of their carrier is a rare event. An illuminating explanation of this fact may be the existence of complex polyfactorial modes of inheritance. One must assume that the genetic system underlying species specific behaviour is structured in such a way that single mutations can drastically alter it rarely or not at all. Where several genes interacted, cummulatively single changes in the gene system would result only in quantitative changes in behaviour. A single mutation event could never entirely extinguish the behavioural difference. Thus far the discoveries in behavioural genetics indicate that evolutionary changes in behaviour patterns arise in general step by step with complex alterations in a system of genic interactions which is most effectively stabilised'.

This point is further emphasised by Jinks and Broadhurst (1974): 'Rothenbühler's dissection of the hygienic behaviour of honey bees as dependent on the action of two major genes* is an example which is cited with deserving frequency. But such cases are rare, especially in the animal kingdom, and we are usually faced with variation which is gradual and continuous, that is, quantitative in kind and which, moreover is sensitive to environmental manipulation to an extent which the actions of genes of major effect are often not. The reason for this state of affairs is not far to seek — discontinuities due to major genes are relatively rare. The more usual situation is one in which many genes, each having an effect which is minor but supplementary to one another, act together on the resultant phenotype. That techniques for the analysis of genes of major effect — the classical Mendelian analyses — came to be developed first is not surprising for such cases naturally came to light by their prominence'. And again, . . .'so you can see the essential feature of the biometrical approach to be the idea that variation is governed by multiple factors both genetic and environmental. The genetic contribution is regulated by numerous genes which are inherited in a Mendelian way which have effects similar to one another, supplementing each other and small as compared with the total variation due to all causes, heritable or non-heritable. In this way, smooth continuous variation of the phenotype results from discontinuous quantitative variations of the genotype and of the environment. In general the effects of single genetic factors will be too small to be followed individually, and the same will be also true of many micro-environmental factors. An immediate consequence of the multiple gene control is that the balanced effect of many genes, some having a positive, increasing effect on the measure and others having a negative, decreasing effect, determines the genotype contribution to the phenotype. Hence various combinations of genes may make the same contribution, indeed the more genes included in the polygenic system governing a particular trait the greater the number of possible combinations of genes that will on balance make precisely the same contributions to the phenotype. Further this multiple control results in the apparent paradox that genotypes which produce identical phenotypes may differ among themselves by as many genes as do genotypes which produce widely different phenotypes'. Many examples too complex to quote here are given in the publications from which these citations are taken.

We therefore have to use what can be called an interactionist analysis of genetically determined situations. Too much of our conventional thinking about individual genes comes from highly exceptional situations, owing to their greater prominence and ease of analysis. It seems indeed that it is dangerous to use the concept gene at all in the context of complex emergent functions such as behaviour. It is therefore unfortunate that the idea of the 'selfish gene' just like the concept of the 'criminal chromosome' XYY referred to earlier, is beginning to work its way into popular mythology. The idea that genes strive to perpetuate themselves in evolution was originally stated by J.B.S. Haldane (see Maynard Smith, 1979), but the all too vivid phrase the 'selfish gene' was introduced by K.W. Dawkins (1977) in his highly readable book of that title. In particular he proffers a rather cavalier concept

---

* Rothenbühler found that the disease known as foul brood in bees was the result of the defect of two genes which controlled two fairly complicated hygienic rituals. This certainly indicates the over-riding importance of a single gene, or rather of its biochemical product, in each of the two modes of behaviour, but does not imply that the normal mode of behaviour is itself the exclusive product of a single gene function. Simply, one would suppose that the defect of one gene is not compensatable by other parts of the genome, and this gene is also poor in alleles which might have led to quantitative differences and a graded rather than an absolute tendency to defect.

of the nature of the gene; as he says disarmingly 'I prefer to think of the gene as the fundamental unit of natural selection and therefore the fundamental unit of self-interest. What I have now done is to define the gene in such a way that I cannot really help being right'. Surely it is more judicious to define the gene as what it actually is in higher organisms at least, as far as present knowledge goes, that is, a bounded bit of DNA which codes for a precise protein. Anything more than this, as Dawkins himself implies, entails a circular argument. The sociobiologist E.O. Wilson (1975), falls I believe into this trap. He is reasonably explicit as to the importance of some sort of interactionist interpretation of gene function, saying for instance . . .'future population genetics seems destined to concentrate more on whole chromosomes, their recombination properties, the intensity of epistatic interactions amongst interlinked loci, and the effects of homozygosity on chromosomes of various lengths' and a little later: 'The adjustments of one locus theory on which this and most branches of theoretical population genetics still rests now to the new locus interaction theory is a task for the future. It remains for sociobiologists to exploit both levels as opportunity provides'. The word 'level' here is I feel misleading as the single locus formulation is not an alternative, but in the vast majority of cases simply inapplicable. So later he writes as follows, which I feel to be enjoyable as rhetoric but unacceptable as argument 'the hypothalamic–limbic complex of a highly social species such as man 'knows', or more precisely it has been programmed to perform as if it knows, that its underlying genes will be proliferated maximally only if it orchestrates behavioural responses that bring into play an efficient mixture of personal survival, reproduction and altruism. Consequently the centres of the complex tax the conscious mind with ambivalence whenever the organism encounters a stressful situation. Love joins hate; aggression, fear; expansiveness, withdrawal, and so on, in blends designed not to promote the happiness or survival of the individual, but to favour the maximum transmission of the controlling genes'.

As Waddington (1975) has emphasised, the units which are worked on by synchronic social interactions and diachrononic evolutionary trends are not genes but phenotypes: that is, the resultants of all the necessary interactions between the genes of an individual.* What one can describe as diachronically conditioned phenotypes will include also modifications to the functioning of the genotype introduced by environmental experience, as in Lagerspetz's non-aggressive aggressive mice or culturally conditioned humans.

I feel that in using a more sophisticated genetic approach the explanatory value of the selfish gene concept in accounting for altruistic behaviour simply evaporates. All that is demonstrated is that altruistic behaviour is the product of the totality of the personality of an animal. Nevertheless I do not wish to undervalue in any way the insights of ethologists and sociobiologists on their own ground, and their importance for evolutionary theory, but only to criticise

---

* The total quantity per cell of DNA (that is of possible genomal material) available in lower animals and indeed in plants is entirely comparable with that in higher animals including man; an estimate of the actual number of genes in man, or in the mouse, is between 10^5 and 10^7. If most gene effects with any influence upon behaviour or indeed on evolution are polygenic and interactional, one could deduce that a highly evolved species as compared with a less evolved species would show in its genotype perhaps nothing very remarkable at a single gene level, but a rather more sophisticated and well adapted interactional system; evolution of higher animals at least, being not so much a matter of mutating genes as of the more subtle organization of interacting systems. Indeed there is no reason to suppose that Darwin or Shakespeare had access to any 'genes for intelligence' other than those already present in Cro-Magnon man in the Palaeolithic, many of them perhaps being present in pre-human hominids as well.

what I feel to be a simplistic interpretation in terms of genetic mechanisms applied to individuals: as I have tried to show, the complexities of the genetic system make any naive analysis in terms of genes inapplicable.

When we come to questions of human behaviour, the ability of humans to respond to the environment, not just through simple sensibilia, but by language and culture, takes them even further from any direct genetic control. It is arguable that what Karl Marx said in 1848 has had far greater selective effects upon human phenotypes than any sort of genetically based selection process. The pattern of genetic interactions at the evolutionary level of a species such as man is such that, on the onset of sophisticated social intercourse, in particular by way of language and writing, quite fundamental modifications of phenotype can occur. So malleable is the animal genetic apparatus that its whole pattern or bias may be altered by interaction with the environment. This may be in the form of possible messages transmitted to an individual by maternal RNA in the ovum embodying some of the experience of the previous generation, or of imprints via the nervous system of an individual's own experience, or in man of culturally conveyed diurnal experience of other humans interacting with him. All these, and their possible effects in flipping the individual's development into one or another 'chreodic pathway' (Waddington, 1972), serve to dilute almost to vanishing point the influence of gene-ordained biochemistry.

The heart of the problem lies in the fact that we are dealing not with a chain of causation but with a network, that is, a system like a spider's web in which a perturbation at any point of the web changes the tension of every fibre right back to its anchorage in the blackberry bush. Network causation, in which partial causes are in effect unbounded or at least non-numerable (it is a pity that the word 'innumerable' has been

stylistically degraded to mean just 'a lot') leads to probabilistic conclusions. Small causes, as by genes or experiences some distance away from what might be supposed the main chain of causation, can have large outcomes in switching pathways.

How does this bear upon the problem of Free Will? I suggest that Free Will is a resultant of the complexity of a network system. This would not forbid a measure of free will to lower animals but human phenotypic behaviour can draw upon such an enormous range of influences, from the genes, to the pathways established in the nervous system, to the intellectual influence brought to bear by cultural interaction, that the complexity is orders of magnitude greater. At some stage in the development of this complexity, freedom becomes an emergent property. At this stage, our capacity for choice, which is what we are trying to link to our genotype, is not at all determined by chemically defined gene products but by the total surface of our network systems, which includes all our past experience. In fact it is determined by what we are; something which humans have always believed intuitively without having to bother with chromosomes, genes or whatever.

The area of ignorance which I have tried to adumbrate is not merely that between the genotype and the phenotype, though we certainly know little enough here, but also involves the nature of individual freedom. The interface which a human presents to the world is a product of so many and so complex interacting forces that it is not open to scientific analytical methods, which deal with units that are not unique. So if the gap in knowledge of man between the operations of the genotype and the behaviour of the person is not merely unbridged, but in principle, unbridgeable then our ignorance will remain ineluctable. Perhaps in the future someone will invent a sort of psycho-computer to deal with it, but I don't know, I really don't know.

References

BECKER, F.W. (1974) In *Genetics of Behaviour*, p. 274 (Abeelen, J.M.C., ed.). Nord Holland Press.

DAWKINS, K.W. (1977) *The Selfish Gene*, p. 34. Paladin.

FRANCK, D. (1974) In: *Genetics of Behaviour* (Abeelen, J.M.C., ed.). p. 36. Nord Holland Press.

JACOBS, P.M., BRUNTON, M. and MELVILLE, M. (1965) Aggressive behaviour, mental subnormality and the XYY Male. *Nature, 208,* 1351.

JINKS, J.L. and BROADHURST, C.M. (1974) In: *Genetics of Behaviour* (Abeelen, J.M.C., ed.), p. 4. Nord Holland Press.

LAGERSPETZ, K.M.J. and LAGERSPETZ, K.Y.H. (1974) In: *Genetics of Behaviour* (Abeelen, J.M.C., ed.), p. 342. Nord Holland Press.

MAYNARD SMITH, J. (1979) The limitations of Evolutionary Theory. In: *The Encyclopedia of Ignorance,* (Duncan, R. and Weston-Smith, M., eds.), p. 239. Pergamon Press, Oxford.

VON BERTALANNFY, L. (1977) *General Systems Theory*, Penguin University Books; a most stimulating and relevant work, which unfortunately I did not come upon until this article was in proof.

WADDINGTON, C.H., Determinism and life. In: *The Nature of Mind*. Gifford Lectures 1971/72, p. 33. Edinburgh University Press.

WADDINGTON, C.H. (1975) *The Evolution of an Evolutionist*. Edinburgh University Press.

WILSON, E.O. (1975) *Sociobiology*, p. 13. Harvard University Press.

CONTRACEPTION

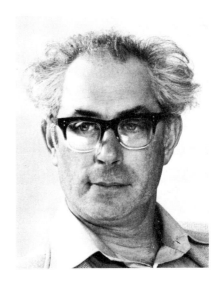

Jack Cohen

Senior Lecturer in Reproduction, School of Biological Sciences, University of Birmingham.

His research activities have involved feather and hair growth and pigmentation and the general principles of development. Recent research has concerned the fate and function of excess spermatozoa in female mammals, and the development of antisperm antibodies as a contraceptive technique. His present interests include social aspects of sexuality and the relationships between development and evolution.

Ignorance about contraceptive methods, mechanisms and practices is an impossibly large canvas, and I will restrict this article to a few areas. Even in these areas it will be necessary to lay some of the foundations in reproductive biology; for much of our failure in the development of contraceptive techniques and in the application of those which we have results from misunderstanding or ignorance of the basic facts.

First, we should look at the 'natural' controls of human multiplication. This leads to consideration of the following questions: do technical methods of contraception reduce births further than these natural methods, or are we stopping the same babies by other

means? How do the natural methods operate, and can their mechanisms be successfully integrated into a technical affluent society? Are the motivations for technical and other contraceptives different from previous natural controls, so that a different breeding pattern might emerge?

Second, consideration of the modes of action of contraceptive techniques relates to some areas of reproductive ignorance. This leads to questions about the concepts of failure rate and suitability of the technical methods, and especially about the longer-term methods presently being developed. Finally, the current moves towards 'involuntary' methods, especially sterilization and injectables, for some parts of the population will be considered briefly in relation to technical controls in a 'free' society.

This subject is in great contrast to most of the topics in the first two volumes of *The Encyclopaedia of Ignorance*. Most people have very little personal experience relating to the Big Bang, quarks or even evolution, but nearly all of the readers of this article will have had experience of potentially fertile sexual intercourse. Most will have had experience of several contraceptive techniques, some technical and some natural. Most of us, too, are at least marginally curious about how other people manage these affairs, and the figures for our society are available (Table 1) and probably fairly accurate. In contrast, our ideas about the 'natural' state of human reproduction are often limited to the 'life is savage, brutal and short' catch-phrase or to imagination of idyllic South Seas grass-skirted beauties; anthropological studies of the more sober aspects of reproductive practice have not enjoyed the press coverage of more salubrious descriptions. Nevertheless, we must consider the less exciting aspects in order to gain a background against which to view the practices of our own society.

In the 'wild', 'natural' or 'primitive' state, human breeding systems are usually said to produce births about every three years to most fertile women.* Pregnancy and lactation alternate and menstruation is rare: most of the ovulations are followed by pregnancies. This means that nearly all sexual intercourse is necessarily infertile, related to recreation rather than to procreation. Even when fertile couples have intercourse at ovulation, pregnancy is not as likely as in wild or domestic animals; a chance of $1:4$ or 5 is usual, and we do not know why or how. Furthermore, more than half of human fertilizations abort naturally and do not result in babies. Human fecundity is, therefore, naturally low, producing babies at about 3–4 year intervals.

In contrast, in nearly all actual human communities, however wild or uncivilized, there are constraints on sexual behaviour which result in even fewer offspring than such total lack of inhibition would produce. Few societies permit pregnancies to the unmarried and there are usually many other social categories who must abstain from heterosexual intercourse or employ non-fertile or contraceptive tactics. Apart from the dubious cases of those folk (e.g. the Trobrianders) said not to have realized the connection between sex and pregnancy, such tactics must also be in common use in all human cultures; not only in illicit relationships, but also in the many circumstances where offspring would be socially or economically embarrassing, people contrive to have sex without producing babies. Social constraints promote such contrivance and usually combine with the low natural fecundity and naturally high infant and juvenile mortality to produce reproduction of the population instead of its multiplication; that is to say, two parents of this generation produce two parents in the next, on average, and the population fluctuates about a mean. Sometimes such populations do increase consistently, but with repeated catastrophic drops as plagues, poor harvests or droughts take their tolls (a saw-tooth oscillation), but this is unusual on a long time scale. It is much more common to find social constraints which effectively prevent the population rising much beyond that which can be continuously sustained, using a great variety of tactics, including venereal diseases and infanticide.† The major non-social constraints on multiplication in these societies are poor nutrition, frequent and extended suckling, slow growth (causing late menarche) and chronic disease, all of which reduce the number of ovulations. Other diseases combine with nutritional deficiencies to cause miscarriage, perinatal death and much juvenile mortality.

The extent to which non-social and social constraints operate varies both between societies and within each society. The usual modern story is of advances in public health

---

* See Short (1976).

† See Douglas (1966).

TABLE 1. Use and failure rates of various contraceptive methods

Method	Unplanned pregnancies/100 woman-years (births)	Method[1] related failure rate, %	Range of[1] failure in use, %	Use in United[2] Kingdom, 1976, fertile, %	World[3] usage 1970, millions	World[3] usage 1977, millions	World[4] usage 1978, millions
Voluntary sterilization ♀ and ♂	0.1 or less	Less than 0.1	Less than 0.2[5]	13	20	80	15–30
Oral contraception, combined Pill.	0.5–3.0 (1.5?)	0.1–0.4	0.7–10.0	28	30	55	50–80
Condom (+ spermicide)	3–5 + (3?)	1.5–3.0 (1.0)	3.0–45 (5)	16	25	35	15–20
Intra-uterine contraceptive devices, IUCDs	2–3 (1?)	1.0–3.0	0.4–5.4	5	12	15	15
Other technical methods (diaphragm, cap, spermicide, etc.)	4 + (2?)	1.5–3.0	2–30	8?	30?	35?	37?
Periodic abstinence (rhythm)	10 (5?)	5–10	0.3–47	10?	?	?	?
Prolonged lactation	?	NA	NA	5?			
Abortion	NA	NA	NA	2? (see Table 2)	Probably between 1–10		50–100

All percentages are of (probably) fertile couples who are not actively seeking pregnancy. [1] Tyrer, B.L. and Bradshaw, L.E. (1979) Clinics in Obstetrics and Gynaecology 6 46. [2] OPCS. [3] IPPF 1979. [4] WHO, 1978, quoted in Djerassi. [5] Usually because of unprotected intercourse too soon after vasectomy. NA = not applicable.

and community medicine which reduce the death rate, slightly increase the birth rate and so lead to an increase of the population by these extra births, until starvation culls at the new higher level. There is a widespread view that death rate/birth rate is a useful measure of the increasing population, and that food supply is in some sense the natural limit to human and animal populations.[1] The survival of more children because of medical and agricultural advance or aid is seen as the major cause of population increases in the modern Third World and it is also clearly the case that very many people are dying of starvation. It is therefore very easy to argue that cutting the birth rate by contraceptive education will help to bring the population down to the food supply.

There are, however, fallacies in this argument which cast doubt on the diagnosis as well as on the supposed cure. First, to talk of reduction in the death rate is as semantically empty as talking of doctors saving lives; the death rate is always equal to the birth rate, but variably delayed — and doctors only put death back a little. In 1976 and 1977 in England and Wales more people died than were born, but this only reflected the high birth rate after the First World War and the fashion for later pregnancies in the late seventies. It did not presage a down-turn in our population, because none of the age group most concerned with our next generation were born in 1976–7 and few of them died then. Similarly, change in the adult death rate has little effect on population growth, compared with survival of a large cohort of juveniles to breed in their turn. Birth rate has not gone up to cause an increase in births; this large number of births is a result of juvenile survival 10–15 years before (the rate may not have changed). Introduction of contraceptive technology does not reintroduce control of birth rate: it adds a new complication to a developing problem.

The second fallacy, that food supply is the natural constraint on human (and animal)

population, has been widely held at least since Darwin read Malthus. But the natural increase of human populations is held to much lower levels than would be expected from the food supply, primarily by cultural constraints which are formally similar to the behavioural constraints used by all higher organisms to regulate their numbers.* Cultural systems which permitted uncontrolled increase may have been lost because the peoples practising them died out from plague or starvation or were converted to more provident ways by conquest or even slavery (this is a kind of inverse social Darwinism!). In any event, most peoples now reduce their fecundity by social constraints, ranging from the late (virgin) marriage and mandatory high alcohol intake of much Irish peasantry to the 'sex is dirty' of some of the Victorians and the 'exposure' of female children by several ancient Mediterranean peoples. The motivation may not be explicit, but the constraint is effective. Continuing this theme into the proposed cure for the production of too many babies, which starve, such social constraints work effectively using only the natural non-technical tactics such as withdrawal, oral or other non-fertile sexuality, and especially abstinence. (Even 'rhythm methods' work by abstinence — sometimes.) France, despite the reputation for sexual adventure and expertise, has retained a very low population growth since the 1900s, and technical contraception simply cannot have been a major factor in this restraint. With cultural motivation, people can plan their families without technical aids; without such motivation, the offer of technical aids is not accepted. We cannot know, therefore, if the introduction of technical methods has reduced population or population growth,[2] because we have good evidence that people can plan babies without them. There are two separate issues here which are both important to our ignorance of contraception: we do not know to what extent the introduction of new methods to developing countries could curb the growth in population

* See Hawthorn (1976).

and we do not know how many babies in our own society are stopped by technical methods which would not have been stopped by older tactics.

The situation in developing countries, if we are to be sceptical of the 'technical fix' solution for the reasons already argued, is totally different from that in our own society. If it is the case that people regulate their populations, by whatever culturally acceptable means are to hand, to levels which do not expose them to culturally unacceptable levels of deprivation (their culture, not ours!), then we should ask what limits are removed by exposure to our technical society so that their population then increases. The simple answer in this new frame is that the cultural constraints worked together with disease and deprivation to regulate breeding down to replacement reproduction; when disease and deprivation were removed, cultural constraints were inadequate by themselves to restrain multiplication. Change in lactational practices, suggested by Short to be the major response which increases fecundity, is seen by him as related to nutrition rather than culture. However, this suggests that people act only mechanically, without regard to the results of their actions, that negative feedback is not a part of the cultural control system. Experience suggests that this is not the case for most human social systems. One can envisage parts of the family planning system which *are* regulated by result, but also parts which are not. For example, the time spent suckling the previous child is very sensitive to the general level of nutrition and delays the next one, regulating the fecundity appropriately; whereas adoption of bottle-feeding need not be related to overall nutrition but only to advertising. However, the early arrival of the next child, for whatever reason, would bring in cultural programmes to prevent or delay further births; it is very difficult to envisage human beings who cannot relate future deprivation to present sexuality. Why do they have more children despite the problems these are sure to bring? Can it simply be that present pleasure is worth more than future misery, at least to the man who forces his desires on the woman?

Some information that would begin to give answers in this area could perhaps be gleaned from the differences between the birth rates of different sub-cultures, for example religious groups or economic classes exposed to the same public health measures, food availability and new technology. Examples of this, in so far as the different sectors may be said to experience innovation equivalently, can be found in India,[*] in several island communities and in the oil-rich Arab states, but the most illuminating examples could well be immigrant communities attempting to maintain the old ways in the midst of new plenty. Unfortunately, there is no general pattern; sometimes all strata multiply (Irish in America), the more affluent may have more children (many Asian communities in Africa) or the affluent may multiply less than the indigent. However, nearly all communities are having fewer children than previously.[†] This emphasizes both that people (even Third World people) do seem to control their multiplication and that we cannot yet generalize about the causality of the control. We do not even know whether generalization is possible in this area. To believe that the introduction of new forms of technical contraception to other societies, or of voluntary or even coercive sterilization, will encourage or permit lessening of multiplication in any human group implies that extra children are both involuntary and regretted. In most cases this belief, while comforting to paternalist political philosophy or to compassionate meddling, has no objective basis.

Are we as ignorant of the causality in our own society? Perhaps we are, but there is a general consensus relating fertility (fecundity) both to attitude and to social class.[‡] What we do know of our own society is that the social constraints of yesteryear are disappearing and that the new motivations relating to fertility patterns are determined more by contemporary than traditional forces. These

---

* See Benjamin (1977). † See Halsey (1977).
‡ See Sai (1966).

contemporary forces do not form part of a balanced fertility pattern and it is common in all 'advanced' societies for the traditional sexual mores to be lost. For example, cultural prohibitions about early, frequent or extra-marital intercourse are disregarded or flouted by part of the population. Unintended pregnancies increase and their previous cultural assimilation into forced marriages does not occur, so these often produce unintended children who reproduce the situation in their turn. Because such advanced societies have regulated public health and usually have some form of aid or welfare programme the extra babies can grow up to contribute to the underprivileged sections of that society. To the extent that this occurs in or contributes to a recognizable group within society, that group will multiply faster than the rest. If the technology can be maintained during this increase (as Malthus denied) there may be little apparent problem — public standards relating to acceptable population densities will change. However, if the increase of numbers in this group meets limits of food, earning ability or general competence within society, then the extra children will aggravate the problems these people already have. They are already unable or exploited and the more complex technological fixes of their society are beyond them or not available to them.

Technology provides new technical methods of contraception for those who have lost the cultural constraints on their reproduction, but among these is the very segment of affluent society which cannot reliably use barrier methods or remember the pill; if they could, they might not need to. This is the classical positive feedback or 'deprivation cycle' — more children result in more poverty, in which more babies appear. This view replaces questions of 'how many?' with questions about 'which?', considerably less fashionable in present ideologies. The explanation of excess births in our society, then, could be seen as the converse of the situation in the Third World. Here, removal of the cultural

practices which previously restricted fertile intercourse now permits more accidental pregnancies; there, removal of some biological constraints on fecundity permits the same number of acts of intercourse to produce more children. Even this simple-minded anti-thesis could explain the variation in fecundity between segments of the same population, constrained either by culture or by resources. If there is such a variation in the fecundity of any reproducing population, we should enquire whether the imbalance is reproductively stable. There are many natural examples of such reproductively stable variation. At one extreme, wolves are like bees in that only one pair (or one female) in the pack has cubs which grow up. Even in rabbit colonies (when they are at a high density) there are many females whose offspring are nurtured inadequately and which therefore fail to contribute to the future of the colony. Rabbits and many other mammals are like the grouse worked on by Wynne-Edwards' team in that there is in each generation a large proportion of non-breeders.* There have been many attempts to show that the human variations in fecundity that I have suggested above are not reproductively stable in this way, but are progressive so that the more fecund part of the population ('them') is contributing more to the future than the more temperate, responsible or intelligent group ('us').[3] That such a fecund proportion will automatically contribute progressively more to the future has been accepted as axiomatic, but counter-examples with a little spurious authenticity can easily be invented: it might be the case, for example, that the deprived children of feckless mothers were very much more likely to be homosexual or infertile for other reasons. If we could find cases of human stability despite such reproductive bias, this would give much support to those who believe that such change is not progressive. Medawar[†] countered the claims of the eugenicists of the thirties, who feared a decline in general intelligence because the unintelligent

*See Medawar (1960).   † See Wynne-Edwards (1978).

manifestly had more children than they did, by comparing the results of intelligence tests on Scottish school children in the early thirties with those of a similar group in the fifties. The mean IQ had, if anything, gone up slightly. Unfortunately, this example is very poorly controlled; teaching methods could have improved so that less able children attained the same proportion of right answers, for example. More worryingly, if the tests were renormalized on a contemporary population (at least to modernize the question range) all that the comparison can show is that arithmetic was consistent over twenty years; we cannot know if the children were more stupid, just as we cannot know if they were taller if the groups were calibrated by comparison with average height! That Medawar, one of our most subtle and able thinkers, chose this example suggests that more objective or convincing evidence for stability is not available. This non-availability does not mean that ability is declining because less able people cannot avoid having babies while able people can and usually do, but some hard comparisons would be comforting.[4]

We have briefly considered the reproductive questions relating to the usage of family planning by natural or technological societies and we can turn to the mechanisms of the various methods. Before we do so, however, there is a general problem which should be considered, for this area of our ignorance of contraceptives is in some ways the most important. Contraceptive techniques are commonly given a failure rate, which is usually presented as 'pregnancies per hundred woman-years'. This method of presentation makes a very big assumption as well as avoiding the difficulties of distinguishing patient-related failure (e.g. women who forget to take the pill) from method-related failure (e.g. pregnancies which occur with an IUD (intra-uterine device). Even this latter distinction is by no means an easy one to draw from any real figures, as will easily be imagined from

the examples given. In Table 1, I have given some informed guesses about the relative contributions of method failure and patient failure of several methods, but have omitted the complication that different doctors or counsellors achieve different ratios. This is especially so, of course, in the more or less technical versions of the rhythm method, when fertile intercourse is avoided by abstinence, and ovulation needs to be predicted. Most importantly for the cryptic assumption introduced above, different doctors assign the same sort of patient to different methods, and still achieve different failure rates. Thus in almost all cases we cannot have figures from unselected patients for the assessment of failure. Some figures from communist countries, in which women were assigned randomly to different methods, are difficult to interpret for other reasons. The IUD may be least subject to this selection (at least in some circumstances) and could be expected to have no patient-related failures. Further, variations between fitters in expulsion rates, pregnancy rates and the extent of response to discomfort, heavy bleeding and pain may be controlled to some extent in a small family planning service. The patient-related failures (not noticing loss, especially) can therefore be allowed for (see below). Two pregnancies per hundred woman-years is an average-to-good figure for this method — it gives the average woman less than one chance in five of one unplanned pregnancy during her reproductive life (age 16—36 of high fertility, minus two children). The cryptic assumption in this figure is implicit in that very statement: is the 'average woman' at risk, or is there a small population for which the IUD is less effective? Because the occurrence of a pregnancy with one method nearly always results in a change of method for that person, it is very difficult to determine whether failure rates reflect variation among people or a stochastic process at work for each person. Clearly, if the failure reflects differences among people then such differences should be sought in order to advise people about methods; if there are inherent possibilities of failure with method, on the other hand, these could be balanced against risks of side effects in the improvement of the method. Since we cannot know whether the incidence of failure reflects variation in usage, susceptibility or counselling, or whether it reflects a reduction of fertility not quite to zero, any consideration of the mode of action of contraceptive techniques should at least consider the possible mechanisms of failure.

Barrier methods seem, at first sight, to provide examples whose failure can be attributed only to failure to use them properly — the other end of the spectrum from the IUDs. However, even when used with spermicidal creams they probably have a real method-related failure rate. They do not usually prevent all spermatozoa from passing whatever barrier they present, except possibly when used with a technical skill and a clinical responsibility not commonly found before sexual intercourse. It is not known why so many spermatozoa are ejaculated (2—3 hundred million). If a large fraction of them can fertilize, then a very small leakage around any barrier could generate a small but noticeable failure rate. Contraceptive creams must compromise between effectiveness and toxicity, so that here too there is room for ineffective prevention: the survival of a tiny proportion can still leave a lot of sperms! So, although we might consider the barrier methods to exemplify the binary state — if used properly they work perfectly, and any failure must be attributed to user error — in fact they may exhibit a spectrum of user and method failures like other methods. (A classic piece of ignorance was, however, demonstrated by the doctor from the Indian subcontinent who, when being instructed by my Family Planning doctor wife about condoms, asked 'But can they fit them themselves, or must they be fitted by a doctor?'!)

The opposite pole from the barrier methods would seem to be the IUD, the 'coil';

here there would seem to be no room for user failure (see above). Once inserted, the device should function without conscious action by the woman. However, again the situation is not so clear, particularly if the person who fits the IUD is also considered as a 'user'. A small proportion of IUDs are extruded or otherwise lost from the uterine cavity, mostly in the first months after insertion. The woman is usually instructed to monitor the continued presence of the threads, which hang through the cervix into the vagina, during this time; at the same time she is usually warned that her early periods will be heavy and possibly more painful but that this should settle down within six or so cycles. Some pregnancies certainly result from unnoticed expulsion, but there are others which result from less appropriate or less successful methods adopted after unsatisfactory beginnings with the coil. There is at least a fair possibility that a proportion of women are not rendered very infertile by some IUDs, as suggested above. The mode of action of this method is still not generally agreed, although in most women sperm transport is not prevented and the incidence of extra-uterine (ectopic) pregnancy is comparable with that resulting from unprotected intercourse. (This latter figure is becoming uncertain, however, as ectopic pregnancy rates are rising all over the world.) It is proposed, therefore, that fertilization is usually of normal (unprotected) incidence but that implantation of the blastocyst fails, so that pregnancy is not established. There is considerable concern among those concerned about the sanctity of human life and those who are reluctant to adopt a biological (or other non-binary) usage for 'human', that this method of birth control may be 'abortion', but there is no agreement among such people as to a course of action if this should be the case. The question seems rather less important to me than the question of whether all women have a certain ('2%') chance of an accidental pregnancy or whether there is a small group for whom this method is unsafe and less effective.

We know more about the effects, and especially the side effects, of the contraceptive pill than of any other medicament in history. Its major hormonal effects are in pituitary and hypothalamic feedback loops (in experimental animals and people) to prevent ovulation: but even effects on earwax are well documented, so I shall not mention them further here. The areas which are in doubt, such as the incidence of loss of libido or morbidity or the efficacy of low-dose progestagen-only pills, are so full of data that further number-quoting will not help.* Our major problem here is to find a suitable control group with whom to compare women on the pill. Should it be 'natural' women, alternating pregnancy and lactation, or should it be the usual women in western society, having a succession of highly unnatural menstrual periods? Should the risks be compared with those of the same types of women using another method, with a factor for the proportional chance of having a baby because the other method is less reliable? Interestingly enough, because the (usual) pill is in many respects a mimic of pregnancy (even the male/female ratio of babies in primiparous pill users is nearer that of multiparous women) the western woman on the pill is more 'natural' than the cycling spinster! This choice of an appropriate group for control is probably less a matter of ignorance than of politics, or at least of public relations; but there is nevertheless a lack of publicly-agreed data on benefits and drawbacks and therefore decisions, both personal and political, must be made in ignorance.

Among the most interesting political questions are those related to the injectable hormonal contraceptives, which result in involuntary contraception for a protracted period after injection and cannot be removed like the IUD. Some of these synthetic hormone preparations, notably Depo-Provera, act in some of the same ways as the low-dose progestagen-only pill, but have the disadvantages that the initial dose is necessarily rather high, 'menstrual' bleeding is irregular, and that fall-off in contraceptive effectiveness varies between women. In some cases, and perhaps particularly in Third World villages (where, for example, pill-taking cannot be hidden from husbands), this kind of protection is much less risky than the alternative (pregnancy) and does not produce more babies with their risks too. There has been much comparison of 'risks' which assumes that the control population (western women) should be the same for all populations, but this must be subject to the same questions as controls for the pills. Depo-Provera is considered to be safe in the UK for two sets of circumstances: for women whose husbands are awaiting sperm-free semen after vasectomy and for those who have received vaccination against Rubella (German measles). Most family planning staff in the UK are in favour of a wider use, especially for so called 'domiciliary' cases pending sterilization, and the use of Depo-Provera in developing countries seems satisfactory.[5] There are many new methods of injectable (usually implantable) hormonal contraception now being developed which meter the dose much more evenly and can even be removed as easily as IUDs. It is still not known whether these will be acceptable alternatives, but they are unlikely to be more toxic than other hormonal contraceptives because the carriers are simple polymers of lactic acid or urea, into which they are degraded and which are both already present in the tissues. 'Acceptability' of contraceptives is a peculiar business.[6]

Such long-term contraceptives (it is anticipated that a year or even five years could be usual) grade into sterilants via a series of immunological methods now in the research or testing pipeline. These use antibodies against hormones or against the membranes of eggs or spermatozoa instead of affecting the endocrine system directly. The anti-hormone methods have had a bad start, associated

---

* See Potts (1977).

with some premature 'testing' on a small population of women in India while trials with lower primates were giving worrying results. This involved using or eliciting antibodies to the characteristic human hormone of pregnancy, human chorionic gonadotrophin (hCG); other work, avoiding the common properties which hCG shares with other reproductive hormones, is showing more promise but more slowly. In my opinion, this will be trumped by two other antibody-based possibilities, both of them repeating 'natural experiments' in human infertility and therefore considered not to be associated with obvious side effects. Antibodies against the special egg membrane (zona pellucida) through which the fertilizing spermatozoon must pass are very effective at preventing fertilization in experimental animals and have been implicated in the sterility of many women. The eliciting or injection of such antibodies in women should soon give us more information about this possiblity. A second kind of antibody-mediated sterility is that caused by antibodies to the spermatozoa themselves, found in many infertile women.[7] Attempts to induce such infertility were described as early as 1900, but until the '70s there were no methods of distinguishing infertility-producing antisperm antibodies from the normal complement of antibodies which coat supernumerary spermatozoa and which are also found in all fertile women. Now that this can be done reliably by several techniques, it remains to be discovered whether all women can make the abnormal antibodies or whether all those who can do so have already produced them in response to spermatozoa delivered by the usual route. Such antibodies, if at least most women can be persuaded to make an effective kind, might well require constant stimulation by spermatozoa; revocation of the sterility might be achieved by avoidance of spermatozoal contact (but not of course sexual intercourse) for a period of some months, for it does seem that women who have this kind of sterility may become

fertile after a year or so of successful use of condoms. (There is some surprising evidence to suggest that the antifertility effects of these so-called anti-spermatozoan antibodies may be attained by the prevention of normal implantation of an embryo instead of by preventing fertilization.) This kind of situation, in which action must be taken to revoke a sterilization in order to produce a child, can easily be seen to be a eugenic scenario by those who point to the dysgenic effects of ineffective contraceptive use by the poor, stupid or otherwise 'them' sub-groups. I will return to this point after consideration of some points relating to more permanent sterilization techniques.

Vasectomy and tubal ligation are, in a sense, organic and permanent barrier mechanisms. Both occasionally revert naturally to tubal patency and so have a real method failure rate, but this is not very puzzling. Much more puzzling in such a well-known technique as vasectomy, well accepted and apparently both safe and successful, is that we are ignorant of the fate of spermatozoa in the vasectomized man. They are certainly produced in something like the normal numbers, at least in the months following the operation, before the antisperm antibody level rises and sperm production declines. Suggestions that they are phagocytosed or lysed have little support. More seriously, we do not know whether there are side effects, clinical or even social. Alexander has recently studied vasectomized rabbits and monkeys and she has shown rather more atheroma (fatty deposits in the arteries) in vasectomized animals on a high-cholesterol diet than normal males on the same diet — on normal laboratory animal diets the difference is not seen. We do not know whether men show any similar effects. Social changes related to the existence of a large population of 'safe' vasectomized men may pose new sociological questions. These have not yet made themselves obvious in other than 'trendy' company, but neck-ties with 'V' or 'IOFB' ('I only fire blanks') are sometimes seen already. Vasectomy may change sexual habits as much as the pill if a large identifiable infertile male group is created. A similar group of oviduct-tied women would not be expected to pursue sexuality so overtly, and the social effect of female sterility by this method is little different from that of the IUD; so social change initiated by these women would not be expected.

Abortion is the contraceptive method, or at least the birth control method, which excites revulsion in most people; it is crude, contrary to the pro-life philosophy of most medical personnel and is being legalized progressively in all non-Islamic countries. In the United Kingdom abortions are becoming increasingly common in very young and in older women as well as in the median fertile population (Table 2). There are many moral and ethical issues, ranging from the questions of pre-implantation loss associated with the IUD to the problems associated with the delivery of near-viable foetuses and their destruction by the same personnel who must care for scarcely older premature births. There is, however, one issue to which I may draw attention here, as it is really an issue about whose basic elements we lack information. It concerns the obverse of the 'right of a woman to do as she likes with her own body' argument and concerns the preferences of the medical personnel involved, especially the auxiliary staff who usually have no real choice in their assigned tasks. (Although they may complain legally, few do in these days of difficult employment.) The principal surgeon is often well paid for his socially necessary but very unpleasant involvement, but the woman concerned has also taken her mistake, error of judgement, contraceptive method failure — foetal human being, not 'piece of tissue' — to other people to deal with for her. It is usual in our society for some to specialize in dealing with the woes, accidents or inabilities of others, and this is proper in a caring society; but the existence of the service inevitably encourages its use both by the 'clients' and by the social service concerned, so that thresholds fall and any regularized service becomes commonplace. (Compare, for example, the change in attitudes to disposal of pet dogs and cats since the RSPCA and PDSA have provided a socially acceptable route). We can never discover the original attitudes of those brought into the abortion schemes, for it is a well-recognized ability of people to adjust their standards to the requirements of their lives. This production of a group of less sensitive medical personnel may be a useful or a regrettable consequence of the expansion of the abortion services, but we cannot judge of its utility, efficacy or ethics until we have more information about those directly involved. It is usual to employ the phrase 'voluntary abortion' but this is itself misleading — only the mother and the surgeon volunteer.

In conclusion, we are ignorant of all the major aspects of our contraceptive involvement. We do not really have much idea of the regulation of the family size in ancient or contemporary non-technical societies, except that prolonged lactation and juvenile death are very important factors. Comparison of high birth rates in contemporary Third World technologies with apparently similar rates in some segments of affluent technical societies is certainly misleading, and I have tried to contrast the likely causality: Third World increase is due to survival of juveniles to breed, not to an increase in births per woman; in affluent societies it could be due mostly to a real increase in births per woman as previous social sanctions lose their power to compel and are replaced by technical methods which are beyond the consistent capabilities of much of the population.

Because of the assignment of different kinds of patient to different methods, separation of method failure from patient failure, or especially of stochastic failure from patient susceptibility, is very difficult; it may be possible only in the more authoritarian

200 J. Cohen

TABLE 2. Incidence of abortion by year, place and age

Situation	Abortions	Abortions as a percentage of live births (approximate)	Source
London, 1937		20	Potts et al., 84, T4
France, 1937	3–500 000	100	Potts et al., 90, quoting D. Glass
Yugoslavia, 1967 (urban industrial)		180	Potts et al., 116, T11
Yugoslavia, 1967 (rural poor)		64	Potts et al., 116, T11
England and Wales (legal abortions)			
1961	16 000		
1967	25 000		
1970	90 000		Potts et al.
1973	170 000		
1975	140 000		
United Kingdom 1979			OPCS 1980
Under 16s	3376		
16–19	28 655	50	
20–34	67 927	15	
35–44	16 767		
Over 45s	514	50	

Pott, M., Diggory, P. and Peel, J. (1977) *Abortion*, Cambridge University Press.

medicine of the communist countries. So the choice of methods for each patient or the political choice for a large category or even country must be made in ignorance of the real advantages and drawbacks. However, the general movement from acute to chronic methods requires that these baselines are drawn well in advance of political decisions.

The very important question of which group in modern societies is contributing more of its children, its culture or its hungry mouths to the future of our world can only be answered by drawing a distinction between stable and progressive reproductive strategies of the various contenders. The simple fact that black people or the middle classes or sex-obsessed poets are having more offspring tells us very little: although the offspring of blacks would be expected to be black, their culture may be very different from that of their parents, while the offspring of the poets may be brought up in a great variety of milieux and contribute thereby to many sub-groups in society. Important as the genetic contribution is, its transmission through to subsequent generations will depend primarily upon which culture it interacts with during development, for human beings are primarily cultural animals. Thus we cannot make pronouncements about the dysgenic effects of the poor, the unable or the clumsy having more unintended babies. Even if they are, this is only temporary, for the new generation of contraceptive methods is nearly upon us. The new, more permanent, methods will make it easier not to have babies than to have them, so the eugenicists will have their prejudices aligned with those of the social services for the first time since Malthus.

There is a further conclusion which, for many people, transforms the development of these new freedoms in sexuality, especially the freedom to separate recreation from procreation but also the separation of irresponsibility from pregnancy and poverty; it transforms freedom into licence. This is the danger of venereal diseases, long the second punishment of the lusty (after pregnancy). That there is now an increase of various venereally transmitted diseases in the UK is generally agreed, but that it relates to more promiscuity is doubtful, and that this supposed extra promiscuity was 'caused' by the pill is not at all clear. The competition among journals, books, television and film for portrayal of modern sexuality in the search for drama has led to models for teenage behaviour which combine the less attractive properties of the billy-goat, the temple whore and the preying mantis. Such evidence as there is suggests that the young are now less affected by these lascivious models and may be returning to a more genuine attitude than us older folk. Perhaps when those in a position to determine the priorities of medical research find themselves exposed to this risk of disease via their pleasures, we may find that venerealogy becomes a well funded and more prestigious discipline. The prospect of sexual intercourse again becoming an art form is very attractive. Hopefully, it will return to the aesthetics of earlier times, but with modern medicine to separate its sensuous pair-bonding functions from its reproductive functions and to protect against disease.

Finally, there is the most important question. Will the development of present methods — and new methods — of contraception avert a population explosion? The answer must, I fear, be 'No' for many of the reasons already presented. Because of the number of children already surviving and who will breed and whose children will themselves survive to breed and survive, the Earth's human population threatens to double by the year 2030. The largest part of the present population will be past breeding by then, so the next generation's cultural constraints may use the new contraceptive technologies to enter the new millennium. In some places, at great cost, they will survive and reproduce our kind.

References and Further Reading

DOUGLAS, M. (1966) Population controls in primitive peoples. *British Journal of Sociology,* **17**, 263–273.

GLASS, D., quoted by BENJAMIN, B. (1977) Social and economic differentials in fertility. In: *Heredity and Environment* (Halsey, ed.), 131–144, Methuen, London.

HALSEY, A.H. (ed.) (1977) *Heredity and Environment.* Methuen, London. Especially papers by Halsey, Hawthorne and Benjamin.

HAWTHORN, G. (1976) Some economic explanations of fertility. Reprinted in: *Heredity and Environment* (Halsey, ed.) Methuen, London.

MEDAWAR, P.B. (1960) *The Future of Man.* Methuen, London.

POTTS, M., SPEIDEL, J.J. and KESSEL, E. (1977) Relative risks of various means of fertility control when used in less-developed countries. In: *Risks, Benefits and Controversies in Fertility Control* (Sciarra, Zatuchni and Speidel, eds.), 28–51, Harper and Row, New York.

SAI, F.T. (1976) The needs of the developing world. In: *Contraceptives of the Future* (Short and Baird, eds.) pp. 57–68, Royal Society, London.

SHORT, R.V. (1976) The evolution of human reproduction. In: *Contraceptives of the Future* (Short and Baird, eds.) Royal Society, London, pp. 3—24.

WYNNE-EDWARDS, V.C. (1978) Intrinsic population control: and introduction. In: *Population Control by Social Behaviour* (Ebling and Stoddart, eds.) Institute of Biology, London, pp. 1—22.

For the general reproductive cases, see Chone, J. (1977) *Reproduction*. Butterworths, London.

NOTES

1. Most elementary biology books have this error, but so do some good more advanced texts, e.g. Hogarth, P. (1978) *Biology of Reproduction*. Blackie, Edinburgh, pp. 155—158.

2. There is, of course, a plethora of good case histories of the uptake of technical methods and of down-turning rates of increase; see *Birth Control, and International Assessment,* edited by Potts and Bhiwandiwala. MTP Press, 1979. But compare this with the avoidance of the question in Berelson, B. (1976) The impact of new technology. In: *Contraceptives of the Future* (Short and Baird, eds.) Royal Society, London, pp. 25—35. The real question is not answered in either.

3. As well as papers by Shockley in the USA and Enoch Powell in the UK, let me quote Barnes, A.C. (1977) Social concerns in fertility control. In: *Risks, Benefits and Controversies in Fertility Control* (Sciarra, Zatuchni and Speidel, eds.) Harper and Row, New York. "Is it fair to ask the younger generation of Americans to practice strict fertility control and limit their families to one or two children and still admit 300 000 to 400 000 highly reproductive immigrants annually?".

4. Polygamic cultures, in which only a proportion of men become fathers, are not quite trivial examples here. See the analysis of relative genetic fitness of different types in Konotey-Ahulu, F.I. (1980) Male procreative superiority index (MPSI): the missing figure in African anthropogenetics. *British Medical Journal,* **281**, pp. 1700—1702.

5. The matter is under consideration in many countries. For a brief introduction to some of the questions (suitability of beagle bitches as human models, legal problems) see King, T.M., Burkman, R.T. and Atienza, M.F. (1977) Other dosage forms and routes — injectables — medorxyprogesterone acetate. In: *Risks, Benefits and Controversies in Fertility Control* (Sciarra, Zatuchni and Speidel, eds.) Harper and Row, New York, pp. 257—262.

6. Malcolm Potts, particularly, has pointed to the risks we accept in other athletic or aesthetic pursuits, usually more by two or three orders of magnitude those of sexual recreation; see, for example, Potts, M., Speidel, J.J. and Kessel, E. (1977) Relative risks of various means of fertility control when used in less developed countries. In: *Risks, Benefits and Controveries in Fertility Control* (Sciarra, Zatuchni and Speidel, eds.) Harper and Row, New York.

7. Various aspects of this are discussed in Cohen, J. and Hendry, W.F. (eds.) (1978) *Spermatozoa, Antibodies and Infertility*. Blackwell Scientific Publications, Oxford. Other issues are raised in Djerassi, C. (1980) The Politics of Contraception. Norton, New York. See also continuing series of publication by WHO and the International Planned Parenthood Federation (IPPF).

FOETAL DIAGNOSIS

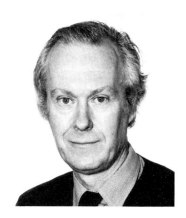

Jack Insley

Consultant Paediatrician and Clinical Geneticist, Birmingham Maternity Hospital.

Honorary Senior Clinical Lecturer, University of Birmingham. His main published works have been in relation to human chromosomal defects and, more recently, to the aims of and problems created by ante-natal diagnosis.

We now expect handicapped children to survive. This is partly because of the general improvement in health in Western societies following public health measures, better nutrition, a positive attempt to prevent neonatal death and the introduction of antibiotics. Only the most seriously abnormal die in the early weeks or months of life. In the circumstances the prevention, or at least the diagnosis, of foetal disease or malformation early enough in pregnancy to correct the defect, seems an eminently respectable objective for an advanced society which controls its conception, accepts termination of pregnancy and keeps its families small. Parents, brothers and sisters who have loved but lived with a seriously handicapped child for any length of time are usually the most anxious to avoid the repetition of such a catastrophe in other children and it was with such families in mind that the initial advances in early antenatal diagnosis were made. The aim then seemed clear – it was to recognize and terminate foetuses that were abnormal. The conditions sought included mongolism (Down's syndrome) which can be recognized by examining the foetal chromosomes, and to this was added a number of rare inborn errors of metabolism which are detected usually by examining the performance of specific enzymes in cells and amniotic fluid. The diagnosis of sex was also an early achievement which could indirectly be used to identify boy foetuses in families with diseases confined to males. The determination of amniotic fluid alpha-foetoprotein (AFP) for the diagnosis of spina bifida followed. The only treatment available for these groups was, and still is, termination.

Rhesus (a red blood cell antigen) incompatibility is the only foetal condition amenable to active treatment in the curative sense. Intra-uterine foetal blood transfusion will often prevent death in those most severely affected with anemia and may be repeated until the baby is mature enough to be delivered.

Even when the matter has been considered at length before pregnancy and the risk of defect is known to be high, termination of pregnancy may have long-term emotional effects on the parents, especially the mother. Amelioration may come from counselling before and after termination and by a careful follow-up programme, but the information on the best way of achieving this is still being sought. The anxieties are naturally increased when a test used to look for one particular condition reveals either an 'abnormal' result of possible significance or demonstrates another disease or malformation about which little is known. The agony is further increased

TABLE 1. Incidence of Birth Defects

Groups of conditions	Incidence live births	Proportion (as percentage) in theory	Diagnosable in foetus in practice
Severe mental retardation	10/1000 (3—5/1000 at 3 yr)	30 (?)	8 (?)
Blindness	severe 1.3/1000 partial 1.3/1000	nil	nil
Profound deafness	1/1000	nil	nil
Severe congenital abnormality	20/1000 (include congenital heart disease 6.6/1000 and spina bifida 1.42/1000)	7*	4.5

* Assumes all cases of spina bifida recognized.

The decision whether or not to embark upon such investigations can lead to much anxiety for parents, especially when the pros and cons, risk figures of all kinds and the nature of the diseases sought, have not been considered previously. The optimum time and method of imparting this information when screening is contemplated has yet to be found.

for some parents who clearly recognize that the available tests such as the amniotic fluid test for spina bifida cannot measure the severity of the handicap.

The aim of this chapter is to define the advantages and limitations of the tests that are available and then map out the present frontier between those conditions where diagnosis is possible and those where at present it is at best incomplete or at the worst unattainable. For the latter a simple list of handicaps and handicapping conditions and the degree of our ignorance as far as their intrauterine diagnosis is concerned is laid out in Table. 1. The former group is amenable to more detailed analysis, for investigation has provided knowledge, some surprises and a great number of unanswered questions. Techniques used to approach the foetus, laboratory tests and foetal diagnosis are as follows.

Tests on Maternal Blood

Blood taken and examined early in pregnancy can be tested for past or established infection with syphilis, and to determine whether there is immunity to Rubella. Serial tests may be used in certain mothers to show evidence of current infection but, even if this is so, it is impossible to tell whether the foetus is affected or not. Blood may also be screened after the 16th week of pregnancy for a high serum alpha-foetoprotein — an indicator of foetal neural tube defect. The blood of rhesus negative women is examined repeatedly through pregnancy for the presence of antibodies against the Rht antigen.

Amniocentesis and Amniotic Fluid

Current techniques demand that the lie of the foetus, the position of the placenta and the pool of fluid be visualized with ultrasound immediately before the needle is inserted through the maternal and abdominal and uterine wall into the amniotic cavity. The 20 ml of fluid which are withdrawn (that is 10% of the total at 16 weeks, 7.5% of total at 18 weeks) contain cells which can be cultured and examined for their chromosomes and chemistry, and a supernatant fluid for its chemical constituents. The principal complication (about which there is little controversy) is abortion with a risk proportional to the number of attempts to tap the fluid and the experience of the operator. The mother herself runs a negligible risk. On the other hand it is not clear whether needling the foetus — which undoubtedly does happen — is always without risk and whether there are possible long-term effects following the removal of amniotic fluid. Three sizeable surveys have been reported from the USA (NICHD Study Group, 1976) and Canada (Simpson *et al.*, 1976) but only in the United Kingdom survey (MRC Working Party on Amniocentesis, 1978) is there a suggestion that there may be more than transient problems following amniocentesis. In this series the birth weight and the gestation of the babies tested were a little lower than the control group and a higher proportion of the tested babies suffered and in some cases died from a respiratory illness at birth. Autopsy confirmed hyaline membrane disease — a disorder resulting from the immaturity of the lung and, in particular, the alveolar cells responsible for surfactant production. The United Kingdom study also suggests that limb deformity — principally talipes equinovarus and, less clearly, congenital dislocation of the hip, is more commonly found in the tested group and might be ascribed to unusual foetal compression *in utero*, perhaps from lack or loss of amniotic fluid. On the other hand the other foetal deformities which are usually to be seen following pregnancies where for some reason or other the amount of amniotic fluid is greatly reduced, are not reported in the series but this may simply reflect a less serious disturbance.

Examination of amniotic fluid cells for chromosomal disease

The indications for chromosomal analysis of foetal cells are currently as follows:

1. Women over 40 years of age (and where facilities are available the age limit has been lowered to 35 years).

2. Where one parent has a chromosomal re-arrangement. The common inversion within No. 9 chromosome is considered as a normal 'variant' and is an exception to the rule. Low priority is given to the Robertsonian translocation between chromosomes No. 13 and 14.

3. In pregnancies which follow the birth of a child with Down's syndrome (trisomy of chromosome 21) and some other aneuploidies (loss or gain of one or more chromosomes).

Although such indications are clear, the actual risk of abnormality to the individual foetus within the group is often far from precise. While the lack of data is partly to blame, there are already well-substantiated contradictions in records which exist. This is very apparent in the comparison between the recorded risk of Down's syndrome in foetal life as ascertained by foetal cell culture and at birth in comparable groups. The incidence is 1.5 to 2.0 times higher in the foetal group than that which occurs at birth.

Other important dilemmas are:

1. It is not known how far paternal age influences the conception of a foetus with Down's syndrome.

2. The recurrent risk of trisomy 21 appears to be greater in mothers below 29 years of age at the time of the birth of the child than those over 29 years of age. Further data are sought to confirm this. There are no plausible explanations.

3. The risk of conceiving another foetus with a chromosomal disorder following the birth of one child with aneuploidy appears to be increased. A figure of 1.7% recurrence risk has been suggested. Further data are needed and the nature of the trigger in these families is as yet unresolved.

4. Other well-recognized aneuploidies, especially those affecting the sex chromosomes, e.g. 47 XYY, may be unexpectedly discovered in amniocentesis specimens. Although there can be no ambiguity about the

diagnosis, the true nature of the disease is not known. A prospective clinical survey based on chromosomal analysis of all babies born in an Edinburgh hospital by the MRC Population Cytogenetics Unit has unfortunately been unable to collect adequate data yet. The difficulties encountered in such a review, particularly when the chromosomal diagnosis has to be withheld from the parents, cannot be underestimated.

5. At least 1/250 of the general population has some form of balanced chromosomal re-arrangement. For the commoner forms — particularly the Robertsonian translocations — the risk of producing a liveborn child with unbalanced chromosomes is known but for most rearrangements the risks can only be guessed.

6. There is a suggestion that in families with a Robertsonian or balanced translocation or an inversion, there is an excess of balanced carrier segregants and unexpected chromosomal anomalies in the children of carrier parents.

7. The risk of a subsequently malformed infant to couples, one of whom is a translocation carrier (ascertained because of repeated spontaneous abortions) is not known.

8. The unexpected appearance of a de novo balanced translocation in a culture produces a dilemma for parents and counsellors alike. Unfortunately, data suggest that 1/8 of such infants may be mentally and possibly physically handicapped. The implication is that existing techniques of chromosomal analysis are still unsophisticated enough to define minute losses of chromatin.

9. Some foetal cell cultures reveal chromosomal mosaicism, usually for an extra fragment. When it only involves a single cell clone it is probably the result of a culture artefact but in some cases it has been found in clones from more than one culture plate. The question, usually unanswered before such foetuses are terminated, is whether the baby

---

* Risk of an 'unbalanced' foetus now estimated as 3.8%. European Collaborative Study (August 1981).

would have been normal. If the fragment is subsequently found in the culture of the foetal tissues the answer is almost certainly yes.

10. The potential use of foetal cells and chromosomes to determine the effect of foetal exposure to environmental agents or the detection of 'chromosome instability' syndromes, e.g. Fanconi's syndrome and X-linked fragile site (Renpenning syndrome) has yet to be explored.

The more practical needs as far as the consumer is concerned are to bring the time of testing earlier into pregnancy, reduce the waiting time between tests and answers, and find an alternative to amniocentesis.

Amniotic Fluid Alpha-Foetoprotein and Neural Tube Defect: Screening for Neural Tube Defect

The failure of the primitive neural plaque to invaginate and bury itself completely as a tube (later to develop as the brain and spinal cord) encircled by bone, muscle and skin, is recognisable as a neural tube defect. The most serious is anencephaly, where the brain is under-developed and exposed through the open skull. The baby dies before or shortly after birth. Encephalocele is a less serious expression but brain — usually covered with a membrane or skin — protrudes through a bony defect at the back of the skull. Failure of the spinal cord to develop as a tube and the surrounding tissues to envelop it is known as spina bifida. It is usually 'open', so that cerebrospinal fluid leaks and is visible. It may occasionally be covered with skin — a closed lesion. A combination of poor neural development and tethering of the cord to local tissues results in a variable but usually serious degree of paralysis of movement and sensation below the level of the lesion (usually on the lower back), urinary and bowel incontinence and hydrocephalus — blockage of the fluid produced inside the brain with consequent

stretching. Hydrocephalus usually results in some degree of mental retardation. Death when it occurs in spina bifida follows infection, progressive hydrocephalus or chronic renal failure.

There are a number of factors which make the prevention and eradication of spina bifida of paramount importance. In the UK it is the commonest severe malformation compatible with a life span of many years and, although the incidence is falling, improved neonatal care has meant that fewer die in the early weeks of life. Unfortunately, efforts to improve the quality of life of these children by intensive surgical and medical care has done little more than prolong the lives — on one follow-up only 3% submitted for surgery were considered to be able to lead an entirely normal life. Attention is currently being focused on antenatal diagnosis and increasingly, on prevention by giving vitamins (particularly folic acid) before conception takes place.

Antenatal diagnosis depends on the examination of chemicals or cells mainly (private to foetal life) which leak out through the open wound into the amniotic fluid. These include the foetal protein, alpha-foetoprotein (AFP), a specific neural enzyme acetyl cholinesterase and certain rapidly growing cells which are thought to have their origin in neural or related tissue. Real-time ultrasound is also used to visualize breaks in the spinal column or skull and detect internal hydrocephalus and this technique may in time supplant amniocentesis. While such tests are freely available for families 'at risk' routine amniocentesis of the general pregnant population is not feasible. On the other hand, screening by the estimation of serum alpha-foetoprotein between the 16th and 18th weeks has been established in many areas of the United Kingdom.

A radio-immune assay is needed to determine the minute amounts of AFP in maternal serum and does so accurately but, because of the considerable overlap in levels obtained between normal and affected, it should be considered as an unreliable screening test. Its implementation reflects the severity of the problem. The usual practice is to scrutinize all pregnancies when the serum alpha-foeto-protein is found to be 2.5 times the median. Even so, only 75% of cases are netted and the false positive rate is 90%. Fortunately, the combination of amniocentesis and ultrasound reduces the danger of terminating normal pregnancies but the detection rate can only be improved by lowering the cut-off point and so submitting many more pregnancies to detailed scrutiny.

Maternal serum AFP is thought to be foetal in origin but little is known of the factors which control its transfer into or disappearance from the maternal circulation. In the foetus the rate of production per unit mass reaches a peak before the 20th week and thereafter the total circulating AFP remains steady with foetal growth, gradually falling after the 32nd week when its place is taken by the adult albumin. Maternal levels also rise to a peak beyond 34 weeks and then fall steeply. If the level in maternal blood is in direct proportion to foetal production, then high maternal levels should be, and indeed are, found in twin pregnancies. But why it should rise with a spina bifida foetus regardless of whether the lesion is open or closed is a mystery.

Amniotic fluid AFP may also be high in the presence of other lesions apart from spina bifida. These include exomphalos-, gastro schisis, congenital nephrosis and foetal death. Fortunately, the number of false positive high amniotic fluid AFPs is very small but they are occasionally found and, in the past, have led to the termination of normal foetuses. The use of high-definition ultrasound and the examination of the fluid for other indices of neural tube defect should now prevent mistakes.

Chemical Tests on Cultured Cells: Tests on Inborn Errors of Metabolism

A very small number of conditions, nearly all inherited in an autosomal recessive fashion,

TABLE 2. Single Gene Disorders (published 1980 figures)

Mode of inheritance	Number of conditions listed*	Diagnosable through amniocentesis	Diagnosable through foetal blood sampling	Diagnosable foetoscopy and/or ultrasound	Linkage
Autosomal dominant	736 (+ 753)[†]	—	—	? limb deformities some bone dysplasias[‡] some facial defects	1
Autosomal recessive	521 (+ 596)[†]	33	4	some bone dysplasias[‡] skin	1
X-linked recessive	107 (+ 98)[†]	4	2	—	—

* McKusick: Mendelian Inheritance in Man (1978) 5th Edition. Johns Hopkins University Press.

† Figures bracketed refer to probable but unconfirmed gene disorders.

‡ Most bone dysplasias 'inherited' in AD fashion are new mutations.

can be recognized chemically from the examination of the supernatant and/or cultured cells taken from amniotic fluid. The more common inborn errors of metabolism, including cystic fibrosis, congenital adrenal hyperplasia* and phenylketonuria, cannot be diagnosed in this way. Table 2 puts the matter in perspective and shows that only a very small proportion of inherited genetic diseases can be recognized with this technique.

The carrier status for such diseases can only be determined in a few instances and only regularly offered to families 'at risk' when foetal diagnosis is available. Such tests can also be used to 'screen' families or populations at risk but once again only when antenatal testing is available and is requested. Tay Sach's disease amongst the Ashkenazi Jews and β-thalassaemia amongst Mediterranean populations are examples.

Foetoscopy

The visual examination of a foetus through a foetoscope (a fiberoptic telescope) allows malformation or deformities of individual parts to be recognized. The face, limbs and front of the body are most easily seen, the back is less accessible as the foetus flexes to fit the contours of the uterine wall. Blood samples can be taken from foetal vessels in the cord or on the placenta. Certain haemoglobinopathies, haemophilias, white blood cell and platelet disorders and enzyme deficiencies have been diagnosed. The diagnosis of Duchenne muscular dystrophy (see below) has proved unreliable. Biopsies of skin for the diagnosis of icthyosis and epidermolysis syndromes have been reported and recently liver biopsy has been successfully accomplished.

The present foetoscopes have a diameter of between 1.7—2.7 mm but the optimal instrument size has yet to be established, while flexible instruments are expected to have advantages. The most serious maternal complication is amnionitis (1%). Early foetal loss rates may be as high as 10% with an additional prematurity rate of 11%. When foetal death does occur, it usually follows exsanguination or spontaneous abortion. Premature birth amongst the survivors remains an important problem, partly because the mechanism which sets it in motion is not clear and partly because death or handicap in the survivors are common sequelae in those born before the 28th week even when there is sophisticated neonatal care. The complications of premature birth are even more pertinent for those families which come from poorer countries for testing. Such is the price for a test in which foetal viewing can fail (13%) or blood samples are unobtainable (3%).

Many unresolved questions remain. A question mark hangs over the new applications for the future of the technique unless the complication rate falls appreciably. Ultrasound already provides some alternatives to direct foetal viewing and, as knowledge increases, diagnoses which cannot be made on foetal blood or other tissues will be possible by other means.

Foetal Imaging and Ultrasound

Foetal imaging can be obtained by introducing radio-opaque dye into the amniotic cavity or by using X-rays and ultrasound. The disadvantages of contaminating the amniotic fluid with foreign material have prevented the widespread use of the former, whilst the relatively late ossification of the foetal skeleton rarely makes foetal skeletal radiography of much use before late pregnancy. The most rapid and promising advances in the detection of foetal abnormality have come from the application of ultrasonography using both β-wave reflected and real-time ultrasound.

* Diagnosis by estimation of 17-hydroxyprogesterone reported 1981.

The ultrasound techniques can pinpoint the week of conception, plot the subsequent growth of the foetus and examine it for any possible morphological defects. Detection of these defects has to a great extent been confined to pregnancies known to be at risk — principally those with neural tube defects and renal tract abnormalities, especially polycystic kidneys. However they are now also applied more generally in some groups, that is to groups of pregnancies where the recurrence risk of a particular defect is low (< 5%) and in some centres for general screening of the pregnant population. The gradual move towards screening has produced occasional but predictable difficulties in interpretation.

Central nervous system (neural tube defect, isolated hydrocephalus, microcephaly)

As machines and operators improve, neural tube defects are diagnosed with increasing confidence but the physical severity of the lesions, especially when the defect is small, cannot always be gauged. Anencephaly is unlikely to be missed by 18 weeks and some centres consider that screening for spina bifida is more accurately carried out with ultrasound than by serum AFP.

Isolated hydrocephalus (that is unaccompanied by spina bifida) is the result of blockage somewhere along the drainage system inside the brain. The brain fluid is produced within small caverns (ventricles) in each half of the cerebrum and then passes on through central chambers to the base of the brain. It bathes the brain and cord and is absorbed back into the bloodstream by the arachnoid granulations — which lie between the skull and the brain. Blockage of the system at any point leads to collection of fluid and progressive stretching of the brain and skull known as hydrocephalus. Hydrocephalus can be recognized during foetal life by measuring the size of the ventricular system but individual experience and accuracy do not allow the technique to be used with confidence in screening for isolated hydrocephalus (inci-

dence 1/2000 live births).

Microcephaly — small brain (and skull) — is a more common problem. Some degree of mental retardation is usual. There are numerous recognized causes including a variety of genetic types. Recurrence risk of unexplained microcephaly in a sibship is relatively high (at least 8%). It is theoretically detectable by ultrasound but in practice there is not yet any useful information about the pattern of growth of the microcephalic skull.

Skeleton

There is an increasing number of reports describing the diagnosis of skeletal defects and bone dysplasias, particularly when limb length is markedly reduced. Certainty in diagnosis has usually come well after the 20th week of pregnancy.

Heart

The four chambered heart becomes visible after 20 weeks and by the end of the second trimester gross abnormalities involving the intracardiac septa can be found. The benefits of screening 'at risk' pregnancies, where there is a previous child with congenital heart disease (maximum recurrence risk about 3%), where there is maternal diabetes or a known teratogenic agent has been taken, have yet to be assessed.

Gastrointestinal system

Omphalocele and gastroschisis (the bowel lies outside the abdominal cavity, either enclosed in a sac — omphalocele — or free as in gastroschisis) can be differentiated and its size assessed. Some of these lesions can be successfully operated upon after birth. Upper intestinal obstruction — principally duodenal atresia — can be seen and the common association with Down's syndrome confirmed or refuted by amniocentesis but diagnosis may only be achieved late in pregnancy. Ultrasound may also inadvertently reveal ascites and oedema of foetal tissues from the middle of pregnancy onwards but the cause of the problem is not easily resolved unless Rhesus disease is known to be present.

Urinary system

Defects in the urinary system are rarely discovered before 20 weeks and are usually represented by fluid-filled cavities. As the foetal bladder empties every 90 minutes or so defective bladder filling or function can be viewed. However, the accurate interpretation of these findings is not always easy and their presence not always confirmed postnatally. Attempts to treat obstructive lesions by trans-uterine drainage have not been useful.

The diagnosis of renal agenesis (total absence of the kidneys) still presents difficulties for, while the presence of renal shadows will confirm normality in pregnancies at risk, an absence cannot be interpreted accurately as the converse, nor can bladder filling and emptying, although helpful after 20 weeks, provide a certain diagnosis.

The complications of ultrasonography

Ultrasound in doses of 1000 times or more than those used for pregnancy diagnosis can disrupt cells and produce chromosomal damage *in vitro* but no ill effect physical or mental has yet been found in those exposed to ultrasound in foetal life. However, it should be remembered that the long-term effects of ultrasound, if there are any, have yet to make themselves known and are currently the subject of further study.

Conditions for which there is Imperfect Diagnosis

Duchenne muscle dystrophy

Duchenne muscular dystrophy, which affects 1/3000 boys, leads to progressive and incurable muscle weakness and wasting. This results in a wheelchair existence by eleven years and usually death by seventeen years from bronchopneumonia or heart failure. One third of these boys are also mentally back-ward. It is usually inherited from a mother who is a carrier (but usually unaffected — some may be a little weak), but a proportion of cases arise from a new mutation and, in that case, there is no family history of the disease. Electromyography and muscle biopsy help in the diagnosis of the disease after birth but the underlying enzyme disorder is not known. Diagnosis in life is confirmed by an estimation of creatine phosphokinase (CPK) concentration — an enzyme released by damaged muscle.

Foetal muscle at 18 weeks shows little or no changes of dystrophy though an increase of eosinophilic fibres with intracellular calcium has been described. Not surprisingly the level of CPK in foetal blood obtained at foetoscopy is not significantly raised and consequently does not provide a diagnosis. At present the best that can be achieved is the determination of odds that a female relative of an affected boy is a carrier. If the woman is a carrier half her boys are likely to be affected. Unfortunately, the only existing foetal test is for sex with the consequence that at least half the males aborted for this disease would have been unaffected.

Dystrophia myotonica

Dystrophia myotonica is a slowly progressive familial muscle disease that usually presents during adult life. The first sign is one of tiredness on walking and climbing accompanied by difficulty in releasing the hand grip and letting go of objects. Yet mothers who are themselves very mildly affected can give birth to children who are not only weak from birth but may also be mentally retarded. An additional intrauterine effect has been postulated to account for this phenomenon. Although the underlying chemical component has yet to be discovered, the gene for the disease and that for the secretor substance are known to be closely linked on the same chromosome. As secretor status can be estimated from body fluids and amniotic fluid, antenatal diagnosis can be achieved as long as the secretor status between affected and non-affected members of the family differs. But, even in informative families this indirect technique is only 75% accurate.

Bone dysplasias

The underlying cellular or enzyme defect for most inherited bone dysplasias is unknown and foetal bone biopsy has not been attempted. Diagnosis can be hazarded by limb measurement using ultrasound. Some conditions such as achondroplasia may not always show a clear clinical abnormality at birth and may be more difficult to diagnose in early intra-uterine life. The success rate of this technique has not been determined.

Conditions for which there is no Diagnosis

Table 1 lists the main groups of handicapping conditions. Many of these are not amenable to antenatal diagnosis.

Mental retardation

Even if every foetus had its chromosomes examined and all abnormals were terminated, only thirty per cent of severe mental retardation would be prevented. The remaining seventy per cent of cases represent a very heterogeneous group, of which a small number can be categorized into specific conditions or syndromes. These are not amenable to foetal diagnosis. In practice amniocentesis is restricted to women over 35 years and assuming that one hundred per cent take up the service only eight per cent of children with mental retardation will be detected during foetal life.

Blindness

The eye is not amenable to scrutiny. About 1.3/1000 of children have blindness. A further 1.3/1000 only have limited sight.

Profound childhood deafness

Although a response to sound can be obtained late in pregnancy such techniques are not applicable earlier. Incidence of profound deafness is about 1/1000 live births.

Congenital malformation

Of the 20 cases per 1000 live births 6.6/1000 have congenital heart disease and 1.42/1000 spina bifida. Although the four-chambered heart can be seen with increasing clarity with ultrasound, major defects in the heart are rarely recognizable before 20 weeks of pregnancy. In practice, spina bifida is the only malformation actively sought in this group.

Genetic Disease (those Inherited through a Single Defective Gene)

Table 2 lists the number of recognized single gene disorders and the numbers amenable to antenatal diagnosis.

Disorders inherited in an autosomal recessive fashion (including inforn errors of metabolism)

At present only 30–40 conditions inherited in this way can be diagnosed in the foetus with confidence. Diagnosis usually depends on cell culture and subsequent chemical analysis and can only be accurately carried out in a few specialised laboratories. The most common inherited disease in the Western world — cystic fibrosis — still eludes diagnosis and even carrier detection has yet to be formally established.

The detection of haemoglobin beta chain abnormalities such as β-thalassaemia and sickle cell disease can be obtained by foetal sampling following foetoscopy, the disadvantages of which have already been defined. The technique is unlikely to be applicable in the third world countries where these diseases are prevalent.

Disorders inherited in an autosomal dominant fashion

Certain malformations affecting limbs or

face can be detected by foetoscopy and/or ultrasound but the more common and serious disorder of Huntington's chorea cannot be predicted accurately before or even after birth.

Ultrasound, foetoscopy and the search for linkage between the loci for dystrophia myotonica and secretor have to date been the only useful techniques for the detection of disorders inherited in this way.

Disorders inherited in X-linked recessive fashion

Complete foetal detection is possible in a small number of disorders including the haemophilias, the Lesch-Nyhan and Menke's syndrome. For the other disorders the abortion of male foetuses thought to be at risk is all that can be offered.

General Aspects

There is little doubt that with a radical improvement in the techniques used to detect foetal abnormality many of the existing unknowns would disappear, though it is perhaps unfair to suggest that very early abortion must necessarily be acceptable to those who want babies. At present the short and long-term effects on parents exposed to the anxieties and decisions imposed by foetal screening and termination are just beginning to be understood. At the same time there is a suggestion that timely counselling will prevent lengthy and perhaps lifelong agony over the termination of a wanted child.

At present tests used in foetal diagnosis are relatively crude and time-consuming with sometimes delays of some weeks between the physical test and the final result. Termination may be delayed beyond the 20th week of pregnancy. The use of cell sorters to separate and collect foetal cells from the maternal circulation for testing is still in the experimental phase. It may prove an effective and accurate method for the detection of male pregnancies and for screening out chromosomal and biochemical defects before the 12th week of pregnancy but the logistics of the problem are overwhelming. In the meantime ways have to be found to make foetal diagnosis generally acceptable, possibly by introducing the concept in the school years. Such programmes are frequently advocated by health care teams but their effectiveness is still to be determined.

The arguments for pressing ahead with foetal screening programmes are partly humane, eugenic and economic. Of these the economic argument is perhaps the one most prone to criticism because figures on survival and the effects of surgery and medical treatment are constantly changing. Retrospective analysis is unpopular in medicine but at present is unavoidable in such circumstances. Effective life tables can only be constructed after a lifetime and must necessarily reflect the past rather than the present.

References

Birth Impairments. (1978). Office of Health Economics, London.

DONNAI, P., CHARLES, N. and HARRIS, R. (1981), Attitudes of patients after 'genetic' termination of pregnancy. *British Medical Journal* **282**, 621.

McKUSICK, V.A. (1978), *Mendelian Inheritance in Man. Catalogs of Autosomal Dominant, Autosomal Recessive and X-linked Phenotypes.* 5th Edition. Johns Hopkins Press. Baltimore.

NICHD (National Registry for Amniocentesis Study Group) (1976), Midtrimester amniocentesis for prenatal diagnosis: Safety and accuracy. *Journal of the American Medical Association* **236**, 1471.

Prenatal Diagnosis — Past, Present and Future (Report of an international workshop). *Prenatal Diagnosis.* Special Issue. John Wiley, 1980.

Prenatal diagnosis of genetic disease in Canada: report of a collaborative study (1976). *Canadian Medical Association Journal* **115**, 739.

Report to the Medical Research Council by their Working Party on Amniocentesis. An assessment of the hazards of amniocentesis (1978). *British Journal of Obstetrics and Gynaecology* **85**, Supplement No. 2.

SIGGERS, D.C. (1978) *Prenatal Diagnosis of Genetic Disease.* Blackwell Scientific Publications, Oxford.

HUMAN PREGNANCY: AN IMMUNOLOGICAL MYSTERY

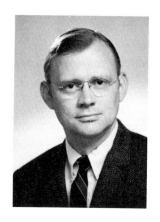

W. Page Faulk

Professor of Immunology, University of Nice, France and Director of the Human Embryology and Pregnancy Foundation, London.

He was formerly the Director of the Blond McIndoe Centre for Transplantation Biology, East Grinstead Sussex and Research Professor, Royal College of Surgeons of England.

Edward McCrady[†]

Introduction

Recognition systems which identify and eliminate alien cells and substances have played an important role in evolutionary survival. Even in the lowest multi-cellular phyla (the Porifera (sponges) and Coelenterata (jelly fishes)), cells of different tissues and from different species, after being dissociated and scrambled together, will recognize their proper companions and reassemble in an orderly fashion to form functional and viable individuals of pure species. Allograft rejection phenomena have been demonstrated in invertebrates as well as in all classes of vertebrates from lamprey eels to man, but when biparental embryos began to attach themselves to maternal tissue, an evolutionary paradox arose. After hundreds of millions of years of natural selection favouring more efficient processes of recognition and rejection of alien intruders, the mammalian mother found herself called upon to accept and nurture an allogeneic blastocyst within her body. Survival of the species thus required rejection of all other invaders, but tolerance and protection and even sacrifically generous support for this unique exception.

There has been no shortage of speculative attempts to explain away this paradox, but most serve only to redefine the dilemma in terms of increasing immunological sophistication.

Dismissal of the centrality of immunity in human reproduction, on the grounds that the success rate of embryonic implantation so far exceeds that of any other graft as to make graft—host analogies in pregnancy unilluminating, is largely based upon anecdotal data. A recent study using urinary human chorionic gonadotrophin (hCG) as the diagnostic index of pregnancy revealed that at least 43% of normal women who conceive, subsequently abort, usually during the first month suggesting that successful pregnancies are more infrequent than has been hitherto considered (see Miller and colleagues, 1980, for details). In addition, there are many data which support the idea that immune processes are invoked to maintain normal gestation. Four of these lines of evidence are (a) the vast amount of immunopathology associated with the materno-foetal interface (reviewed by Faulk & Johnson, 1980), (b) blocking antibodies in placentae, (c) the absence of blocking factors in the blood of chronic aborters and (d) cytotoxic effects of maternal leucocytes upon trophoblastic tissue.

Viewed in this light, the immune system is much involved in pregnancy, but some incompletely understood interplay between gestational and immunological functions enables the embryo, in a sufficient number of cases, to escape maternal immunosurveillance and rejection. If this ability is mediated by a gene product, the gene or genes might most advantageously operate in extra-embryonic tissues, for only these come into physical contact with maternal tissues. Identification and control of such genes might greatly benefit several areas of human biomedicine which presently do not enjoy the success we should hope for, an obvious example being clinical transplantation. That foetal products can be useful in transplantation has been demonstrated by the use of amnion as a preparatory aid in skin grafting as well as by the marked inhibition of immune recognition caused by certain chemical fractions of human syncytiotrophoblastic membranes. Although gene products from extra-embryonic cells may be useful in transplantation, the same products elaborated by malignant cells could have disastrous effects. This is demonstrated by the observation that many human tumor cells maintained in vitro manifest human trophoblast antigens on their plasma membranes, suggesting that these products may have allowed the abnormal cells to escape their own body's immunosurveillance by means of the embryo's ploy.

If immunology is important in normal pregnancy, its failure may account for certain obstetrical misfortunes, the causes of which are presently unknown. An example of this is pre-eclamptic toxaemia (PET), a relatively common disease of unestablished etiology which is characterised by high blood pressure and abnormal kidney function during the third trimester of pregnancy. A role for extra-embryonic products in the control of allogeneic reactions would however be more important at, and immediately following, implantation, and it is of interest that this is when most pregnancy failures occur. Maternal blocking factors usually appear during the second trimester and a failure to produce such factors has been associated with spontaneous abortion. Whether diseases of the third trimester are simply late clinical manifestations of early immunological imbalances is not known, and no careful studies have been undertaken to determine if maternal immunity is involved in a spectrum of foetal disorders, such as congenital malformations. Certainly there is ample evidence to show that congenital defects of the central nervous system can be caused experimentally by the passive transfer of certain antibodies, but there is as yet no clear example of this in human medicine.

The Materno-foetal interface and extra-embryonic membranes

In human beings, the materno-foetal interface is the plasma membrane of the syncytiotrophoblast, as this is the only surface in contact with maternal blood (for a useful text on the human placenta, see Boyd and Hamilton, 1970). Ultrastructural analysis of this interface reveals syncytiotrophoblastic microvilli which age, break away into the intervillous spaces, and are swept by maternal blood through the uterine veins, inferior vena cava, and heart to lodge eventually in the maternal lung. In other words, the human mother is transfused with allogeneic membranes, the effects of which are unknown. In addition, aggregates of syncytiotrophoblastic tissues called syncytial sprouts have been recovered from maternal blood, disclosing another source of intravenous barrage of extra-embryonic, allogeneic tissue from the conceptus into the pregnant female. Perhaps even more astonishingly, stromal trophoblastic buds have been reported to sink into the villi and enter the umbilical circulation of the embryo without any known effect upon either development or immunity. The implications of such reports are sufficiently serious to merit confirmation of the observations before comment on the possible role of trophoblastic traffic into the foetus. Nonetheless, under classical conceptions of graft–host immunobiology, one would not expect systemic immunization of donor or recipient to function beneficially for the graft. As an understanding of trophoblast development is essential to appreciate its role at the materno-foetal interface, some of the events which precede implantation and trophoblast formation will be discussed before considering the role of extra-embryonic membranes in the ontogeny of immunity.

Like all sexually reproducing species, the human embryo begins as a single egg cell or ovum which becomes fertilized in the upper part of the fallopian tube by a single spermatozoon and promptly begins a series of mitotic divisions called cleavages. The resulting cells, called blastomeres, have been shown by many experiments on other mammals to be completely unspecialized. That is, if separated and allowed to proceed independently each can produce a whole individual with a complete set of appropriately specialized tissues and organs. This cluster of totipotential, or protodermal cells is described as a morula. It is held together and protected by a thick, non-cellular gelatinous cover called the zona pellucida and swept toward the uterus by cilia lining the maternal oviduct. After about four days it arrives at the uterine fundus where the zona pellucida vanishes within twelve hours by an unknown process, and the morula floats freely in uterine fluid for another 64 hours, after which it becomes converted into a unilaminar blastocyst by an ill-understood process called cavitation. A split appears between the outer layer of cells and the inner ones at a point which is thereby identified as the vegetal pole of the embryo and the split spreads in all directions from there until it has detached the surface cells from the inner cells everywhere except at the opposite or animal pole (Fig. 1A). Accumulation of fluid in the cavity, called the blastocoele, by endosmosis or active secretion, or both, stretches and flattens the outer cells everywhere except where they remain attached to the inner cell mass at the animal pole (Fig. 1B).

For more than half a century, many embryologists were committed to the idea that embryonic and extra-embryonic materials were separated by the first cleavage. They named the outer layer (Figs. 1A, 1B) the trophoblast and thought that it gave rise to all extra-embryonic tissues such as the chorion, the amnion and the primitive yolk sac. This latter structure was called Heuser's membrane and was regarded as being mesodermal. Some authors imagined the trophoblast to be the source of the allantoic mesoderm and blood vessels of the placenta.

These ideas seem to have been discredited by recent observational and experimental data. Briefly, it has been shown that each of the first two blastomeres of the rat is totipotent, and subsequent studies revealed that the four- and eight-cell stages of the mouse are also totipotent. In fact, the inner cell mass has been separated from the outer layer and it has been shown that the inner cells do not lose their totipotency until sometime between 69

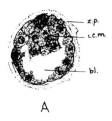

A

Fig. 1A. Fifth day human unilaminar blastocyst with inner cell mass (i.c.m.) and blastocoele (bl.) which has formed by cavitation. Outside cells are surrounded by the zona pellucidum (z.p.).

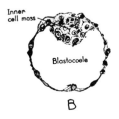

B

Fig. 1B. Sixth day human blastocyst with flattened chorionic ectoderm.

and 93 hours of tissue culture after the two-cell stage in the mouse (see Spindle, 1978, for details). During this period they are even capable of regenerating an outer layer as well as producing a chorion, amnion, yolk sac, allantois and all organs of the body, but the outer cells in culture give rise to nothing but

ectodermal vesicles. For a diagrammatic representation of the extra-embryonic membranes, see Fig. 2. The results of these experiments seem to deny any theory of separation of embryonic and extra-embryonic material during early cleavage. Though the origin of the trophoblast is still a subject of lively debate, in the North American Opossum there seems little doubt that the corresponding cells are simply non-medullary ectoderm, and many embryologists now agree that the trophoblast in mammals is ectodermal in origin.

Implantation and beyond

On the seventh day the embryo usually makes contact with the maternal mucosa and promptly responds in two ways; firstly, the cells of the chorionic ectoderm which touch

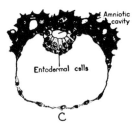

C

Fig. 1C. Seventh day human blastocyst showing endoderm (entoderm), medullary plate and non-medullary ectoderm now differentiated into amniosomatic cells (surrounding amniotic cavity), syncytiotrophoblast (dark tissue at animal pole) and its cytotrophoblastic progenitor.

the uterine epithelium immediately anchor themselves by inserting pseudopods between the uterine epithelial cells, and secondly, the cytotrophoblast begins to produce a new tissue called syncytiotrophoblast in which all cell walls vanish and nuclei are scattered at random through a continuous cytoplasm (Fig. 1C). A single layer of endodermal cells becomes recognizable below the medullary plate and amnio-somatic ectoderm which collectively complete the inventory of the inner-cell mass on the eighth day.

During the tenth and eleventh days, the contiguity between amnion and cytotrophoblast remains undisturbed, but the proliferative frenzy of the endoderm, instead of coming to rest after completing the primary

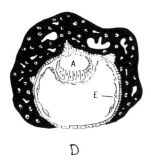

D

Fig. 1D. Ninth day human blastocyst showing extension of the syncytiotrophoblast (dark tissue) and increase in the number and size of its lacunae. Most of the chorion is now converted into cytotrophoblast. Note also the extension of the endodermal lining (E) of the blastocoele towards the vegetal pole, and expanding amniotic cavity (A) with its amniosomatic ectoderm.

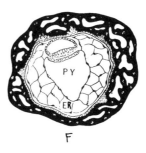

F

Fig. 1F. Eleventh day. Complete endodermal reticulum (ER) partially enclosing interconnected subdivisions of the primary yolk sac (PY).

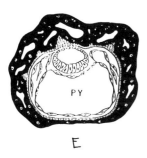

E

Fig. 1E. Tenth day. Bilaminar blastocyst with complete primary yolk sac (PY) and beginnings of the endodermal reticulum. Note extensions of the cytotrophoblastic layer into the darker syncytium to begin formation of the trophoblastic villi.

During the ninth day, endoderm proliferates beyond the medullary plate until it has completely lined the vesicle (Fig. 1D), converting most of the blastocoele into a primitive yolk sac (Fig. 1E).

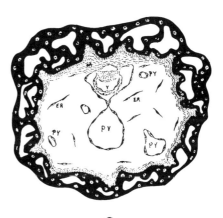

G

Fig. 1G. Thirteenth day. Extension of mesoderm (M) beneath the cytotrophoblast to form the connective tissue cores of the villi. These soon vascularize to form complete trophoblastic villi. The primary yolk sac (PY) has collapsed and the endodermal reticulum (ER) is beginning to disintegrate, and all of the PY fragments are absorbed except for the portion immediately beneath the medullary plate. This remains as the definitive yolk sac (Y).

yolk sac, continues to shed cells which form a tenuous reticulum between its well formed lining and the cytotrophoblast (Fig. 1F). Until recently, the lining of the primitive yolk sac was called Heuser's membrane, under the impression that it was mesodermal and derived from the trophoblast. However, it has now been shown that trophoblast cannot give rise to anything but trophoblast, and the results of an important study by Luckett (1978) of all stages of yolk sac development in man and monkey make it seem clear that Heuser's membrane is endodermal and that the cavity it encloses is primary yolk sac and not extraembryonic coelom. During the thirteenth day, most of the primary yolk sac disappears except that portion most closely associated with the medullary plate (Fig. 1G) which is retained to give rise to the definitive yolk sac, gut and allantois. Finally, as the shrivelling primary yolk sac and its reticular extensions shrink away from the cytotrophoblast, they are replaced by mesoderm which by the fifteenth day has spread from the primitive streak and become continuous around the outside of the amniotic and definitive yolk sacs, separating for the first time the amniotic ectoderm from the cytotrophoblastic layer.

The somatic portion of the amnio-somatic ectoderm rolls out upon and adheres to the embryonic body as the latter enlarges, leaving the amniotic portion as the inner lining of the amnion, the outer surface of which is the extraembryonic mesoderm just mentioned. The amniotic sac thus formed (Fig. 2) is commonly called the 'bag of waters'. It contributes several protective and supportive services that are thought to be important in foetal survival. By providing complete immersion in a private pond, the amniotic fluid equalizes the pressure in all directions, and diffuses evenly over the entire body mechanical forces which might be injurious if concentrated locally. The same fluid environment includes lubricants which reduce the probability of adhesions of parts in contact with

each other. The mesodermal layer of the amnion includes smooth muscle fibres, the periodic contractions of which cause gentle rocking motions, further reducing the probability of adhesions. These mechanical services of the amnion have been recognized for many years, but an important immunological function of the somatic ectoderm also deserves attention. The somatic ectoderm which covers the embryo's third branchial arch as well as a

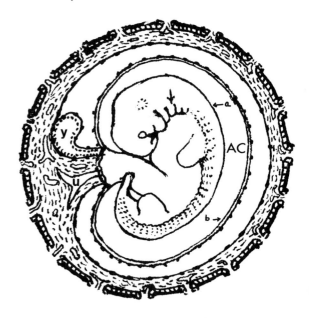

Fig. 2. Thirty-fifth day of human development. The amniosomatic ectoderm has now differentiated into its two derivatives; (a) the somatic ectoderm which has unfolded upon the surface of the body and body stalk as they have taken shape, and (b) the amniotic ectoderm which has remained as the lining of the amniotic cavity (AC). The outer (mesodermal) layers of the amnion approaches and soon forms contact with the corresponding layer of the chorion (i.e. the outermost shell). The yolk sac (Y) is reduced to a vestige closely applied to the cranial side of the primordial placenta. The endodermal lining of the allantois has not grown for the last two weeks and is now hidden within the base of the umbilical cord as an extension of the bladder, but the allantoic or umbilical artery (u) is well developed. The arrow points to the 3rd branchial arch and groove which supplies the ectodermal components of the thymus. The outside covering with villus twigs is the chorion.

groove that adjoins the arch on the caudal side (Fig. 2, arrow) makes a contribution to the thymic cortex, and this bit of ectoderm is essential to the development of another structure of unknown function within the thymus gland known as Hassall's corpuscles. This idea is supported by studies of hairless or so-called 'nude' mice with abnormal thymus glands, where abortive development of the ectodermal component of the thymus in the embryos of these animals has been shown to result in abnormal Hassell bodies and profound immunological deficiencies. The thymus thus produced is not extra-embryonic in either origin or final location, but it cannot play its central immunological role without somatic ectoderm plus a supply of stem cells from an extra-embryonic source, the foetal yolk sac.

The foetal yolk sac in some fishes and in all reptiles, birds and mammals (i.e. in all Amniotes) is an extra-embryonic extension of the midgut. In birds and mammals, it is known to give rise to stem cells which migrate first to the foetal liver and then to the central lymphoid organs, the thymus and the bursa of Fabricius (or its mammalian equivalent), in which they mature and diversify and from which they seed to the peripheral lymphoid structures to form the cells of the immunological system. The details of this cell traffic were first worked out in chickens by using chromosomal markers and parabiosis, but it has been possible to confirm some of the details in mice and some others in man by the use of karyotype analysis of the lymphocytes which repopulate transplanted thymus glands in nude mice and in patients with the Di George syndrome, an uncommon form of immuno-deficiency disease in which, among other defects, the thymus gland is rudimentary. Though the yolk sac in man is vestigial — the mother having rendered food storage obsolete by taking over all commissary functions herself — there is a stage in human development when it is robust enough to carry on its historic role of harbouring all of the primordial germ cells until it releases them through the umbilical cord to their final home in the mesodermal genital ridges. Similarly, it has not relinquished its role as a primordial source of blood cells, including those providing immune protection.

The last extra-embryonic structure to be considered is called the allantois. This was originally a storage depot for nitrogenous waste in cleidoic eggs (i.e. eggs enclosed within a relatively impermeable casing), but it progressively became overloaded and distended as the period of gestation grew longer. It was originally only a urinary bladder, but as it expanded outside the body wall it made contact with ectodermal chorion, the trophoblastic surface of which was closely applied to one of the following; (a) the uterine mucosa, (b) endothelium of the mother's capillaries, or (c) maternal blood, depending on the extent of the trophoblastic invasion achieved in different species. Here the turgid bladder found relief as its effluent gained access to maternal blood from where the mother's kidneys removed it and disposed of it externally. The mammalian allantoic placenta thus arose as a waste disposal plant, and the connections which served this function admirably enabled it also to tap the maternal supplies of nutrients, oxygen, and immunoglobulins for the embryo at an early stage of development. Interestingly, in chickens the bursa of Fabricius and the allantois both arise from the hind gut, but whether cells of the allantoic mesoderm in mammals are associated with B-lymphocyte development has not been explicitly investigated. The nearest approach is a study by Melchers & Abramczuk (1980) of precursor B-lymphocytes in the blood of mouse embryos. These investigators followed a definition of pre-B cells as being those which, upon adoptive transfer together with antigen into irradiated syngeneic recipients, will not yield an immediate B-cell response of antigen-specific, immunoglobulin-secreting, plaque-forming cells, but will do so after a period of several days in the host. They also extended the definition to include precursor B-cells in bone marrow and in foetal liver which show delayed *in vitro* responsiveness to the B-lymphocyte mitogen lipopolysaccharide.

The search for cells thus identifiable in the blood of embryonic mice revealed that they can first be detected at day 10, and become most abundant at day 12, thereafter rapidly disappearing. The search for their source revealed that the earliest pre-B cells detected were in the placenta, and a later wave appeared between days 13 and 19 in

foetal liver. Neither yolk sac nor liver contained pre-B cells at the time they first appeared in the placenta. Finally, they appear in bone marrow, and continue to come from both bone marrow and liver throughout life. Melchers and Abramczuk did not mention that the placenta of the mouse and of nearly all mammals is an allantoic derivative from the hindgut near the site of origin of the Bursa of Fabricius in birds. Until, and unless, contrary evidence is found, we interpret these observations as supporting our hypothesis that the mammalian equivalent of the Bursa

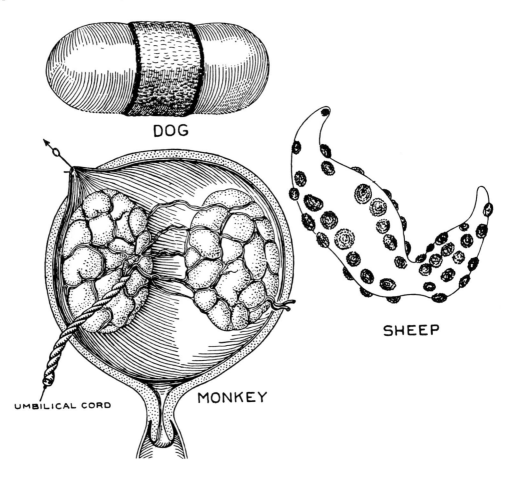

Fig. 3. Anatomical differences in placentae from 3 different mammals exemplifying the concept that the evolution of viviparity developed somewhat along the lines of a general idea without a precise blueprint. Such gross dissimilarities are also mirrored in structure and function; denying the extrapolation of experimental results in placental research from one mammal to another. (Modified from Corner, 1944).

of Fabricius of birds is the allantois, and that the splanchnopleuric mesoderm adjoining its endodermal lining is the earliest site of maturation of stem cells from the yolk sac into pre-B and B-cells.

Studies of Animal Models in Materno-Foetal Immunity

Basic physiological processes have usually been investigated by using analogy with animal models, and in problems relating to other organ systems this has often been a valid and useful approach. However, unlike livers, kidneys, etc. which generally have followed parallel, conservative lines of evolution, placentae seem to have developed more independently, almost as though an idea was offered without a blueprint (Fig. 3). Indeed, even gross anatomical aspects differ so much that it is sometimes difficult to recognize similarities, placentae from dogs, sheep, and monkeys being cases in point. In addition to gross differences, there are also histological variations, most placentae being assignable to one of four basic histological types based on the nature and extent of interaction between placental and uterine tissues. However, the usefulness of this system of nomenclature is more apparent than real, for humans, mice and guinea pigs all have haemochorial placentae, but the microanatomy of placental tissues from these three mammals is strikingly different.

In the placenta, there are major physiological differences which prevent confident extrapolation of results from one species to another. Immunoglobulin transfer provides a good example, for most haemochorial placentae allow the specific passage of certain immunoglobulin classes, while none of the ungulates allows any antibodies to pass from mother to young before birth (for review, see Brambell, 1970). Even physiological similarities may be deceptive,

for while both man and guinea pig transmit maternal IgG to the foetus, IgG transport in the human placenta is via a unique receptor (called the Fc receptor, for it binds to the so-called Fc fragment of IgG molecules) on syncytiotrophoblastic membranes drained by allantoic veins, while in the guinea pig the passage is across vitelline veins from the yolk sac. Other basic differences among haemochorial placentae include the presence of specific receptors at the maternofoetal interface. For example, human placentae are an excellent source of insulin receptors but this is not the case with rats. Another receptor on the trophoblast which has been suggested as being important in human reproductive immunobiology is that for transferrin (for a fuller description, see Faulk & Galbraith, 1979) but it is not found in the mouse, whose placenta is also haemochorial. At this point, it is important to mention that trophoblast receptors can differ in the same animal in different areas of the trophoblast. Human transferrin receptors are found on the syncytiotrophoblast at the materno-foetal interface within the placental bed, but are not present on the cytotrophoblast of the amnio-chorionic membrane.

Although it is presently poorly understood, many immunologists would speculate that the deportation of trophoblastic material from placenta to maternal lung is very important in the immunology of pregnancy, and such speculation is supported by a report that the flux of trophoblast membranes in certain abnormal pregnancies is in excess of that found in normal pregnancy. Nonetheless, trophoblast deportation has to date only been described in one other mammal, the chinchilla. In summary, animal models are certainly important, but it would seem that Alexander Pope's admonition that 'the proper study of Mankind is Man' is particularly appropriate in the field of materno-foetal immunity.

Allotypic Antigens in the Graft–Host Analogy of Pregnancy

Many mothers produce antibodies to antigens within the human leukocyte system (HLA) but there is no human condition in the embryo or foetus which is caused by maternal anti-HLA, even though the antibodies are IgG, and as such are transported into the placenta. Maternal immunization to incompatible HLA antigens probably results from the leakage of HLA-positive cells into the intervillous spaces through placental tears, for there is no evidence that human synctiotrophoblast membranes bear antigens of the major histocompatibility complex (for original report see Faulk & Temple, 1976). Other incompatible allotypic antigens stimulate immune responses in the mother which are potentially damaging to the foetus, and some of these have been extensively investigated; the most well studied example is that of antibodies to the D or Rhesus antigen. Because human placentae lack D antigen, maternal IgG antibodies can pass unimpeded through chorionic villi to be collected in the umbilical and foetal circulation where they encounter and destroy D-positive erythrocytes, causing the clinical syndrome of erythroblastosis foetalis. Babies so affected were often referred to as 'yellow babies' due to their extensive jaundice. Erythroblastosis foetalis was a major cause of braindamaged infants and thus led to the waste basket diagnosis of 'Cerebral Palsy'. A hint of the potential of basic research in human reproduction is given by this disease, which has been virtually eliminated. Other circumstances in which the mother is immunized transplacentally by incompatible allotypes to cause distress in the baby such as neonatal thrombocytopenia, await similar therapeutic innovations.

One reason that maternal antibodies to antigenic groupings on foetal immunoglobulins do not cause serious clinical disease is that they do not in fact reach the foetus. They bind and precipitate their antigens within the mesenchymal stroma of chorionic villi and in that state they are not free to enter the foetal circulation. This observation is supported by a report of an activated fragment (C1q) of the first component of human complement being found around foetal stem vessels, as this molecule is known to fix and co-precipitate immune complexes. In addition, those complexes which are not co-precipitable by complement will, in all probability, be bound by Fc receptors, both placental endothelium and Hofbauer cells being a rich source of Fc receptors.

A concept thus emerges of maternal IgG antibodies which enter but never leave the placenta, suggesting that there is a sink for immune complexes within the connective tissues of human placentae. Consideration of the placental sink also reveals why maternal antibodies to D-antigen cause disease in the foetus and antibodies to HLA do not, for D-antigens are not found in placenta, yet HLA antigens are present on all cells of chorionic villi except the trophoblast. This suggests that maternal antibodies to allotypic antigens cause foetal disease only when they are not immunoabsorbed onto antigens within the placenta.

Trophoblast Antigens in Materno-Foetal Biology

The point at which rejection is initiated in most grafts is the operational interface between recipient and graft. That is, the point of contact between representatives of the recipient's immune system and antigens which that system recognizes as being nonself. Although several such interfaces can be anatomically defined in human pregnancy, they all share the common feature that the foetal component is trophoblastic. None of the histocompatibility related antigens has been convincingly identified at the haemochorial interface in humans, but a great deal more work remains to be done before one can be too sanguine on this point. Cells obtained from trophoblastic neoplasms do manifest HLA, albeit only those loci which are representative of the paternal haplotype (see Shaw *et al.*, 1979 for an illustrative case). Presently, it is only possible to report that human syncytiotrophoblastic tissues do not manifest histocompatibility-related gene products on their plasma membranes, although they might retain the capacity to do so under certain experimental conditions.

Inasmuch as the trophoblast forms the materno-foetal interface in human pregnancy, some investigators have begun to focus on structural components of the trophoblastic plasma membrane as being of possible importance in reproductive immunobiology. A useful method has been published for the preparation of syncytiotrophoblastic microvilli, and the characterization of several proteins and glycoprotein subunits at the interface have been detailed. We have described serological criteria for the definition of unique trophoblast antigens (TA) termed TA_1 and TA_2 (Faulk and co-workers, 1978), and these findings have been extended by several different groups, and one can expect new and exciting developments in this aspect of materno-foetal immunobiology in the future. We have also shown that both antisera to TA_1 antigens as well as the antigens themselves are potent inhibitors of the mixed lymphocyte culture reaction *in vitro* (for key papers, see McIntyre and Faulk, 1979a and b), a reaction which is widely held to be an equivalent of the *in vivo* phenomenon of the passage of foetal lymphocytes into the maternal circulation during normal pregnancy.

Summary and Conclusions

Information in this compendium challenges contemporary knowledge by pointing out that immunity evolved through hundreds of millions of years to produce our present complex system of immunosurveillance, yet reproductive patterns in mammals resulted in a process that required the co-habitation of self and non-self antigens throughout pregnancy. How this could have happened is shrouded in the puzzle that it did not diminish maternal immunity for infections, but in some poorly understood way seems to have devised a trick to exempt extra-embryonic tissues from rejection. One way of approaching this question is from the viewpoint of transplantation biology in which the site of rejection is the interface of self with non-self antigens, but, embryologically speaking, only extra-embryonic tissues make contact with maternal cells in the host—parasite relationship of human pregnancy. Thus, is there something peculiar about extra-embryonic tissues in the realm of allogeneic recognition and rejection reactions?

The tissue responsible for intra-uterine co-habitation is a specialized syncytium derived from chorionic ectoderm called syncytiotrophoblast, and when this structure is cultured *in vitro* it gives rise only to ectodermal vesicles, even though it is a product of the totipotential tissues of the morula. A puzzling question about the transplantation analogies of this extra-embryonic membrane is related to the observation that it is formed by the embryo yet it produces microvillous buds that break away from the placental bed without causing any of the evidences of rejection or inflammation in the genetically different mother. Not only syncytiotrophoblast but other extra-embryonic tissues such as amnion, allantois and yolk sac seem to enjoy an as yet unexplained role in the materno-foetal relationship of human pregnancy, although mounting evidence indicates that these structures are very important in the development and diversity of the immunological system.

The comparative state of ignorance in our present understanding of the role of extra-embryonic membranes in the transplantation analogies of human pregnancy is amplified by the anatomical reality that scant hope is held for progress in the delineation of their contribution in human reproduction from experimental studies done in other animals. This is because the placenta, amnion, yolk sac and allantois vary so much in their gross anatomy, histology and physiology from mammal to mammal that investigations to understand gestation in the human probably have to be done on human tissues. This is, for example, manifest in the trans-placental passage of immunity from mother to foetus: This process occurs transplacentally in some and in others via breast milk, both routes being utilized in human mothers. Another curious aspect of the human placenta is that maternal antibody responses to incompatible foetal antigens inherited from the father are immunoabsorbed onto antigens present within placental connective tissues, these antibodies never reaching the developing embryo. This extraordinary phenomenon has given rise to a concept of a placental sink for some maternal antibodies, and it is only when foetal/paternal antigens are not present within the sink that the antibodies are allowed to pass unimpeded into the foetus and cause their particular biological or pathological effects.

One of the central questions about human reproduction which has been periodically approached with the development of new technology is whether trophoblast membranes at the materno-foetal interface manifest characteristic antigens that are capable of escaping maternal recognition and rejection reactions. The concept of tissue-specific trophoblast antigens has given rise to an idea that vaccines might be developed to trophoblast products to control human reproduction, the idea being that immunization could stimulate a condition of maternal immunity that would either deny implantation or trigger immunological rejection of the blastocyst by processes similar to those responsible for the rejection of foreign tissue. A small step towards clarifying this issue has recently accrued from the observation that a structural component of the trophoblast is capable of exerting control over the *in vitro* equivalent of transplantation rejection *in vivo*, and it is possible that careful study of this reaction will cast light on the role of extra-embryonic membranes in transplantation analogies of human pregnancy.

Acknowledgements

We are grateful to Dr. John A. McIntyre for reading and commenting on the text.

This work was supported in part by the Medical Research Council, Action Research and the East Grinstead Research Trust.

References

BOYD, J.D. and HAMILTON, W.J. (1970) *The Human Placenta*, The Macmillan Press, London.

BRAMBELL, F.W.R. (1970) *The Transmission of Passive Immunity from Mother to Young*, North-Holland Publishing, Amsterdam.

CORNER, G.W. (1944) *Ourselves Unborn*, Yale University Press, New Haven.

FAULK, W.P. and GALBRAITH, G.M.P. (1979) Trophoblast transferrin and transferrin receptors in the host—parasite relationship of human pregnancy, *Proceedings of the Royal Society (B)*, **204**, 83—97.

FAULK, W.P. and JOHNSON, P.M. (1980) Immunological studies of human placentae: Basic and practical implications, *Recent Advances in Clinical Immunology*, **2**, 1—31.

FAULK, W.P. and TEMPLE, A. (1976) Distribution of B_2-microglobulin and HLA in chorionic villi of human placentae, *Nature*, **262**, 799—802.

FAULK, W.P., TEMPLE, A., LOVINS, R. and SMITH, N.C. (1978) Antigens of human trophoblasts: A working hypothesis for their role in normal and abnormal pregnancies, *Proceedings of the National Academy of Sciences, USA*, **75**, 1947–1951.

LUCKETT, W.P. (1978) Origin and differentiation of the yolk sac and extra-embryonic mesoderm in presomite human and rhesus monkey embryos, *American Journal of Anatomy*, **152**, 59–98.

McINTYRE, J.A. and FAULK, W.P. (1979a) Antigens of human trophoblast: Effects of heterologous anti-trophoblast sera on lymphocyte responses *in vitro*, *Journal of Experimental Medicine*, **149**, 824–836.

McINTYRE, J.A. and FAULK, W.P. (1979b) Trophoblast modulation of maternal allogeneic recognition, *Proceedings of the National Academy of Sciences, USA*, **76**, 4029–4033.

MELCHERS, F. and ABRAMCZUK, J. (1980) Murine embryonic blood between day 10 and 13 of gestation as a source of immature precursor B-cells, *European Journal of Immunology*, **10**, 763–767.

MILLER, J.F., WILLIAMSON, E., GLUE, J., GORDON, Y.B., BRDUZINSKA, J.G. and SYKES, A. (1980) Foetal loss after implantation, *Lancet*, **II**, 554–556.

SHAW, A.R.E., DASGUPTA, M.K., KOVITHARONGS, T., JOHNY, K.V., LeRICH, J.C., DOSSETOR, J.B. and MACPHERSON, T.A. (1979) Humoral and cellular immunity to paternal antigens in trophoblastic neoplasia, *International Journal of Cancer*, **24**, 586–593.

SPINDLE, A.I. (1978) Trophoblast regeneration by inner cell marses isolated from cultured mouse embryos, *Journal of Experimental Zoology*, **203**, 483–489.

TRANSPLANTATION BIOLOGY

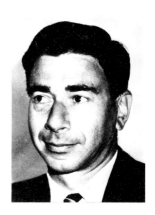

R.Y. Calne, F.R.S.

Professor of Surgery, University of Cambridge.

He is also an Honorary Consultant Surgeon, Addenbrooke's Hospital, Cambridge and a member of the Court and Council of the Royal College of Surgeons. Professor Calne is a general surgeon with a particular interest in vascular surgery and transplantation surgery.

The successful grafting of plants, even across species provided they are relatively close, has been practised successfully in horticulture since early times. When thoughts of surgical grafting of tissues for the treatment of human disease began to emerge there were no reasons to believe that the observations in plants would not be applicable to animals. Such a happy outcome was not to be. Despite the fact that Baronio in 1800 showed that free grafts of skin from one part of an animal to another part of the same animal would take permanently, whilst grafts from a different animal would be destroyed, there were to be numerous subsequent attempts at both intra- and inter-species grafting before it became quite clear that no matter how good the technique, the graft would be destroyed unless it came from the same individual (or an identical twin who is biologically the same individual).

In the 1940s Gibson and Medawar (1943) showed that this process of graft destruction had the characteristics of an immune reaction. It is similar to the immunity that follows infection with the measles virus, when subsequent contact with measles results in rapid virus elimination. Thus if a graft from individual A to individual B (which may be destroyed in a week), is followed by a second graft from A to B, the 'second-set' graft will be destroyed in a day or two.

In the subsequent decade much work was undertaken to define the details of this rejection process. The microscopical appearance of a rejected graft suggested that lymphocytes were involved, since many of these cells infiltrated the grafted tissue before it was finally destroyed. (Lymphocytes are a class of white blood cells. There are two types of lymphocytes: T-lymphocytes and B-lymphocytes. The T-lymphocytes are concerned with Cell Mediated Immunity [for example in the host's response to a measles virus], transplantation rejection and the regulation of the immune response. The B-lymphocytes are antibody producing cells.) An important new concept arose from the results of experiments by Billingham, Brent and Medawar (1954) who showed that if the developing embryo or, in some species the neonatal individual, was given a graft before its immune system was fully developed, it was unable to reject the graft and would subsequently accept further tissue from the same donor. This artificial graft acceptance was known as 'immunological tolerance' and, although not directly applicable to grafting in patients, its demonstration was an important stimulus for further research. For the first time, it had been possible to obtain permanent graft survival from one individual to another in the same species, even when these individuals were not related.

With this historical background certain other known factors need consideration:

(1) Blood transfusion — The existence of different blood groups on red blood cells and reliable laboratory methods of typing for these blood groups enabled routine blood transfusion and a complete new era of surgery to evolve. Unfortunately, matching for these red blood cell groups did not enable grafts of other tissue such as skin and vascularized organs to be accepted, although if these blood groups are deliberately transgressed, graft destruction may be more rapid than if they are matched.

(2) Corneal Grafts — It has been known for a long time that corneal grafts are usually, but not invariably, successful. Failure of a corneal graft is accompanied by ingrowth of blood vessels into the normally bloodless cornea.

(3) The lack of rejection of dead grafted tissue — for example, blood vessels that have been soaked in Formalin or alcohol, steel pins that have been used for repairing fractures.

Putting these observations together it was apparent that in order to elicit a rejection reaction, tissue needed to be living and provided with a blood supply and the factors (antigens) responsible for rejection were additional to red blood cell antigens. Since the effector path of graft destruction appeared to be directed primarily by lymphocytes, a variety of different agents that damaged lymphocytes were investigated to see if they would prevent graft rejection. The two most effective that have been used in clinical transplantation in the past twenty years are the anti-leukaemia drug Azathioprine (Imuran) and corticosteroid drugs (Prednisone). With much trial and error, relatively safe dose combinations of these drugs can produce remarkably good results in organ grafting, e.g. the results of kidney grafting are shown in Table 1. It can be seen that the source of kidney donation is of great importance. The closer the relationship of donor to recipient the better the results.

Table 1. Kidney transplants — functioning grafts

	1 year	5 years
Sibling	75%	60%
Parent	70%	50%
Cadaver	50%	30%

Thanks to the pioneering efforts of Dausset, Terasaki and Van Rood the most important antigens involved in graft rejection were found on white blood cells and reproducible methods of defining these antigens were developed. Work on so-called 'transplantation antigens' has proliferated and now occupies numerous scientists in hundreds of laboratories throughout the world. It has been shown that these human leucocyte antigens (HLA) which constitute part of the major histocompatibility complex (MHC) of genetic material, are contained on a portion of one chromosome, the sixth chromosome in man. It has been found that special patterns of antigen (tissue-types) correlate with certain diseases, whose nature had previously been completely obscure. This, however, has nothing to do with tissue transplantation. When the tissue types are used for selection of appropriate donors of kidney grafts, it has been found that within a family the tissue typing is extremely important and there is a one in four chance of the HLA antigens being identical between brothers and sisters. A graft that is identical for the MHC has an extremely good outlook. Nevertheless, the immunosuppressive drugs Azathioprine and corticosteroids have still be be given in most cases. Much effort has been made to try and find more effective and safer drugs to prevent rejection and a promising new agent is Cyclosporin A. It is a derivative of an earth fungus and extremely powerful and non-toxic as an immunosuppressive agent in a variety of different animals receiving organ grafts. In man it is also very promising but much more difficult to use, because of side-effects that were not apparent in animals.

This is a very sketchy background of current knowledge of transplantation biology. The essentials for rejection are antigenic incompatibility between donor and recipient. The foreign graft is recognized by the immune system and is treated as if it were an invading virus or bacterium and the reaction that causes destruction of the tissue involves lymphocytes (Fig. 1). If the lymphocytes are destroyed totally there can be no rejection of the graft, but the patient would be deprived of immune defences and would succumb to simple, usually non-fatal diseases, such as chickenpox and influenza. What we would like to be able to do is manipulate the immune system so that it will ignore the life-saving organ grafts but still be otherwise

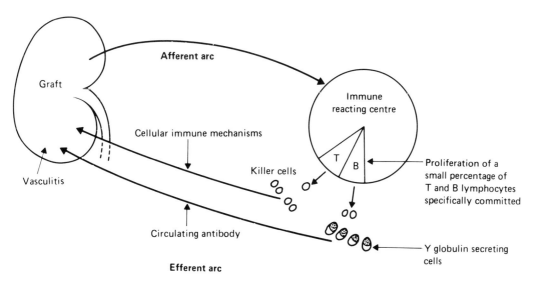

Fig. 1. Interactions between the host's immune system and the transplanted graft.

normally reactive. Such a simple objective sometimes is achieved in patients without our understanding the mechanisms involved. For example, some kidney grafts where the donor has been unrelated and of a poor tissue match to the recipient, have nevertheless functioned for ten years or more and kept patients in good health with only modest doses of Azathioprine and corticosteroids.

It is clear that more knowledge is required concerning the chemical nature of transplantation antigens – how they are recognized as foreign and how the body reacts against such foreign antigens. Despite volumes of scientific reports that would fill whole libraries on this subject, one has to admit that the precise details of these phenomena are not understood and our ignorance is spectacular. Part of the trouble is that with each new probing analysis made by research workers, instead of the phenomena resolving as clearly understood interactions, what appeared at one time to be a simple straightforward reaction is now shown to be exceedingly involved.

In fact the immune system appears to have a variety of different components which interact with each other in a way not dissimilar to the interaction of neurones in the brain. For example, there are a variety of different chemical structures in grafts which may behave as antigens. The macrophage scavenger cells in the blood may be necessary to process these antigens and present them to certain special types of lymphocytes, some of which respond by producing chemical circulating antibodies which destroy the graft; others proliferate to form a new population of special killer lymphocytes which infiltrate the graft and destroy it accounting for the microscopical appearance of a rejecting graft. Such a simple chain of reactions, however, could lead to an unbridled action of the immune system and therefore there are very discrete and careful controlling mechanisms which prevent this. For example there is another population of 'suppressor' lympho-cytes which instead of causing destruction of grafted tissue, actually inhibit that process. Some lymphocytes produce 'enhancing' antibodies which interfere with graft destruction. Other lymphocytes, while not actually partaking in the graft destruction, are necessary for the rejection process to occur, the so-called 'helper' cells.

A picture of the immune system as a complicated armed force with different components, not all of them aggressive, is probably only a sketchy impression of what will eventually be found. In theory, even if the whole picture were clearly defined, the interactions might be too complicated for us to manipulate it in a predictable and safe manner. A whole new armamentarium of therapeutic modifiers of the immune system might need to be developed. It is very important to recognize these fundamental defects in our knowledge. At least by doing so we are not under the illusion of comprehension, but realize the enormous amount of further understanding that is still required.

Having looked at the process of rejection and accepted, with due humility, our lack of knowledge, we are similarly unable to explain the good results that can be obtained in clinical organ grafting using very crude immunosuppressive agents. This perhaps is not too pessimistic a state of affairs as far as patient treatment is concerned. We are likely to develop better empirical immunosuppressive agents and the more effective they are the better will be the results of organ grafting, and by reason of their effectiveness they probably set the stage for natural acceptance of the graft. Such positive observations may be easier to study than the more basic understanding of mechanisms.

If a drug like Cyclosporin A is relatively effective and non-toxic as an immunosuppressant, it must be modifying the immune response in the direction we would theoretically also like to be able to do, provided we ever gain sufficient knowledge to proceed in a logical way at discrete immunological manipulation. Thus, by studying the cellular immunology both *in vivo* and *in vitro*, of patients treated with modern, effective, immunosuppressive drugs, it should be possible to learn more about the components of the immune system that are concerned with graft rejection. For example, if a Cyclosporin A treated patient had a deficiency of 'helper' cells circulating in their blood, or if the helper cells were unable to exert their normal biological role, this would point to a specific attack on the helper cells as being a profitable target for further development of immunosuppressive agents.

A similar argument might be advanced, but in a different direction, if it were found that Cyclosporin A stimulated the production of specific 'suppressor' cells which inhibited rejection of the grafted organ. The more basic immunology that is understood, even in artificial models removed from clinical organ grafting, the more points of manipulation would be revealed for application to man. Although it is dangerous to make any predictions in science, I would doubt that there would be a sudden, enormous advance as is envisaged by the popular term 'breakthrough'.

More likely, there will be a slow but steady nibbling away of the defences permitting improved understanding and care of patients to evolve.

References

BILLINGHAM, R.E., BRENT, L., MEDAWAR, P.B., *et al.* (1954) *Proceedings of the Royal Society, B,* **143,** 43.
GIBSON, T. and MEDAWAR, P.B. (1943) *Journal of Anatomy,* **77,** 299.
MOURANT, A.E. (1977) Why are there blood groups? In: *The Encyclopaedia of Ignorance,* Vol. 2. (Duncan, R. and Weston-Smith, M. eds.). Pergamon Press, Oxford.

COMBAT WITH PARASITES

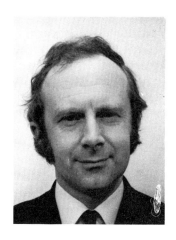

Keith Vickerman

Professor of Zoology, University of Glasgow.

His principal interest is in Protozoa. He was awarded the Royal Society's Tropical Research Fellowship for his work leading to understanding of the complicated life cycles of sleeping sickness trypanosomes in terms of their mitochondrial and antigenic adaptations. He is a member of the World Health Organization's Expert Advisory Panel on Parasitic Diseases.

It is difficult for dwellers in temperate climes to realise the stranglehold that infectious disease still maintains on the lives of those living in the tropics. In rural communities in particular, tropical diseases can affect every aspect of human life. When they do not kill, these diseases disable and debilitate — sometimes the entire population of a particular area. By increasing the effort required for human survival, they result in stagnation of social and economic progress.

Many of these diseases are caused by animal parasites — protozoa, roundworms and flatworms. These pathogens may be several orders of magnitude larger than the viruses and bacteria which are the main agents of infectious disease in the developed world. Animal parasites are also set apart as infectious agents by their independent mobility and the sheer complexity of their genetic, metabolic and structural organization, and these factors contribute to their extraordinary cunning when it comes to avoiding the host's defensive reaction to their presence.

Although parasites usually stimulate a vigorous immune response on the part of their host, complete acquired resistance to them is almost unheard of. What immunity there is simply serves to keep parasite numbers down in the case of protozoa which multiply in their hosts, or to prevent further infection in the case of helminths (parasitic worms) which usually do not multiply. This is largely because parasites are masters of the art of evasion when faced with host attack and this evasion can have serious consequences for the host. In the first place, sustained or repeated evasion may greatly prolong the course of the infection, hence the chronic nature of many parasitic diseases, and their debilitating effects. In the second place, the host's immune response may become greatly disordered or exaggerated, so that in the end the host damages itself more than the offending parasite. And lastly, the ineffectiveness of the host's response in demolishing the parasite may mean that trying to protect the host against infection by vaccination is impossible.

Because it is important to continue trying to ameliorate the misery caused by parasitic diseases the battle between host and parasite has come under increasing scrutiny in recent years. This has been facilitated by the possibility of analyzing mechanisms of attack and defence on either side at cellular and molecular levels. It is my intention in this article to survey some of the weaponry and subterfuge employed in this intimate combat, bearing in mind that contriving eventual victory for the human host is the reason for studying the strategies. As befits this Encyclopaedia of Ignorance, it will become patently obvious that in most cases we do not know much about the weapons employed, about the way in which they are employed or, indeed, in some cases whether they are being employed at all!

I propose to consider three questions which reflect major areas of our ignorance: (1) How are parasites killed off by the host; (2) How do parasites avoid the host's immune response; and (3) Is it possible to tip the scales in favour of the host?

(1) How are Parasites Killed by the Host?

Our understanding of the way in which the human body attempts to defend itself against parasites is to a large extent based on inference from experimental host-parasite systems, where a laboratory animal substitutes for the human host. Quite often a related parasite is used as a substituted for the human pathogen as not all parasites of man will infect laboratory animals. The human malarias, for example, will not. We also extrapolate from artificial *in vitro* situations (for example, a contrived encounter between a parasite and known components of its host's defence mechanisms) to the *in vivo* situation. Parasitologists are aware of the cloud of doubt that envelops such inference but can do little about it.

The mechanisms mediating resistance to disease causing organisms can be classified as either natural or adaptive. Those involved in natural immunity are largely the same as those responsible for reacting in a non-specific way to tissue damage with the production of inflammation. Many parasites by virtue of their size and destructive activities cause obvious damage. It is therefore all the more remarkable that many parasites do not induce inflammatory reactions in the tissues. The dysentery amoeba, *Entamoeba histolytica* (Fig. 1a) causes ulcers in the colon but moves on to the liver where it destroys parenchymal cells. Liver damage normally provokes quick mobilization of the leukocytes to the site of the damage but here there is a weak or no inflammatory reaction. Why? We know that the surface of Entamoeba can activate complement — a series of enzymes present in the serum which, when activated, produce widespread inflammatory effects, as well as lysis (breakdown) of the activating cell or pathogen by puncturing tiny holes in its bounding membrane and leaving it to die of ionic and osmotic imbalance. Another example, equally mysterious, is the filarial nemotode (roundworm) *Onchocerca volvulus*, whose larvae (Fig. 1h) wander into the eye causing blindness. They can readily be observed moving in the cornea where they incite no leucocyte infiltration although this does occur

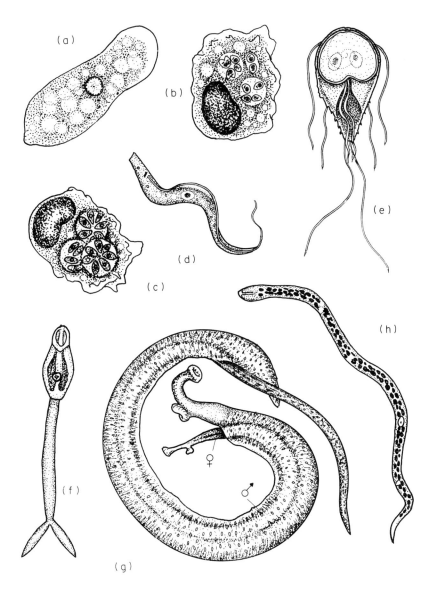

Fig. 1. Parasites of man. a, the dysentery amoeba, *Entamoeba histolytica* (✕ 1000); b, c, macrophages with vacuoles containing (b) tiny aflagellate *Leishmania mexicana* (✕ 750) and (c) *Toxoplasma gondii* (✕ 750); d, sleeping sickness parasite, *Trypanosoma brucei*, bloodstream form (✕ 2200); e, *Giardia intestinalis* (✕ 2000); f, cercaria stage of blood fluke *Schistosoma mansoni* (✕ 75); g, adult *Schistosoma mansoni*, male worm with female lying in a deep groove in his body (✕ 15); h, microfilaria larva of roundworm *Onchocerca volvulus* (✕ 600).

after the death of the larva. Are such parasites able to produce factors able to antagonize or inactivate the mediators of the acute inflammatory response? We do not know.

The nematode parasites, unlike active protozoa and flatworms, do not present a living surface to their hosts but a secreted cuticle. In some nematodes the cuticle activates

238

K. Vickerman

complement directly (by the so-called alternative pathway), that is without the help of antibody (which triggers the so-called classical pathway), while in others it does not and Onchocerca larvae may be in this second category. Many parasites seem to go to pains to conceal their complement-activating surface when they enter a mammalian host. Thus the sleeping sickness trypanosomes (Fig. 1d) put on a thick glycoprotein coat, with no exposed carbyhydrate groups, to hide theirs in the salivary glands of their tsetse fly vector, while the cercaria larva of the blood fluke *Schistosoma* (Fig. 1f) loses its complement-activating glycocalyx (coat) when it penetrates the skin to become a tail-less schistosomula.

Fifteen or more serum components make up the complement system and their sequential activation and assembly into functional units lead to three main effects: (1) the release of peptides active in inflammation, (2) deposition of a powerful attachment promoter or 'opsonin' on the activating pathogen which predisposes it to phagocytosis, and (3) membrane damage resulting in lysis. Lysis and phagocytosis are important means of destruction in natural immunity but parasites in their natural hosts are not usually affected by these mechanisms partly for the reasons outlined above but also for unknown reasons. They have no difficulty in overcoming in the first place the non-specific resistance of the host.

Even more intriguing are those protozoan parasites which rely upon phagocytosis to carry them into the next stage in their life cycle — which is often inside the phagocytic cell itself! Such parasites include the sandfly transmitted leishmanias (Fig. 1b) which are parasites of the mononuclear phagocyte (macrophage) system and cause disfiguring skin diseases or fatal anaemia according to the species and whether it has a predilection for skin or visceral macrophages. Other macrophage-dwelling parasites are *Trypanosoma cruzi* the bug (hemipteran)-transmitted agent

of Chagas disease in South America (though it principally parasitizes muscle cells) and *Toxoplasma* (Fig. 1c), a natural parasite of the cat's intestine which embarks on a bout of riotous multiplication when it infects other hosts. These protozoa are avidly phagocytosed by macrophages but somehow fail to awaken the cell's killing mechanism. The 'respiratory burst' that accompanies phagocytosis of susceptible organisms and leads to the generation of toxic oxygen metabolites (hydrogen peroxide and free hydroxyl radicals) does not occur; it is somehow miraculously switched off by the parasite.

Natural resistance mechanisms, for reasons we understand poorly, do not kill parasites. It is the acquired (adaptive) response of the host based on the special properties of lymphocytes of the immune system which leads to parasite destruction. Lymphocytes respond to stimulation with the parasite's antigens; the humoral element is provided by the B ('bone marrow'-derived) lymphocytes secreting antibody while the T ('thymus'-derived) lymphocytes help the B-lymphocytes in the production of antibody or take part in cell-mediated immune mechanisms.

Thus host antibody in the presence of complement rapidly lyses sleeping sickness trypanosomes and opsonizes them so that they are readily taken up by the macrophages in the liver and spleen. We do not know which of these two mechanisms is responsible for clearing the blood in African trypanosomiasis and it may depend on the host species. Malaria-parasitized red cells carry exposed parasite antigens which invoke an antibody response as do the naked merozoites which infect new cells (see Fig. 2). As a consequence both may be destroyed in the same way as trypanosomes. How gut protozoa are eliminated is not known. Thus infections with the most cosmopolitan of human protozoal infections, the flagellate *Giardia intestinalis* (Fig. 1e) are eliminated from the body in a few weeks but by what immune mechanism we do not know. Various explanations have been put forward and include the suggestion that the prevention of parasite adherence is achieved by secretory immunoglobulin (IgA) and their destruction by 'killer' cells which attach to the flagellates and murder them by an unknown mechanism.

Two striking features of helminth infections are eosinophilia — a raised count of eosinophil leukocytes in the blood, and high levels of reaginic antibody (IgE). Eosinophils are undoubtedly of major importance in the killing of helminth parasites, especially in the skin. They will plaster themselves all over an invading schistosomula and disgorge their granules onto its antibody-coated surface. Enzymes (peroxidase) and basic and acidic proteins damage the unique double lipid-bilayer membrane which covers the syncytial tegument forming the outer cover of the worm. This allows the eosinophils to penetrate beneath the tegument and literally skin the schistosomula by prizing off its tegument. Neutrophils and macrophages then descend like vultures on the prey to scavenge its remains.

Despite their different surface structure, (with no living outer layer), larval nematodes are also susceptible to eosinophil attack, whereas adult worms do not invoke much inflammatory reaction. An exception is Onchocerca whose adults are found in nodules in the skin accompanied by eosinophils, though these cells do not seem to be able to make contact with the worms. Why is a mystery, but the drug dimethylcarbazone used in treatment of the disease enables the eosinophils to contact the worms and finish them off.

What the IgE in helminth infections is doing no one knows. One intriguing aspect is that much of it is non-specific for the parasites. IgE binds to mast cells in the tissues. Mast cells then release their vasoactive amines when they encounter the IgE-specific antigen and this results in rapid local inflammation. It has been suggested, but is far from being proved, that this inflammatory reaction may

hinder worm attachment or block entry. The expulsion of worms from the gut, common as an immune phenomenon in many roundworm infections of domestic animals, may depend on such termination of attachment, though in experimental systems expulsion can occur in the absence of IgE. If IgE is a host weapon against helminth parasites we do not know how it is used.

The evidence so far available suggests that cell mediated immunity is responsible for killing those parasites that live in macrophages. The killing is thought to occur through a process of macrophage activation which is initiated by a lymphokine (macrophage activating factor) produced by immune T lymphocytes. Activation of the macrophage presumably results in arousal of its killing oxidative machinery but insufficient data are available to be sure as yet. What is strange is that a given Leishmania species may show quite different capacities for survival in activated macrophages of different host species.

Seclusion of the parasite within the macrophage raises the question of the mechanism whereby its antigen is presented to the lymphocytes to stimulate them. Do parasite antigens leave the macrophage, or does antigen leave when the parasite goes to infect a new cell? In the case of Leishmanias there is the question of whether the parasite avoids leaving the host cell by stimulating it to divide so that the parasites are shared out to daughter cells as though they were cell organelles. Needless to say we do not yet know the answer to this question.

(2) How do Parasites Avoid the Host's Immune Response?

Although the host has mechanisms for destroying parasites through its acquired immune response, many parasite infections are extremely long lived. Infections with *Plasmodium vivax, P. ovale* and the malignant

P. falciparum last 2 to 3 years and *P. malariae* (quartian malaria) can linger on for as long as 50 years. Why does the host take so long to terminate the infection? The answer is undoubtedly in part to do with the parasite's ability to foil host defence mechanisms.

One way to avoid the host's defence is to hide from them in an 'immunologically privileged site'. The red cell, as we have seen, is not such a site but before it embarks on its life in the bloodstream, the malaria parasite undergoes a cycle of development in the liver following its injection by the mosquito at the sporozoite state (Fig. 2). Until recently most malariologists believed that sudden relapses of the non-malignant malarias were

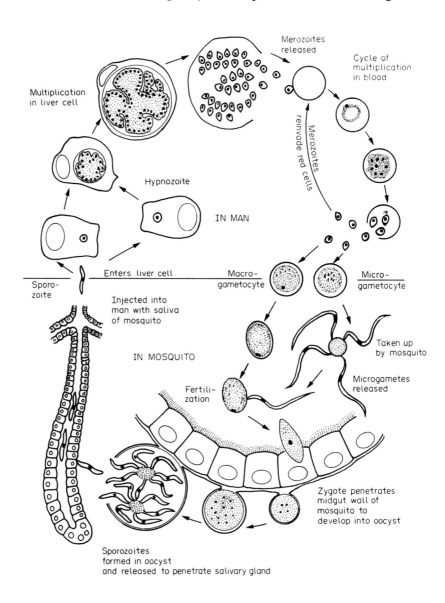

Fig. 2. Life cycle of *Plasmodium vivax*, one of the malaria parasites of man.

due to secondary liver cycles resulting in delayed invasion of the blood. A controversial view which is now gaining favour is that certain sporozoites, having invaded a liver cell, may become dormant 'hypnozoites', slumbering unmolested for weeks, months or years until some unknown signal awakens them. The liver stage excites no detectable immune reaction and the liver cell is presumably a privileged site.

But bloodstream malaria infections can also be persistent. Quartian malaria undoubtedly owes its relapses after several decades not to hypnozoites but to the subclinical ticking over of repeated red cell cycles, as it can easily be terminated by drugs against the red cell stages. One possible explanation is that malaria parasites can change repeatedly the nature of their exposed antigens so that the host has to produce a new specific antibody to each succeeding variant in order to eliminate it. As yet evidence for the occurrence of such antigenic variation in malaria comes only from experimental infections with malaria parasites of mice and monkeys. What is lacking is a suitably convenient test for its demonstration in human malarias. But maybe the human malarias have another method of evasion!

Antigenic variation is, however, well documented in sleeping sickness trypanosomes. Unlike Plasmodium, these parasites do not hide inside the cells of their mammalian host, though they may hide in immunologically privileged sites, for example the testis. Undoubtedly the main factor in parasite persistence is its ability to change the antigenic nature of its monomolecular glycoprotein coat. The host produces a vigorous macroglobulin (IgM) antibody response to each variable antigen type that constitutes the majority of any bloodstream population and when that majority is eliminated, one of the minor types present increases in numbers to take its place. The full antigen repertoire of a particular trypanosome clone has not yet been determined but it is likely to be in the hundreds. Antigenic change seems to occur spontaneously in individual trypanosomes and is not induced by host antibody as was previously believed. What we would like to know is why the change occurs with greater frequency at some stages of the infection than others, for example directly after tsetse fly transmission the rate of change is several orders of magnitude greater than in syringe passaged infections in mice. There is good evidence that transposable genetic elements or 'jumping genes' are involved in the gene-switching mechanism but what makes the genes jump is still unknown despite the large number of biological systems in which transposable elements have been described.

Another blood parasite famed for its changes of clothing is the schistosome. Schistosomes live as pairs (Fig. 1g), male and female, in small veins in the wall of the bowel or bladder. The adult worms appear to evade immune attack by absorbing red cell antigens and transplantation antigens and thus disguising themselves as host tissue. However an alternative explanation would be that the worms mimic the host by synthesizing these substances themselves but gene hybridization studies are beginning to rule this out. At the same time they stimulate an antibody response which can destroy subsequent infections at an early stage by the eosinophil-mediated mechanism described previously. But the young invading schistosomula has several tricks up its sleeve — or rather on its tegument! Different investigators credit it with different tricks and the number of tricks is growing rapidly. Within a few hours of having penetrated the skin the schistosomula is resistant to immune attack. This has been interpreted on the strength of *in vitro* observations as due to: (1) the loss of antigens from the covering membrane and the uptake of serum lipids to develop a hydrophobic surface; or (2) the rapid turnover rate of surface membrane so that bound antibody is quickly shed; or (3) the absorption of host epidermal cell proteins which mask the schistosomula's own antigens; or (4) the development of proteases that cleave bound immunoglobulin.

The schistosomula has no shortage of possible escape mechanisms. But are they all used? As one notable schistosome fan has remarked 'there is an important discrepancy between the amount of detailed description of potential escape mechanisms and our real knowledge of their function during the schistosome life cycle. Schistosomes certainly know better than we do!'

In addition to parasite sequestration, antigenic variation, antigenic disguise and other forms of surface modulation, one other major host response evasion mechanism of parasites has been widely discussed: spiteful disordering of the host's immune response especially to produce immunosuppression. Depression of the host's immune response has been described in malaria, trypanosomiasis and toxoplasmosis; it is not a feature of helminth infections.

Most, but not all, antibody responses can be suppressed by malaria; cell mediated responses are less susceptible. The tacit assumption is that the parasite may be modifying the host's antimalarial responses, but hard evidence for this has yet to be found, and the nature of the responsible parasite components or products has still to be determined. In sleeping sickness the situation is clearer. The massive proliferation of B (antibody-producing) lymphocytes and high macroglobulin (IgM) levels characteristic of the pathology of the disease have been linked with the marked immunosuppression. The trypanosome has been envisaged as a mitogenic stimulus, switching on antibody synthesis in B cell clones in a non-specific fashion ('polyclonal activation') in order to confuse its host. This is because much of the IgM produced is reputedly not specific for trypanosomes and reacts with other antigens such as sheep red blood cells. However this non-specificity, and therefore the entire theory of polyclonal activation is open to question. For example the raised IgM of the serum of a Glasgow medical student who accidentally infected himself with sleeping sickness was almost wholly absorbable with trypanosomes suggesting it was specific for a wide range of variable antigens. In other words, the human host was simply defending himself rather than being manipulated by his unwanted intruders.

Arguments over the nature of immunosuppression in protozoal infections are rife at the moment, but no doubt several mechanisms are involved. Perhaps more question marks exist in this area of immunoparasitology than in any other mentioned so far.

(3) Is it Possible to Tip the Scales in Favour of the Host?

We have seen that the human body's development of protective immunity to parasitic diseases is often slow and incomplete and that in some cases (e.g. sleeping sickness) the symptoms of the disease are due more to the immune response than to the parasite. These observations have long made the prospect of vaccinating susceptible hosts seem a remote one. Yet for reasons outlined earlier the individual protection provided by vaccination is desperately needed to spare a great deal of human misery. In addition, traditional control of tropical diseases by anti-vector measures and drug treatment are breaking down for many of these diseases through the development of resistance on the part of vector or parasite.

In the veterinary world some success in anti-parasite vaccination has been achieved by immunization with irradiated living parasites (cattle lungworm, dog hookworm, bovine schistosomes). Irradiation limits the parasite's viability in the animal but allows it to stimulate protective immunity. But whether a living product would be acceptable for immunizing man is doubtful. Parasite extracts of various kinds run the risk of activating those processes which in the disease itself promote parasite survival but which are such a nuisance to the host, for example immunosuppression.

Recently, however, two exciting developments in biology — the hybridoma and recombinant DNA technologies have raised hopes considerably. The hybridoma technique involves fusing an antibody secreting cell with a malignant myeloma tumour cell to produce a hybrid from which a cell line can be established in culture. The progeny retain the antibody-producing capacity of one parent and the replicating capacity of the other, and secrete large amounts of highly specific 'monoclonal' antibody. Such antibody can be used to extract the corresponding antigen from heterogeneous mixtures such as parasite homogenates. The ability of the monoclonal antibody to confer passive protection against the parasite concerned can be tested and in this way monoclonal antibodies conferring protection against rodent malaria and one of the human schistosomes have already been identified. The next step is to obtain the corresponding protection-inducing antigen. If this can be used to confer protection by active immunization, without activating the damaging effects of the parasite's pathogenic processes, then it has considerable potential for use in vaccination. Recombinant DNA technology can be used to isolate the gene coding for the antigen and by grafting it into the genome of a bacterium using a plasmid vector large quantities of the antigen could be obtained for vaccination programmes.

Conclusions

I hope that enough has been said to make it clear to the reader that we still have a lot to discover about the nature of the weapons employed by the human host in combatting parasites or of the subterfuge used by the parasites in avoiding the blows. Moreover, much of what we think we know is open to doubt. In order to tip the scales in favour of the human host, however, much might be achieved now that we are in a position to identify those components of the parasite that stimulate a protective immune response on the part of the host and separate them from other components that stimulate a non-protective or self-damaging response. There will be difficulties in translating this identification into the development of effective vaccines, of course! The identified protective antigen, for example, may vaccinate against only one stage in the parasite's life cycle, or against particular genotypes or antigenic variants. But by concentrating on the variants of a crucial stage in the life cycle, say the man-invading stage, this variation should not prove insuperable. Although this methodology is still in the experimental stage, the prospect of alleviating some of the misery caused by parasitic diseases now seems brighter.

Further Reading

COHEN, S. (ed.) (1982). *Malaria*. British Medical Bulletin, Volume 38, No. 2. Churchill-Livingstone, Edinburgh.

COHEN, S. & WARREN, K. (eds.) (1982). *Immunology of Parasitic Infections*. 2nd Edition. Blackwell Scientific Publications, Oxford.

COX, F.E.G. (ed.) (1982). *Modern Parasitology*. Blackwell Scientific Publications, Oxford.

METTRICK, D.F. & DESSER, S.S. (eds.) (1982). *Parasites — Their World and Ours*. Elsevier Biomedical Press, Amsterdam.

MOLLER, G. (ed.) (1982). *Immunoparasitology*. Immunological Reviews, Vol. 61.

VAN DEN BOSSCHE, H. (ed.) (1980). *The Host-Invader Interplay*. Elsevier North Holland Medical Press, Amsterdam.

INDEX